Equitation Science

For the horses

Equitation Science

Paul McGreevy, BVSc, PhD, MRCVS, MACVSc

and

Andrew McLean, BSc, PhD, DipEd

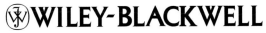
WILEY-BLACKWELL

A John Wiley & Sons, Ltd., Publication

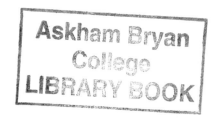

Blackwell Publishing was acquired by John Wiley & Sons in February 2007. Blackwell's publishing programme has been merged with Wiley's global Scientific, Technical and Medical business to form Wiley-Blackwell.

Registered office
John Wiley & Sons Ltd, The Atrium, Southern Gate, Chichester, West Sussex, PO19 8SQ, United Kingdom

Editorial offices
9600 Garsington Road, Oxford, OX4 2DQ, United Kingdom
2121 State Avenue, Ames, Iowa 50014-8300, USA

For details of our global editorial offices, for customer services and for information about how to apply for permission to reuse the copyright material in this book please see our website at www.wiley.com/wiley-blackwell.

Library of Congress Cataloging-in-Publication Data

McGreevy, Paul, 1964-
  Equitation science / Paul McGreevy and Andrew McLean.
    p. cm.
  Includes bibliographical references and index.
  ISBN 978-1-4051-8905-7 (pbk. : alk. paper)   1. Horses–Training.   2. Horsemanship.
3. Horses–Psychology.   I. McLean, Andrew (Andrew N.)   II. Title.
  SF287.M4426 2010
  798.2–dc22   2009048321

A catalogue record for this book is available from the British Library.

Set in 9.5/11.5 pt Palatino by Aptara® Inc., New Delhi, India
Printed and bound in Malaysia by Vivar Printing Sdn Bhd

1   2010

Contents

Preface

This is a book for horse industry personnel, and indeed everyone who spends time with horses and ponies. It will help to ensure that humane, proficient horsemanship becomes more prevalent.

Many equine scientists, veterinarians, ethologists and behaviour therapists share the view that the current lack of science in equitation contributes to the prevalence of undesirable equine behaviours with human-related causes. The number of horses worldwide is large and growing. As a consequence, there is an increasing number of horse-owners, many of whom are new to horse-keeping, with little knowledge of how to train their animal. This has led to a rise in the number of associated horse-welfare problems culminating in high wastage rates. Such problems reflect the uninformed practices, poor training techniques, inappropriate use of training equipment and, in some cases, inhumane handling of horses. In addition, horse-related injuries are a major public health concern, with most occurring while the rider is mounted. Death rates from horse-related injuries are in the vicinity of one death per million head of population and in terms of injuries, horse-riding is more dangerous than motorcycle sports and equally as dangerous as rugby. Improving riders' understanding of horse behaviour and subsequently reducing the number of 'conflict behaviours' horses develop will reduce the prevalence of such accidents. Furthermore, the increasing profile of 'Natural Horsemanship'

and 'horse whisperers' has made horse industry personnel question some traditional practices, prompted them to consider how novel techniques operate and to question how the language relating to horse-training and riding relates to what is known through psychology, ethology and veterinary science. This book helps them in all of these three endeavours.

The title introduces 'Equitation Science', an emerging discipline that aims to provide an understanding of the behavioural mechanisms that underpin the human–horse interface. Equitation science is the measurement and interpretation of interactions between horses and their riders. Our book describes the first equine-training system that is totally based on what is referred to in the behavioural sciences as 'learning theory'. This system explains training at all levels in a refreshingly simple, logical and illuminating way. The objective measurement of variables is important, so this book explains from first principles traditional and novel techniques to reveal what works, what does not, and why. Most importantly, it also explores the welfare consequences of training and competing with horses under different disciplines.

In contrast to the latest generation of horse whisperers, advocates of Equitation Science are not commercial purveyors of techniques, training certificates or merchandise. Equitation science has an extremely promising future since it is more humble, global, accessible and accurate, and less denominational, commercial, open to interpretation and misinterpretation than any formulaic approach. It has the potential to be the most enduring of all approaches used to train the horse.

The authors offer unique perspectives by being able to combine tertiary qualifications in veterinary medicine (PM), ethology (PM), zoology (AM), comparative cognition (AM) and animal welfare (PM) with significant experience in animal-training (AM & PM), elite equestrian competition (AM), clinical behaviour modification (AM & PM) and coaching (AM & PM).

Acknowledgements

We wish to acknowledge the tremendous support we have received over many years from our colleagues in academe and the horse industry. Early attempts to apply learning theory to horse training were made by AM (*Horse Training the McLean Way*) and PM (*Why does my horse ...?*). Since then, the emerging discipline of Equitation Science developed rapidly following discussions between Debbie Goodwin, Natalie Waran and PM following the Havemeyer Foundation Workshop on Horse Behavior and Welfare in Iceland in 2002.

The first workshop on Equitation Science was held at the Royal (Dick) School of Veterinary Studies, University of Edinburgh in 2004 where AM gave practical demonstrations of the application of 'learning theory' in-hand and under-saddle. As a result of the interest of approximately 30 equine scientists at this workshop, it was decided to launch the first symposium in Equitation Science at the Australian Equine Behaviour Centre the following year. Further symposia followed in Milan (2006), Michigan (2007) and Dublin (2008). In addition to the above-named colleagues, those who made notable contributions to the eventual establishment of the current International Society for Equitation Science (ISES) include Machteld van Dierendonck, Carol Hall, Elke Hartman, Michela Minero, Jack Murphy, Hayley Randle, Camie Heleski, Amanda Warren-Smith, Kathalijne Visser and Lisa Beard.

The formation of the ISES is a great step forward for horses and is a direct result of the growing worldwide interest in this area by equine scientists and equestrian professionals alike. The equestrians that we wish to acknowledge include Portland Jones, Manuela McLean, Jody Hartstone, Anjanette Harten, Warwick McLean and Niki Stuart.

For their help with the current text, we wish to thank Bob Boakes, Hilary Clayton, Ruth Coleman, Debbie Goodwin, Carol Hall, Camie Heleski, Machteld van Dierendonck, Katherine Houpt, Kathalijne Visser, Jan Ladewig, Leo Jeffcott, Daniel Mills, Jack Murphy, Niki Stuart, Julie Taylor, Natalie Waran, Amanda Warren-Smith and Mari Zetterquist-Blokhuis; all of whom reviewed at least one chapter each. Lynn Cole, Portland Jones, Lesley Hawson and Catherine Oddie gave invaluable advice on each chapter. Further editorial assistance was provided by Joseph Le Doux, Pierre Malou, Nicola Drabble, Laura Payne and Danielle McBain. The tables that appear in Chapter 3 are drawn from a paper co-written with Catherine Oddie and Francis Burton. The illustrations are largely the work of an outstanding equestrian illustrator, Samantha Elmhurst.

Photographs were supplied by Manuela McLean, Andrew McLean, Elke Hartmann, Julie, Wilson, Julie Taylor, Christine Hauschildt, Amelia Martin, Minna Tallberg, Philippe Karl, Sandy Hannan, Amanda Warren-Smith, Greg Jones,

Jenny Carroll, Pierre Malou, Sandra Jorgensen, Christine Hauschildt, David Faloun, Georgia Bruce, Roz Neave, Susan Kjaergard, Portland Jones, Carol Willcocks, Becky Whay, Cristina Wilkins and Eric Palmer. While we have made every possible effort to contact the rights owners of other images used in this book, there have been cases where it has not been possible to trace the relevant parties. If you believe that you are the owner of an image or images used in this book and we have not contacted you prior to publication, please contact us via the publisher.

Disclaimer:

The book is not a manual and is not intended to endorse any particular gear, technique or discipline. This may explain the representations of sporthorses on the cover. The authors and the publishers do not necessarily condone or recommend riding without the use of safety helmets, and riders are cautioned to take heed of local laws and regulations.

1 The Quest for Knowledge

Introduction

This is a book for everyone who spends time with horses (and by that we mean ponies as well). We want to share our approach to horse management, handling and training in order to move towards the best possible outcome for humans and horses.

Please do not be put off by the word 'science' in the title of this book. We pledge to keep things simple because, if we confuse you, we will have failed: our mission is to reduce confusion when you next interact with a horse. Like all animals, horses learn most effectively when the training methods are appropriate. Inappropriate training practices can also have a negative impact on a horse's welfare and can lead to conflict behaviours that jeopardise the safety of riders and handlers. Equitation Science gives us a way of measuring and interpreting interactions between horses and their riders.

We understand that some readers never really enjoyed science at school and have avoided it with great commitment ever since. To those readers, we say, 'Relax! We are going to make this as easy as possible.' It is worth noting from the outset that we will repeatedly refer to 'learning theory', which is simply a comprehensive term for the ways in which animals learn. It is called 'theory' but, although you may not realise it, it is already universally practised in all animal-training. You cannot avoid it and there is much to be gained by embrac-

ing it. No one owns it. Learning theory establishes clear guidelines and training protocols for correct training practices and methods of behaviour modification. It is truly fascinating, easy to relate to and really quite simple to understand.

Horse-training differs fundamentally from the reward-based training methods used for marine mammals, exotic carnivores and most companion animals because it largely relies on negative reinforcement. During their early training, horses learn that the correct responses result in the reduction of pressure from the bit via the reins when they stop or slow. Pressure from the rider's legs or spurs is reduced when the horse moves forward. To be effective and humane, the application of pressure must be subtle and its removal immediate once the horse complies. This reliance on negative reinforcement (see Chapter 6, Learning III: Associative (aversive)) underlines the need to ensure that training programs are effective and humane. Science can and should step in to measure, analyse and interpret what we do with and to horses.

Some readers may feel that horse-riding is purely an art. Of you, we ask: has science diminished our awe of the universe in any way? Surely, if we can quantify what works, what is relevant and what is mere window-dressing, both horses and humans will feel the benefit. After all, technologies such as kinematic analysis and pressure-detecting devices have been able to refine human technique in a host of other sports from tennis and rowing to boxing and fencing. If we accept that horses work best when riders have good technique, we can see that, as sentient beings, they are more deserving of these advances than any piece of sporting apparatus.

Of course, one could argue that scientists routinely underestimate the emotional intelligence of animals and the profound bonds humans share with them; that the bond between a horse and human is wonderful and that is all we need to know. Unfortunately, this approach attracts interpretations of horse behaviour in human terms and is underpinned by unsubstantiated and often dangerous leaps of faith. As we will see, there can be significant welfare consequences when one overestimates the cognitive abilities of horses.

Science is sometimes accused of objectifying animals, but the emergence of animal welfare science has already created changes in legislation that have improved animal wellbeing. It has shown us how modern diets may prompt obsessive–compulsive disorders; how weaning can affect social relations among animals; and how the behaviour of a breed can be a product of its shape.

Those with concerns about applying a scientific approach to equitation seem to fear the construction of equitation as a science, which is certainly not our intent. Equitation Science represents the scientific *study* of equitation; it does not seek to turn equitation into a science. Scientific measuring of variables is important because it allows riding and training techniques to be compared in order to demonstrate what works and what does not. Equitation Science will also allow us to measure the welfare consequences of doing the wrong thing.

Ideally, equestrian technique combines art and science. The central point here is that once you have got the science sorted out, you can go ahead and concentrate on the art. We warmly invite naysayers to open their minds to some simple principles. When we know better, we can do better – why not seek to know as much as we can? We are not trying to sell a philosophy, but simply wish to pass on to horses and riders the benefits of more than a century of scientific endeavour. Traditional approaches to training animals *must* be challenged to ensure that the methods we now use are both effective and humane.

The quest for knowledge is the foundation of progress. If the medical profession, for example, still clung to the way things have always been done, doctors might still be trepanning foreheads. Nasty! We recognise that feelings and affiliations contribute to the relationships between riders and horses and that they can make a critical difference to the effectiveness of a partnership. The intense and undoubted rapport that exists will continue to complement our understanding of effective approaches to training and will never be threatened by scientific findings. Perhaps one day these feelings will be available for scientific scrutiny and we would certainly welcome this. However, the *physical* interactions between humans and their horses are readily available for study right now. For welfare reasons, understanding these interactions correctly is crucial because, on the one hand, excessive pressure is often being used to signal to horses and, on the other, we cannot expect horses to know what we require of them without at least some cues. What we have learned from still-evolving studies of human behaviour should ensure that, in its infancy, Equitation Science takes the best possible route to maturity. The central point to remember is that Equitation Science measures only the measurable.

Veterinary epidemiologists, whose job it is to describe the spread and impact of disorders, often talk about wastage within a population. This is the percentage of animals or, in the case of working animals, the percentage of potential working days lost through illness or disease. Problem behaviour is the cause of much of this wastage, and in the world of the riding horse it is more significant than many of us would like to imagine. A global improvement in application of learning theory, particularly the timing and consistency of pressure release, would see a significant increase in the number of horses considered to be trainable (see Figure 1.1).

We know that slowness is an aspect of thoroughbreds and standardbreds that can be life-threatening since slow racehorses are culled from the population. If they are mares or stallions, they may have a future in a breeding program – though the merit of breeding from slow parents is obscure. For slow geldings, culling means either re-training for other ridden work or euthanasia. Slow standardbreds in particular face a bleak outcome,

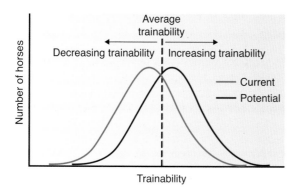

Figure 1.1   Theoretical normal distributions to show how the numbers of horses that cope with training can be increased by using more enlightened approaches. (Reproduced from *Equine Behavior*, copyright Elsevier 2004.)

as their breed is not highly regarded as a riding animal.

Horses are being confused on a very regular basis by less-than-ideal handling and become unusable or, worse, dangerous as a result. For example, Buckley (2007), reporting on 50 out of 84 Pony Club horses, noted that this focal sub-set of owners reported a total of 251 misbehaviour days during a 12-month period. Importantly, on more than half of these days, this misbehaviour was classified as dangerous enough to cause potential injury to horse and/or rider. Generally speaking, horse-riding is more dangerous than motorcycle riding, skiing, football, and rugby (Ball *et al.*, 2007). In Australia, horse-related injuries and death exceed those caused by any other non-human species (domestic or otherwise) (AIHW National Injury Surveillance Unit, 2005).

Among non-racehorses, previous studies indicate that up to 66% of euthanasia in horses between 2 and 7 years of age was not because of health disorders (Ödberg and Bouissou, 1999). The implication is that they were culled for behavioural reasons. Clearly, this level of behavioural wastage is unacceptably high. The likelihood is that many such horses are mistrusted or labelled troublesome. With their reputation for being dangerous preceding them, they are met with an escalation of tension in the rein or pressure from the rider's legs, the very forces they have learned to fear and avoid. Difficult horses go from one home to the next and are often forced to

trial new ways of escaping pressure and satisfying competing motivations.

The sport we focus on in this book is Dressage, which translates as training – and forms the basis of many individual equestrian disciplines, including Jumping and Eventing. Dressage offers the greatest challenges for riders and coaches and the greatest risk of confusion for the horse, since it demands that horses are ridden with constant rein contact.

The performance of the horse under-saddle and the consequent development of riding instruction tend to focus on outcomes rather than mechanisms. Outcomes vary with context and the context of horse-riding can vary radically within one discipline. In dressage, there can be a great divide between competitive riding by modern elite riders and the training undertaken by classical riders. For example, competitive dressage has developed aspects that seem to value 'impressions of power' in the horse rather than 'lightness' in the rider's signalling, outcomes that riding masters of the eighteenth century might find unacceptable (Ödberg and Bouissou, 1999). However, while various equestrian techniques have been discussed at length (e.g. Roberts, 1992), there are almost no data to inform the discussion.

Equitation Science has the potential to address a series of important problems. First, it elucidates the role of negative reinforcement and habituation in the learning processes of horses on which we ride and compete. Second, it addresses the need to measure rider interventions that may compromise horse welfare, which will assist the Fédération Equestre Internationale (FEI) in determining what practices and interventions are acceptable on welfare grounds. For example, devices such as whips and spurs are still used routinely by some trainers. Indeed, at elite levels, spurs and double bridles (which are more severe in their action than regular single bits) are mandatory. Third, and perhaps most important, Equitation Science will educate current and aspiring riders in how best to apply the core principles of learning theory.

Riding manuals have historically by-passed the central tenets of learning theory (Waran *et al.*, 2002). Since the ideals of equestrian technique combine art and science, students of equitation encounter a few measurable variables, such as tempo, rhythm and outline, alongside many more conceptual ones, such as harmony, looseness, respect and leadership (McGreevy and McLean, 2005). This complex mixture, along with the shortage of mechanistic explanations of cause and effect in-hand and under-saddle, frustrates attempts to express equestrian technique in empirical terms; they also account for some of the confusion and conflict that arises in many human–horse dyads. Science has begun to develop systems for measuring and defining many of these mechanisms (de Cartier d'Yves and Ödberg, 2005; Warren-Smith et al., 2007a). Already, it has helped to elucidate breed differences in the way horses perceive their environment (Evans and McGreevy, 2005), identify causes of wastage that relate to behavioural problems (Hayek et al., 2005) and debunk some old myths (Warren-Smith et al., 2005a, 2005b, 2007b).

The application of pressure begins the first time a horse is led and pressure is used continually until the horse learns to respond to light pressures. In the same way, a dog learning to walk on a collar and lead must learn how to avoid any pressure around the neck. A central hypothesis of this book is that the simplest explanation of equine responses to signals from riders is that horses learn to respond to aversive stimuli (pressures). It is desirable to train horses in ways that allow these stimuli to rapidly become as mild as possible. Negative reinforcement is probably unavoidable in current performance-horse-training because the horse is controlled by approximations of various pressures provided by the rider and refined by discriminative training. Therefore, to explain the response in terms of learning theory we are obliged to accept that – however mild these stimuli may be – they *do* follow the rules of negative reinforcement.

Any use of the reins and the rider's legs constitutes negative reinforcement (or punishment). The bit is neutral only in horses that have become habituated to bit pressure and therefore do not respond to it anyway. These horses are heavy on the bit and unresponsive to stop signals. Nevertheless, many riders mistakenly believe that they use mainly positive reinforcement (Warren-Smith and McGreevy, 2008a). At first glance, the distinction between different types of reinforcement may seem academic but incorrect application of learning theory is responsible for some serious

welfare issues. By improving riders' and coaches' basic appreciation of the science that underpins their work, we have been able to engage them in improvements that occupy the cutting edge of equitation. For a scientific riding manual, readers are directed to *Academic Horse Training: Equitation Science in Practice* (McLean and McLean, 2008).

> In some sectors of horse-training, such as the sport of dressage, the cues and signals used to elicit alterations in the mobility and posture of horses are known as 'aids'. This word is antique in origin, derived from the French verb 'aider', meaning 'to help'. The notion that cues in any way offer assistance to horses is anthropocentric and has been abandoned in our text because it nourishes the notion of the 'benevolent' horse, the horse that is a willing partner. Horse-trainers should respectfully recognise that training is an act of equine exploitation rather than equine enlightenment, and modern equitation must take full account of the cognitive processes of the horse.

Equitation Science largely avoids the word schooling and instead considers horses at various stages in their training via instrumental and classical conditioning. This is important because the word schooling appears throughout the equestrian literature. This, of course, demands a definition of schooling. If schooling is the development of new responses then reinforcement is inarguably the process – and in the absence of attractive primary reinforcers, including food, sex, water and company, then negative reinforcement must be at work. When schooling is the maintenance of behaviour, the process may chiefly involve classical conditioning.

Any system of training that aligns with learning theory will result in subtle signalling and therefore, by implication and necessity, an independent seat. Our contention is that 'stop' responses to the bit and 'go' responses to the rider's legs are the foundations that underpin all advanced riding techniques. It is prudent to train riders to sit appropriately from the word 'go' so that the horse does not receive mixed messages as the rider attempts to hang on. We emphasise this principle since it is central to all riders' correct use of negative reinforcement. It would be good to see a return to traditional coaching protocols that required novice riders to learn to balance before picking up the reins. This would avoid the delivery of conflicting signals. For riders, the benefits include safety, reduced frustration, effective control and good results. For horses, there will be minimal confusion, no conflict and a long working life.

This book is essentially an introductory text because there is much still to discover about the way mechanisms of horse-training align with more than a century of studies of learning in laboratory animals. There is also room for considerable caution because there is no laboratory equivalent for the ridden horse – you cannot ride a rat. Without restraining a rat, you cannot easily apply and then release pressure. So, serendipitously, the horse is the very best model of negative reinforcement. Studying its responses to clear signals and confu-

sion will expand our understanding of learning in general. This possibility represents one of the most exciting aspects of Equitation Science.

What we have learned from the evolution of studies of human behaviour should ensure that, in its infancy, Equitation Science can take the best possible route to maturity. The central point to remember is that Equitation Science measures only the measurable. The intense and undoubted rapport we share with our horses will continue to complement our understanding of effective approaches to training and will never be threatened by scientific findings. Far from objectifying the horse in any way, this book emphasises effective techniques and identifies irrelevant and abusive training practices.

2 Cognitive Ethology

Introduction

It is useful to think of a horse in terms of the way it fits into its social group, the domestic setting and its interactions with humans, including the work we require of it. These can be encapsulated by the term umwelt (from the German word for 'environment' or 'surrounding world' (von Uexküll, 1957). Every organism creates and reshapes its own umwelt when it interacts with the world. It is a useful concept as it explains how invasions into a horse's umwelt can have effects in other domains. Physiologically, we can think of a single stressful facet of the horse's world as lowering the threshold at which other events become frustrating (see Figure 2.1). Therefore, a horse that is in an inappropriate social group may be less responsive during training and, equally, a horse that has encountered inconsistent training may be more likely to be distressed by marginally frustrating aspects of its world when not being ridden.

The biological constraints on what a horse can physically do clearly predict what it can be trained to do. Its cardiovascular characteristics affect its stamina and ability to take in oxygen and expel carbon dioxide (Evans *et al.*, 2006). Its musculoskeletal attributes affect its ability to contract and extend its scope over obstacles. In addition, its perception and visual acuity affect its ability to judge the position of hazards (Hall, 2007).

Beyond these physical constraints, there are also cognitive restraints that apply to the horse's ability to process and remember information. These are the limitations to learning and, therefore, limitations on training that we will consider in this chapter. It is interesting to reflect upon strategies that have facilitated survival. They include horses' abilities in making associations between stimuli and weakness in generalising among stimuli. Clearly, on an individual level, such cognitive characteristics can have a critical impact on the work we require of horses. Consider, for instance, the 'will to win', the competitive edge that gives the impression that horses understand the significance of the finishing line and that showjumpers grasp the importance of a jump-off. Whether science will ever define and measure these equine cognitive characteristics remains to be seen (McGreevy, 2007). Even with the most outstanding training programs, with perfect timing and consistency, these constraints may have considerable impact on performance in competition.

The horse in a domesticated niche

While humans have been interacting with horses for many millennia through hunting, it is only relatively recently that horses have become beasts of burden and been used for transport, war,

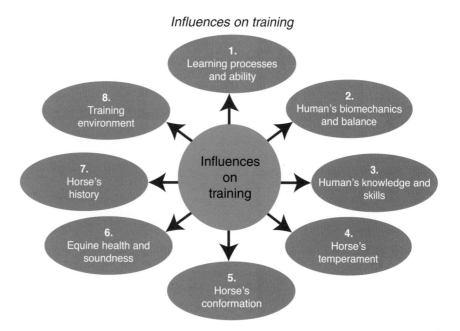

Influences on training

1.
Learning processes
and ability

8.
Training
environment

2.
Human's biomechanics
and balance

Influences
on
training

7.
Horse's
history

3.
Human's knowledge and
skills

6.
Equine health and
soundness

4.
Horse's
temperament

5.
Horse's
conformation

Figure 2.1 Success in horse-training is influenced by at least eight broad variables.

agriculture and, more recently, sport and leisure. Direct evidence suggests that horses were domesticated at around the end of the second millennium BC (Levine, 2005). Since the beginnings of domestication, various techniques for horse-training have been developed and passed on to subsequent generations orally or through literature. All these techniques are underpinned and constrained by the biology of the horse. When it comes to getting the most out of horses in sport and work, we need to be well acquainted with their behaviour. Effective and humane training *always* takes account of the animal's ethology, but training systems, however successful, can only ever partially align with the animal's ethogram (behavioural repertoire). Ethology is primarily the scientific study of adaptive behaviour in animals, as it evolved in a natural environment; applied ethology is the study of animal behaviour in the human domain. Equine ethology is, strictly speaking, limited to the study of horse behaviour in free-ranging contexts (Figure 2.2).

The word 'wild' is deliberately avoided here, as there are no longer any examples of truly wild horses. Przewalski's horses (*Equus przewalski*) were, until recently, considered a separate

species from domestic horses (*Equus caballus*) due to anatomical and genetic differences. They became extinct in their natural habitat in the 1950s (Mohr, 1971). However, from a small nucleus of 13 foundation animals (one of which was a hybrid with the domestic horse), they survive today in captivity and in successfully re-introduced

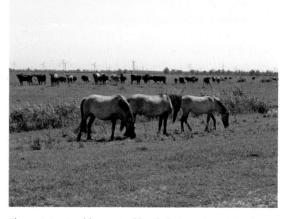

Figure 2.2 Feral horses and herds that receive minimal management, such as these Konik horses in Oostvaarders Plassen, the Netherlands, provide critical information on normal horse behaviour.

free-ranging populations (e.g. in Mongolia; Boyd and Bandi, 2002; King, 2002). The survival story of Przewalski horses is an extraordinary one, and we are indeed fortunate to be able to study them in a variety of contexts. Nevertheless, studies of their behaviour should be treated with some caution since they have emerged from a shallow gene pool that has been filtered through 20 generations of captivity. So, before assuming that present-day Przewalski horses behave as true wild horses, we should acknowledge that some would regard them as survivors of the first stages of domestication. In this text, we use examples of feral caballine (i.e. from *Equus caballus*) horse behaviour rather than Przewalski horse behaviour as benchmarks for what is normal.

It is likely that since domestication, selective breeding may have reduced awareness and, by implication, some learning capacity (Heitor and Vicente, 2007) but the hyper-reactive tendencies of the horse have not been completely eradicated (e.g. a small percentage tend to buck when girth pressure is first applied during foundation training; see Figure 2.3).

So, while it is probable that during the process of selective breeding over four millennia of domestication the associative learning abilities of the horse have not changed, the same may not be true for habituation. Therefore, it has been proposed that the major cognitive change that occurred during selective breeding over the millennia was the capacity for habituation, including to thoracic pressure and possibly other phenomena (McGreevy and McLean, 2007). The domestic horse habituates readily to a wide array of environmental and social stimuli (Miller, 1995). Such an ability to habituate to thoracic pressure may have been maladaptive for the wild horse but has been selected for in the domestic horse.

Perception

The laboratory challenges we design for horses to test learning are constrained by the subject's ability to perceive. For example, when we give horses visual learning tasks, their performance depends upon the features of their visual system. A horse's ability to look at the ground when grazing and simultaneously scan the horizon for potential

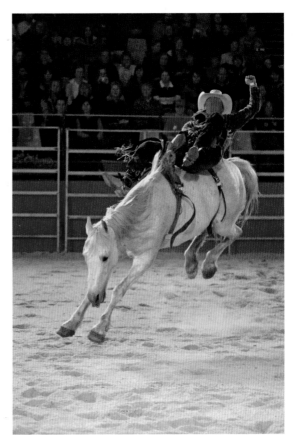

Figure 2.3 Occasionally, horses are selected for their resistance to habituation, such as the family lines of bucking horses used in rodeos. (Photo courtesy of Julie Wilson.)

predators (Harman *et al.*, 1999) may limit its ability to focus attention on a single object (Lea and Kiley-Worthington, 1996). A horse must lower its head to observe stimuli on the ground because doing so projects the image onto the most sensitive area of the retina (Harman *et al.*, 1999). The need for visual surveillance and the necessity to respond in ways that afford the horse a better view of potential threats are attributes that often provide troublesome intrusions in ridden work (Hall, 2007). In terms of vision, horses are classed as dichromats because they have two types of cone photopigment. Consequently, the colours they most easily discriminate are yellow, orange and then blue (Grzimek, 1952; Hall *et al.*, 2005).

Horses have evolved to spend approximately 60% of their time grazing and, as a result, their

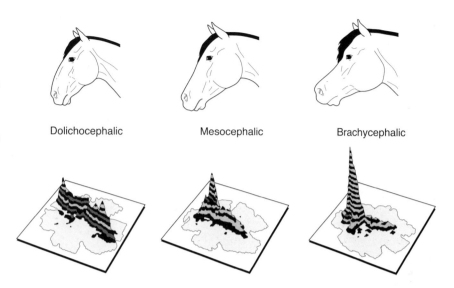

Figure 2.4 Retinal ganglion cell density maps from horses of three breeds with the dorsal part of the retina in the background, ventral in the foreground, nasal to the left and temporal to the right. Each shaded band represents 400 cells/mm². Studies of the retinae of horses with different skull shapes have shown that (at least some of) the neural tissue of morphologically diverse breeds differs.

Dolichocephalic   Mesocephalic   Brachycephalic

eyes are at a set height above the ground, but it is a mistake to assume that all horses perceive the world in the same way. Studies of ganglion cell distribution suggest that skull shape may affect visual acuity (Evans and McGreevy, 2006; see Figure 2.4). Equally, the height of stimuli above the ground (Hall *et al.*, 2003) and relative to the height of the observing animal's head will affect the way in which stimuli are perceived. So, ponies and horses cannot be expected to perceive the same stimuli in the same way and experimental tests with visual stimuli should take into account the head and neck position of subjects.

Heffner and Heffner (1983, 1984, 1986, 1992) have explored the horse's ability to discriminate between sounds of variable frequency and intensity by depriving them of water and rewarding correct responses to stimuli with small volumes of water. They indicate that equine hearing ranges into what humans call ultrasonic, but that sounds need to be louder for horses than for humans. Recently, we have seen the emergence of intriguing evidence of horses' ability to recognise individuals cross-modally, from both their appearance and the sounds of their voices. Horses were shown a familiar conspecific and then heard the played-back call of a different affiliated conspecific. They indicated that the incongruent combination violated their learned associations by responding quicker and looking longer in the direction of the call than when the call matched the herd member

they had just been shown (Proops *et al.*, 2009). The impact of the special features of equine hearing on training is minimal because trainers vocalise in the human range and, in any case, in some equestrian codes, the use of the voice by trainers and riders is either not encouraged or actively forbidden. One interesting exception is the use of the voice to cue transitions on the lunge and in other codes of horsemanship.

Trainers usually report that horses are quick to acquire these cues, so it is worth bearing in mind that if they can be used with consistency, auditory signals are humane. (It is fascinating to note that in 360 BC Xenophon [translated by Morgan, 1962] regarded it as orthodox to calm down a horse with a chirrup, a smooching noise made with the lips alone, and to rouse him by clucking the tongue against the roof of the mouth. Without using terms that have their origins in modern learning theory, he also noted that these behavioural outcomes were the product of classical associations with operant techniques, so swapping the learned cues would also swap the effects: 'Still, if from the first, you should cluck when caressing and chirrup when punishing, the horse would learn to start up at the chirrup and calm down at a cluck.')

It is important to note that many riders describe ear movements (especially alternate pinnae flicking caudally) as evidence that the horse is attending to their signals (see Figure 2.5). There is still much to be studied in this domain. For

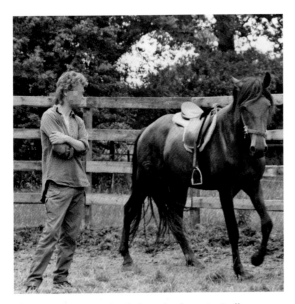

Figure 2.5   Ears moving independently are typically regarded as a sign of attentiveness.

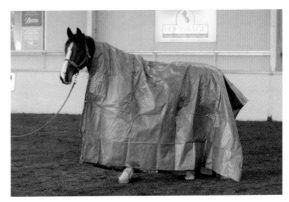

Figure 2.6   Horse with tarpaulin, illustrating the principle of habituation.

example, it is worth pointing out that top show horses and dressage horses may exhibit very different ear movements and we have yet to fathom which offer the best example of equine relaxation or attentiveness. Generally, ears that are constantly pricked forward are associated with fearful behaviour, and the horse flickers its ears loosely forward and back when it is ridden and relaxed (McLean and McLean, 2008). However, there is currently a dearth of empirical data in this domain. An assessment of the significance of ear movements in the ridden horse may assist dressage judges of the future if they are to score a given performance for behavioural legacies of inhumane training.

In general, there is a great deal still to be discovered about equine perception. While vision has received the most attention in studies of equine perception, it has been pointed out that 'senses probably of more crucial importance to the horse's umwelt have been neglected' (Saslow, 2002). For example, olfaction is critical in interactions between horses, but has been the focus of remarkably few studies. The same is true for tactile perception, despite its importance in equitation. Sensitivity of the skin of the ventral thorax (the sides where the rider's legs make contact) and the

mouth has a profound impact on a horse's response to training cues from the legs and reins.

Horse-training always involves some habituation (see Figure 2.6) and some sensitisation (McGreevy and McLean, 2005). A sensitive horse is responsive to the reins and the legs but the requirement in some sports (notably, dressage) to maintain a neutral contact with the horse via the reins and legs offers the ultimate puzzle for trainers. A certain amount of habituation to these cues is necessary for riders to feel the mouth through the reins and the ventral thorax of the horse via their legs. By the same token, pressures beyond the level to which the horse has been habituated must always elicit a response. The fine line between habituation and sensitivity seems narrower in horses with so-called hot-blooded ancestry, including Thoroughbreds, Arabians and their crosses, which are often especially sensitive to pressure. Indeed, some dressage texts refer to not only 'sensitive' horses but also 'hypersensitive' and 'extremely sensitive' horses (Pineo, 1994). Horses at this end of the spectrum present a tighter margin for error during training and are sometimes regarded as less forgiving than heavier, 'colder' breeds.

Ethology

We do well to study the horse's social behaviour repertoire (its social ethogram) when considering how to be effective and remain safe while handling these animals. The agonistic ethogram of the bachelor band (all-male groups found in free-ranging herds) has been described in detail and includes a total of 49 basic behaviours, three complex behavioural sequences and five distinct vocalisations (McDonnell and Haviland, 1995). There are subtle differences in the way horses respond to threats from conspecifics and potential predators. In very broad terms, the main resistances to and evasions of the pressure we apply as riders reflect the horse's anti-predator responses, whereas undesirable responses as we deal with them in-hand are derived chiefly from their sociogram.

Given that all aspects of behaviour are subject to natural selection, ethology is not merely the study of innate behaviours but also the study of how selection, both natural and artificial, has influenced learning processes and capabilities. Natural selection will, for example, have influenced whether or not an animal learns well individually, or learns by observing conspecifics, or both. It will have influenced such variables as relative attention devoted to learning new food-finding techniques versus scanning for predators.

The predisposition of an individual horse to learning and training reflects interactions between the ethology of the horse and the selection of breeds, maternal behaviour, weaning protocols, nutrition, housing, early handling, subsequent training and numerous individual differences. The complexity of the unique background that emerges for each horse as a result of these influences explains why, although the need for fundamental responses (including stop, go and turn) is universal and learning theory can be optimally applied to all horses, an identically rigid structure and time-frame of training can never be imposed on all horses effectively. Fundamental differences between horses lie in the time needed to train a specific quality. Good trainers recognise this and customise their interventions with each horse accordingly (Podhajsky, 1965). That said, to be effective, the mechanisms used in each custom-built approach should be applied with absolute adherence to the principles of learning theory.

Therefore, equine ethology informs not only communication but also equine behavioural needs and preferences, learning processes and motivation. It helps us to predict some of the ways horses *out* of their natural environment (i.e. in the domestic context) might react and cope with various challenges, and how behaviourally flexible, compliant and adaptive they may be.

As such, equine ethology underpins enlightened and effective training but, despite the efforts of some marketing teams, it cannot be used to label a training system or philosophy per se without misrepresenting ethology itself.

Memory and learning

Clearly, memory and learning mechanisms are intimately entwined. Nerve fibres grow by following genetically determined positional cues towards the general target with which they synapse. Then, fine-tuning of the pattern and density of projections is accomplished by the horse's experience. Relationships between synapses are constantly being remodelled through increases or decreases in the size and strength of associations that also lead to the formation of new pathways. Working memory, declarative memory and procedural memory are well understood as is the process of long-term potentiation (LTP), which increases synaptic strength and strengthens pathways (Kandel *et al.*, 2000). What is less clear is the extent of the working memory in horses and if it relates to LTP in the same way as it does in humans.

Memory

A memory is a set of encoded neural connections. The encoding can take place in several parts of the brain and the neural connections can be widespread. The horse's memory is excellent and in some respects may be superior to human memory. While our memory can be altered by our recall, contexts and reasoning abilities, the memory of the horse appears more stable, perhaps because it is unclouded by reflection or projection (McLean, 2001), or perhaps we just have yet to design methodologies that reveal that horses are capable of these (Goodwin, 2007). Wolff and Hausberger (1996) showed that horses could remember precise learned responses without practice for up to a month. However, thinking, analysing and reflecting can corrupt memory. Humans are continuously reflecting (i.e. thinking without 'doing') on some of our memories, retrieving them from storage when we think or tell a story, then later re-storing them again. Importantly, after this process of reflection, the memories are stored a little differently. They are altered by the contexts in which we reflect on them (physical, emotional, perceptual aspects of the moments of reflection). Our elaborate prefrontal cortex, the characteristics of which are uniquely human (Bermond, 1997), is responsible for this reflective ability (Kandel et al., 2000). The absence of tissues with the unique cellular characteristics of the human prefrontal cortex (Kandel et al., 2000; Premack, 2007), the absence of evidence that horses have object permanence (McLean, 2003) and the stability of equine working memory currently suggest that such reflection does not occur in horses.

Learning

As with all species, learning in the horse relates directly to survival requirements and it is generally accepted that it is appropriate to discuss issues of cognition, learning and memory without resorting to the term intelligence (Linklater, 2007). Intelligence aside, the complexity of learning can be mapped out according to a hierarchy of learning abilities from habituation to conceptualisation (see Table 2.1).

Like humans, horses are highly social animals. This explains why horses kept in isolation are more likely to show separation-related behaviours and stereotypies than those kept in group-housing conditions (Cooper and McGreevy, 2002). Companionship is important to horses. So strong is the instinct for togetherness that grooming each other at the base of the neck is almost immediately relaxing. Feh and de Mazières (1993) showed that grooming and stroking horses just in front of the withers (see Figure 2.7) causes a significant lowering of heart rate compared with other regions. Grooming there lowers heart rate and apparently strengthens familial bonds. It is likely to be the optimal site to positively reinforce a horse with tactile rewards. It would be interesting to explore how much of the heart-rate response to wither scratching is learned and how much is innate.

Every horseperson knows that the horse is acutely aware of changes in its visual environment. To the detriment of training, the horse appears to remember far better than the rider 'what happened where'. For example, riders may occasionally notice that the horse goes better on one part of the circle than elsewhere and, gradually, if training is correct, the length of this sector increases. The horse makes associations between the behaviour he is currently doing and where

Table 2.1 Hierarchy of learning abilities

Level	Learning
1. Habituation	Learning not to respond to a repeated stimulus that has no consequences
2. Classical conditioning	Making responses to a new stimulus that has been repeatedly paired with an established effective stimulus
3. Operant conditioning	Learning to repeat a voluntary response for reinforcement or not to repeat a voluntary response to avoid punishment
4. Chaining responses	Learning a sequence of responses to obtain a reinforcement at the end of the sequence
5. Concurrent discriminations	Learning to make an operant response to only one set of stimuli from more than one set of stimuli applied concurrently
6. Concept learning	Discrimination learning based on some common characteristic shared by a number of stimuli
7. Conjunctive, disjunctive and conditional concepts	Learning of concepts that emerge from the relationship between stimuli such as 'A and B' (conjunctive), 'A or B' (disjunctive) and 'If A, then B' (conditional)
8. Bi-conditional concepts	Logical reasoning, such as 'Option A is likely' if and only if 'Option B is present'

Source: Adapted from Thomas (1986) and Murphy and Arkins (2007).

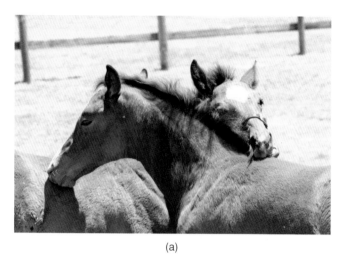

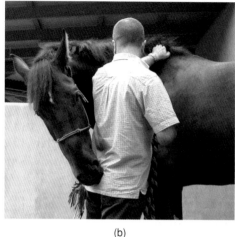

(a)   (b)

Figure 2.7   (a) Horses allogrooming and (b) human grooming a horse's withers.

he is doing it. This context-specific (or place-dependent) learning can be a very useful tool in training (see Chapter 8, Training). For example, some behaviours that are hard to train should be trained in the same place until some reliability emerges. On the other hand, context-specific learning can be a hindrance if, through classical conditioning, the horse learns to exacerbate flight-response behaviours in certain places or contexts. The horse learns tense and fearful responses more rapidly and more indelibly than other responses (McLean, 2004). Sometimes it takes just one or two episodes of a flight response to cause repetition in the same contexts. Fear memories can be suppressed with error-free practice, but when circumstances are the same, the response can return with alarming speed and accuracy. This is known as spontaneous recovery. For this reason it is an essential principle that flight-response behaviours (see Figure 2.8) should be properly identified and training schemes should generally be tailored to avoid them. At the same time, it is acknowledged that horses may detect subtle differences in the behaviour of a nervous human and respond with increased preparedness. Keeling *et al.* (2009) have shown how a nervous human can affect a horse's reactions or responses. They demonstrated how variations in equine heart rate followed very similar heart-rate activity patterns for both handlers and riders. The relationship between these patterns persisted when some individuals were told in advance that an umbrella would be opened sud-denly as they rode or led a horse past an experimenter with the umbrella. Although the umbrella was not actually opened, anticipation of sudden umbrella activity significantly increased the heart rate in both the person riding or leading and the horse when compared with control conditions.

As mammals, horses have brain characteristics that suggest their learning mechanisms may be similar to those of humans (Hahn, 2004). Like humans, they are proficient at trial-and-error learning (learning to perform a reaction through

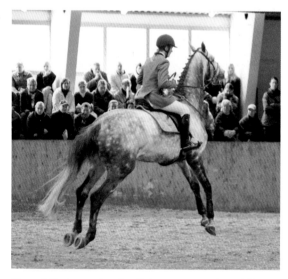

Figure 2.8   Horse showing flight response under-saddle. (Photo courtesy of Minna Tallberg.)

reward), classical conditioning (learning associations between events) and habituation (learning to ignore aversive stimuli that do not hurt). Above these basic learning mechanisms, horses can also learn to generalise stimuli (Nicol, 2002), and they can even learn to categorise objects based on similar physical characteristics (Hanggi, 1999). However, cognitive research to date has not produced empirical evidence that horses can develop abstract concepts (Nicol, 1996). Indeed, there is no peer-reviewed published evidence that horses possess significant higher mental abilities beyond generalising and categorising (Level 5 in Table 2.1). What horsepeople erroneously consider examples of reasoning in their horses turn out to be excellent examples of trial-and-error learning. The pony that fiddles with the gate latch and learns to open it is a typical example. It is clever, but it is not an example of reasoning.

The biological relevance of tasks we have tended to give horses in learning studies has been questioned many times (Bekoff, 1995; McLean, 2001; Nicol, 2002) and although early results from Haag et al. (1980) indicated a good correlation between learning for appetitive and aversive outcomes, later results failed to show this (Visser et al., 2003). Too few studies of negative reinforcement in horses have been conducted (Nicol, 2002), largely because of the lack of technology for measuring pressure as it applies to the horse. Clearly, if equine learning research is to make the results more applicable to equestrian techniques, consistent, easily applied methods of delivering and measuring aversive events, however mild, must be developed. The need for technological advances in this domain is being addressed (McGreevy, 2007) so that we can effectively study learning in the unridden horse. In addition, we must acknowledge that lack of learning performance in the experimental situation may not necessarily reflect lack of learning ability (Lefebvre and Helder, 1997). Furthermore, the insufficient use of discrete subtle signals in equitation generally reflects the inability of the trainers to deliver these rather than any shortcoming in terms of learning or perception by the horse (Creighton, 2007).

In recent years, there has been considerable research into the mental characteristics of horses. Much of this has centred on testing their abilities in

negotiating mazes (Kratzer et al., 1977; Haag et al., 1980; McCall et al., 1981), discriminating various visual stimuli (McCall, 1990; Hanggi, 1999) and acquiring and implementing 'rules' to solve problems (Hanggi, 2003). Researchers have used food rewards as well as avoidance-learning paradigms, and, in general, it has been shown that younger horses learn faster, are more interested in novel stimuli than older horses (Mader and Price, 1982; Houpt et al., 1982) and are more investigative in trial-and-error learning (Lindberg et al., 1999). This may simply reflect the fact that older horses have to 'unlearn' associations and have had more life experience to discriminate between relevant and irrelevant cues. It has also been shown that female horses tend to outperform males in certain rule-learning tests (Sappington et al., 1997) as well as tests with combinations of barriers (spatial detour tests; Wolff and Hausberger, 1996). Finally, horses managed in small groups at pasture learn faster than those housed singly in stalls (Rivera et al., 2002; Søndergaard and Ladewig, 2004).

If establishing relevant tests and gathering together a group of standardised subjects is difficult, then so is extrapolation from a study to other contexts. Although links between learning ability and training ability have been explored in a number of equine studies (Fiske and Potter, 1979; Wolff and Hausberger, 1996), poor correlations exist between an individual horse's learning behaviour and its subsequent performance during different experimental tasks. This implies that we are unlikely to be able to classify horses according to any unified scale of 'intelligence' (Nicol, 2002).

We must exercise caution when interpreting the results of learning studies published to date. Studies of learning in horses have to be carefully designed because horses are easily and inadvertently influenced by humans nearby. For example, Clever Hans (Pfungst, 1965), who was trained to 'count' by tapping the ground with his hoof, was inadvertently trained to stop counting when he reached the right number. His owner and countless spectators convinced themselves that Hans could indeed count, even though they were unwittingly sending him the visual cues (such as looking at his hoof and titling their heads) to stop counting as he reached the right number (see Figure 2.9). This story reminds us that horses can moderate their behaviour as

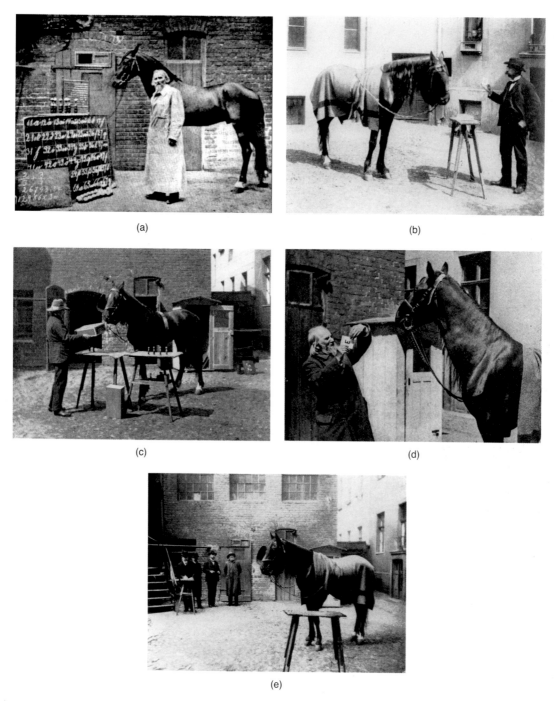

Figure 2.9 The man with the white beard and hair, wearing a long coat (see a and d) is Herr von Osten, who became famous for claiming that his horse, Clever Hans, had been successfully trained to count and to read. Herr von Osten never accepted the criticism of this claim. Instead he helped some of his admirers (shown in b and c) to train and test successors to Clever Hans, as shown in this set of photographs from 1912. In (e) von Osten is on the right of the four onlookers and wearing the hat that – unknown to him – was probably critical in training Clever Hans since it would have amplified the inadvertent visual cue of head tilting.

a result of operator effect, especially if those operators have been training them. This, along with the finding that under certain circumstances, proximity to humans can elicit fearful responses (Lansade *et al.*, 2004), suggests that horses should be isolated from personnel when they are being tested, with observations ideally being made from video recordings. They should not, however, be isolated from conspecifics, since this can induce fearfulness in the horse (Lansade *et al.*, 2004).

Flannery (1997) described horses making higher-order discriminations based on matching shapes that allowed them to generalise this learning under several different conditions. Beyond that, attempts to demonstrate concept formation by horses remain rare in the literature and are so far confined to the conceptual categorisation of objects according to size (among objects; Hanggi, 1999), open or closed centres (among two- and three-dimensional objects; Hanggi, 2003) and hard and soft materials (Watt and McDonnell, 2001). A concept is the 'idea of a class of objects'. Lea (1984) argues that a concept represents an idea, such as common functional properties, rather than physical attributes. Perhaps this is why some horses adopt a flight response when they first encounter a donkey or even a small pony, failing to categorise quadrupeds as potential predators or not. Concept formation, especially in animals that have no language, is a topic of enormous theoretical interest, but there is currently no good evidence that horses have this ability (Nicol, 1996). As with evidence of a lack of spatial memory (McLean, 2004), the relevance of these tasks to the horse's behavioural repertoire merits detailed consideration (McCall, 2007). When concept learning in the three highest levels of learning in Thomas's hierarchy (Levels 6–8 in Table 2.1) is described in horses, the reporting authors note that horses take some time to grasp the concept (McLean and McGreevy, 2004), but having done so, their responses become more rapid and accurate (Creighton, 2007). So, rather than concept learning, this may be what is called learning to learn, the horses having overcome novelty and having learned the salience of various elements in the experimental apparatus.

The outcome of learning studies can depend on the age, reproductive state, social rank and body score, as the benefits and costs of learning may dif-

fer as a result of these variables (Heitor and Vicente, 2007). Certainly, a horse's motor laterality (its left- or right-leg preference) could affect learning, for instance in a maze with left and right turns (Murphy and Arkins, 2007). So, standardising the experimental group for these variables may be as important as standardising the group's prior exposure to learning opportunities, including conspecifics (Søndergaard and Ladewig, 2004), prior training (Le Scolan *et al.*, 1997) and regular handling (which is already biased to the left side by convention; McGreevy and Rogers, 2005).

Perseveration is the term used to describe the behaviours of animals that continue to offer a trained response even when it no longer yields rewards. It is recognised as a feature of stereotypic birds and rodents (Garner and Mason, 2002) but more recently has been reported in horses (Hemmings *et al.*, 2007; Hausberger *et al.*, 2007a). The equine studies in this domain have positively reinforced subjects for pressing levers, so there is a need for caution when applying these findings to the ridden horse that is trained almost exclusively with negative reinforcement. Anecdotally, however, riders do not seem to pick up on any critical differences between stereotypers and other horses with respect to training. Perhaps riders simply fail to notice those horses that are somehow resistant to extinction under a negative-reinforcement training paradigm. If they did, they would surely notice that the cribbers were over-represented among those horses labelled 'forgiving' or even 'stubborn'. Nevertheless, this area merits a detailed investigation.

Equine cognition in equitation

As we will discuss in Chapter 3 (Anthropomorphism), the temperament of a horse is a topic characterised by poorly defined terms but, nevertheless, it is of tremendous importance to riders (Hennessy *et al.*, 2007). For example, it has been found that less-reactive horses perform significantly better in some experimental tasks, possibly because the apparatus itself may distract the more-reactive horses, compromising their performance (Clarke *et al.*, 1996). In addition, social ranking appears unrelated to learning ability in visual discrimination tasks, simple maze tasks and avoidance learning tests. Research repeatedly shows little correlation between a horse's ability in one task and another where the motivations differ. This suggests that any unified scale of 'intelligence' in horses is neither possible nor relevant. Differences in performance between individual horses are much more likely to reflect differences in motivation rather than in intelligence (McLean and McLean, 2008). For example, a less-reactive but highly food-motivated horse may show poor performance in avoidance learning but may be impressive in tasks that involve food rewards, and vice versa. Therefore, it can be concluded that characteristics such as fearfulness and motivation have a significant influence on success or failure in both laboratory and real-life situations (Nicol, 1996).

Aside from the above constraints, perhaps the most important aspect of equine cognition for horse-trainers concerns the presence or not of higher mental abilities. Because of the unique characteristics of the mental life of humans, many people expect to find similar abilities in animals. If insufficient thought is given to the ramifications of cognitive differences between humans (whose competencies are domain general and serve numerous goals) and horses (whose competencies are mainly adaptations of a few specific goals), significant mistakes can be made. Thus, misunderstanding a horse's cognitive abilities has important implications not only for its training program but also for its welfare. There are negative welfare implications in both *overestimating* and *underestimating* mental abilities in animals.

Historically, underestimating an animal's cognitive capacities was a typical viewpoint that elevated mankind above the animal kingdom. Animals such as horses had no intrinsic moral value because they were unable to reason and apparently had no soul. This anthropocentric view gave implicit approval to the abuse of animals. Nowadays, the pendulum has swung the other way and some argue that a closer analysis of the dissimilarities between human and non-human animals is needed to prevent us from confusing similarity with equivalence (Premack, 2007). Until this analysis is fully applied to all aspects of equine and human cognition (including teaching conspecifics, short-term memory, causal reasoning, planning, deception transitive inference and language), the current prevalent tendency will be for the vast

majority of horsepeople to overestimate the mental abilities of horses. The dangers here are more subtle but no less anthropocentric. To suggest, as some lay authors such as Skipper (1999) have, that horses have similar mental abilities to humans is to suggest that there is something more desirable about our own mental abilities. Furthermore, such expectations encourage the use of delayed punishment, which is frequently justified on the grounds that 'he knows what he did wrong'. Overestimating equine cognitive abilities can give tacit approval to poor timing of signals and reinforcement ('he knows what I am asking for, he's just being stubborn!'). It can encourage punishments (see Figure 2.10) that bear little or no relation to the original (incorrect) response and so,

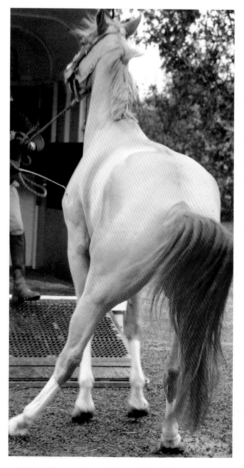

Figure 2.10   The notion of the stubborn horse encourages punishment.

from a learning standpoint, are useless and detrimental (see Chapter 6, Learning III: Associative (aversive), which describes the uses and abuses of punishment).

In the light of our cultural connection with the horse, it is hardly surprising that humans tend to err on the side of overestimating higher mental abilities in horses. To most humans, the horse is a rare mixture of benevolence, beauty and power. So important was the horse to Western civilisation in the past two millennia that most older European cities are adorned with many statues of the horse, primarily as the carriers of leaders (Endenburg, 1999). The horse fought in our wars, it toiled for us and it helped us to build much of the Old as well as the New World. Nowadays, it fulfils our dreams, and still fires our imaginations. Horses are not just pleasure vehicles – much more is expected of them. A horse may be our best friend, our only friend, our child or our partner. The Swiss psychologist Carl Jung (1968) believed that the image of the horse is a powerful symbol in the human psyche. Perhaps this is because the horse has always represented something of a paradox. How could such a big, powerful beast, so capable of rebellion, be typically so tolerant, gentle, forgiving and even patriotic? Most likely, the answer partly lies in the horse's cognitive characteristics and the ways it learns.

It is important to acknowledge that different equestrian pursuits place different demands on horses. This is explored in some detail in Chapter 9, which sets out the ethological, learning and cognitive challenges of various sports and forms of work involving horses. Although many breeds present a genetic predisposition to develop certain skills, representatives of these breeds have refined these skills over an extensive period of structured, guided practice and feedback. Thus, some horses may develop skills in a given type of sport or work and may exhibit what might be regarded as expertise (Helton *et al.*, 2009). Similarly, it is worth pointing out that there are some situations where acknowledging horses' superior sensory abilities allows them to communicate these and influence the rider's decisions. Examples are endurance-riding over unfamiliar land or trail-riding where hazards (e.g. bogs, weak bridges and predators) may be undetected by the rider to the detriment of the safety of both participants (see Figure 2.11).

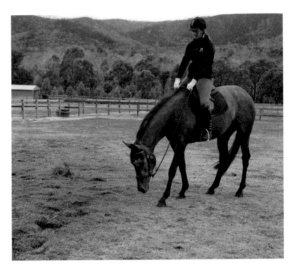

Figure 2.11 It is adaptive for naïve horses to investigate water or marshy ground.

Social learning

In laboratory settings, a variety of species, including chickens, grey parrots, quails, ravens, cats, octopi and chimpanzees, have been shown to pass information about foraging strategies from one individual to another (McGreevy and Boakes, 2007). It makes sense for offspring to learn from their parents and for social animals to learn from one another, for example, what food is safe to consume or, in the case of predators, how to despatch prey. For social animals, synchronising behaviour also makes sense (see Figure 2.12). So, when one animal eats, others are compelled to do so; when one lies down, others may follow. This group effect is known as social facilitation.

At first glance, observational learning seems simple, but it is more complex than it might at first appear. True observational learning requires reasoning and insight to allow exact imitation (Nicol, 1996). It requires animals to see and remember a behaviour sequence, mentally transpose it to their own repertoire, and then perform it. Observational learning of novel behaviour (copying a novel act) has long been considered indicative of some degree of higher mental ability. This form of learning has been researched extensively in horses in four separate investigations (Baer *et al.*, 1983; Baker and Crawford 1986; Clarke *et al.*, 1996; Lindberg *et al.*,

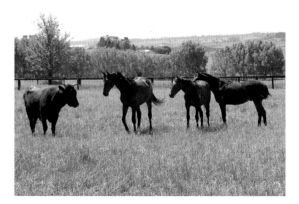

Figure 2.12 Strength in numbers facilitates investigative behaviour.

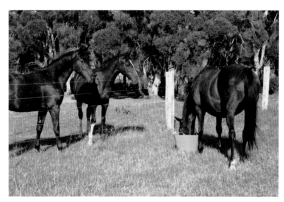

Figure 2.13 The relevance of a bucket to a naïve horse may be enhanced by observation of feeding.

1999) and all published experiments have yielded negative results, although the results of Clarke *et al.* (1996) showed that the presence of a tutor decreased the experimental horse's latency to approach the experimental apparatus. Therefore, using well-trained jumping horses to train young jumpers following behind is not an example of observational learning but rather utilising the motivation of horses to follow one another.

In contrast, observational learning can readily be demonstrated in predators because of the need to teach their young safe killing techniques for large and potentially dangerous prey. For prey species, learning predator avoidance may be more important than food acquisition, and of all cognitive abilities, this is perhaps the most likely to yield evidence of observation learning in horses (D. Goodwin, personal communication, 2007).

When considering the transfer of information between animals, we must distinguish between social facilitation, stimulus enhancement and true cultural transmission. In social facilitation, innate behaviours are initiated or increased in rate or frequency by the presence of another animal carrying out those behaviours. Horses, for example, are more likely to drink when they see others drinking. Stimulus enhancement is the ethological term that describes the ability of one animal (the so-called demonstrator) to draw the attention of another animal (the observer) to the location of reinforcement opportunity rather than an activity per se. A common example arises when a horse rattles a bucket while feeding from it and arouses the at-tention of neighbouring horses. The noise has enhanced the current relevance of the bucket stimulus as a feeding opportunity (see Figure 2.13).

As social animals with excellent vision, one might predict that horses would use observations to improve their biological fitness. With animals that conform to a certain social order, it makes sense that they should be able to learn from pre-trained conspecifics; for example, young farm horses were traditionally harnessed alongside a steady mature plough horse to be taught verbal driving commands. But this is associative and not necessarily observational learning (see Glossary). While horses seem good at responding to socially enhanced stimuli, empirical evidence of observational learning is elusive. Controlled studies in the horse have provided some evidence that stimulus enhancement may result from the behaviour of demonstrator horses as they approach and interact with experimental apparatus that delivers food (Clarke *et al.*, 1996). However, these studies have failed to demonstrate that observational learning enhances an individual's ability to perform an operant task (Lindberg *et al.*, 1999) or make a choice between two feeding sites (Clarke *et al.*, 1996). As such, these studies have challenged the notion that stereotypies can be acquired by mimicry.

Studies in other species demonstrate that animals do not observe all conspecifics with the same enthusiasm. For example, chickens pay particular attention to the feeding strategy of dominant members of the group. It has been pointed out that horses may have evolved to avoid sites where conspecifics have foraged (since these may no longer contain food), and it has been emphasised that designs for social learning studies have so far failed to appreciate the deeply social evolution of horse behaviour (Linklater, 2007). It may be that we have failed to ask the right questions of horses, to ask these in contexts where they are able to learn (Goodwin, 2007) and to ask them of horses that are appropriately related in terms of rank, kinship or affiliation to demonstrators (Nicol, 2002; Murphy and Arkins, 2007).

There is some evidence that learning to follow a human can develop through observation and that relative social rank affects the way observer horses may learn this from potential demonstrator horses (Krueger and Heinze, 2008). In addition, there are reports of cultural transmission of browsing techniques on holly and gorse in family groups of New Forest ponies (Gill, 1988), but in these free-ranging groups, the effects of stimulus enhancement followed by trial-and-error learning cannot be eliminated. However, as the techniques persist in some groups of ponies and are not present in the whole population, this could be analogous to the cultural transmission of sweet potato washing by Japanese macaques (Kawamura, 1959).

Future studies on social learning should focus on the role of the dam as tutor to her foal because vertical transmission of information seems the most likely form of observational learning in a social species (see Figure 2.14). Houpt *et al.* (1982) reported no evidence of foals learning a spatial task from their dams. However, foals that were ex-posed in the first five days of life to humans as they groomed and fed their mothers during a short period (total of 1.25 hours) approached and initiated physical interactions with humans sooner than those subjected to forced handling that included imprinting and haltering (Henry *et al.*, 2005). Studies of this sort may help us to explore how we provide cooperative teaching to equine subjects, for example by interacting with relevant objects verbally (Hothersall and Nicol, 2007). The importance of pursuing this line of enquiry lies chiefly in the notion that any training program or technique instituted by humans could be improved by incorporating appropriate elements of the horse's highly developed social, behavioural and learning repertoire and that, fundamentally, social learning may operate quite differently from mainstream learning theory (Krueger and Flauger, 2007).

While horses show considerable improvement in how quickly they can learn certain things, their performance is nowhere near the levels achieved by some primates and dolphins. These species rapidly learn to apply certain rules to novel problems and can often solve 100% of novel problems at the first attempt (Leslie, 1996). Rule-learning is likely to be more adaptive for a cooperative predator than a grazing animal for which food procurement relies more on memory than higher mental abilities such as planning. In addition, the extra neural circuitry for higher mental abilities requires extra brain tissue, which, as Deacon (1990) showed, is significantly more expensive energy-wise than any other tissue in the body. Evolutionary theory decrees that, like its physical abilities, an animal's mental abilities would be the result of the adaptive forces that it faced, particularly in procuring food, over the eons of its evolution (McLean, 2001).

Free-ranging horses occupy a home-range that they learn to exploit for resources and safety. By using different parts of the range, they can capitalise on the available food and water resources, even using different terrain at different times of year (Olsen, 1996; Linklater *et al.*, 2000). The capacity of horses to return to bountiful grazing spots is a critical contributor to their success in foraging. Horses choose the richest patches when they have recent experience with them, but when they do not have such experience, they adopt a strategy of dynamic averaging that allows them to choose

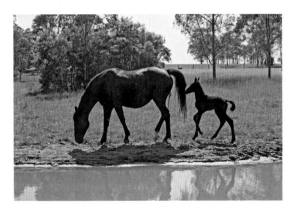

Figure 2.14   The vertical transmission of information from mares to foals merits detailed scrutiny.

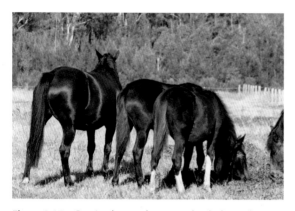

Figure 2.15 Grazing horses do not randomly forage but instead select food on the basis of sight, smell, taste and previous experience of that pasture.

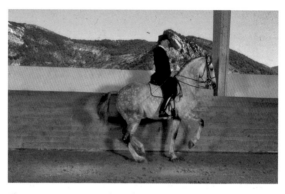

Figure 2.16 Baroque breeds are naturally more upstanding in the forequarters than many modern breeds and are, thus, more easily collected. (Photo courtesy of Cadmos Verlag and Philippe Karl.)

their feeding sites according to the long-term average richness of the available sites (Devenport *et al.*, 2005; see Figure 2.15).

Horses' knowledge of the range facilitates their escape from predators and even biting insects (Linklater *et al.*, 2000). Their daily treks allow them to become familiar with tiny landscape changes, especially visual ones (Hall, 2007) that are avoided or otherwise investigated if they appear innocuous from afar. Horses require considerable spatial representation abilities to migrate when seasonal ecological conditions demand, to be able to navigate between patches of preferred grazing in their home range (Howery *et al.*, 1999) and travel up to 25 km to drink (Stoffel-Willame and Stoffel-Willame, 1999). How free-ranging horses use this to structure their home ranges and form cognitive maps (Tolman, 1948) warrants further investigation (Leblanc and Duncan, 2007), and this is best studied in the niche for which they have evolved (Hothersall and Nicol, 2007). This should allow us to see how cognition in the domestic horse is truly illustrated, exploited and frustrated.

Individual differences

It takes around five years to train a horse to the Grand Prix level. The elements of dressage are difficult for horses to learn and the learning must be accompanied by significant physical development. Particular horses find some aspects of dressage more difficult than others. Certain types of

conformation lend themselves to collection and the analysis of croup:wither ratio covers the most important principles. For classical dressage, where there is an emphasis on collection, a short back and a higher wither-height to croup-height ratio are preferred (see Figure 2.16). Compared with the modern performance breeds (especially the Thoroughbred), the baroque breeds, such as the Lusitanians, Andalusians, Friesians and Lippizaners, are naturally more upstanding in the forequarters and, thus, more easily collected.

There is evidence that selecting for small heads and long legs may inadvertently lead to a population bias to graze with one leg in advance of the other and morphological asymmetry because individuals with these morphological attributes are compelled to reach relatively farther than others for food on the ground (van Heel *et al.*, 2006). This lead preference may compromise balance in performance horses (McGreevy and Rogers, 2005).

Even without the involvement of observational learning, the influence of the parents should not be overlooked, since the influence of the sire has been found to have a significant effect on the training of leading (Warren-Smith *et al.*, 2005b) as well as on spatial tasks (Wolff and Hausberger, 1996). The inheritance of desirable, and indeed dangerous, qualities merits further scientific scrutiny.

The individual differences that characterise equine temperaments have been dubbed 'horsonality' (Visser, 2002). They include features such as laterality, compliance and trainability. Laterality is

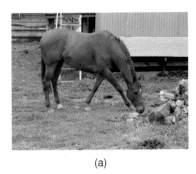 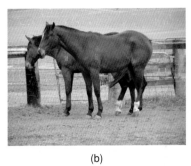 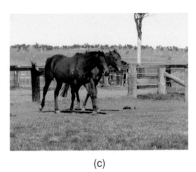

(a)   (b)   (c)

Figure 2.17   Studies of grazing horses (McGreevy *et al.*, 2007) have examined the preference for many lateralised behaviours, including standing (a), flexing (b) and moving relative to conspecifics (c).

of growing interest to equitation scientists as the impact of left- and right-hemispheric dominance and consequent motor preferences becomes more clearly understood. In humans, the right cerebral hemisphere has been associated with emotional responses, including negative effects (nervousness, distress, fear, hostility; Wittling and Roschmann, 1993), while in rodents, left-paw preference and leftward turning behaviour have been associated with heightened physiological stress responses (LaHoste *et al.*, 1998; Neveu and Moya, 1997), suggesting that right brain dominance and speed of arousal may be correlated in these animals. Arousal responses are important in horses because they may indicate what type of work best suits an individual. For example, racehorses must be highly reactive to certain stimuli while many other forms of equitation demand low reactivity (e.g. to be safe in traffic).

Fortunately, it is becoming clear that measurement of emotionality as an outcome of avoidance learning tests is possible and that early detection of this quality in yearlings gives a reliable prediction for life and is more consistent than responses in reward-based (positive reinforcement) tests (Visser *et al.*, 2003). Given the links between laterality and emotionality mentioned above, it may be that, in selecting for differing flight responses, breeders have unwittingly influenced the lateralisation of breeds.

In contrast to species that use thoracic appendages (arms, flippers and paws) for prehension, grazing animals are not directly dependent on a single thoracic or pelvic appendage when

foraging (see Figure 2.17). They graze from a stationary position, moving the head and neck in an arc limited on one side by the presence of the advanced forelimb (McGreevy *et al.*, 2007). After each step, grazing follows an arc medial to the advanced limb. There is no evidence that the head/neck position is a result of one or other eye being preferred for surveillance.

In horses, locomotion is integrated with grazing and, because horses seldom take more than two mouthfuls in one spot before stepping to the next, large areas may be traversed in a single grazing bout (Archer, 1971; Houpt and Wolski, 1982; Fraser, 1992; Francis-Smith and Wood-Gush, 1997). Unless they are disturbed by a threat or displaced by a conspecific, foraging horses look up only when moving from one patch to another and then only long enough to help locate the next suitable food source (on the basis of olfaction and vision).

As the horse moves forward while grazing, its forelegs move alternately, with the hindlimbs following in diagonal couplets. It has been estimated that horses take 10 000 steps per day when grazing (Katherine Houpt, personal communication, 2002), but clearly, this will depend on the quality of the pasture. Based on the premise that horses may graze for up to 16 hours per day, this gives an estimate of 10 steps per minute. The shape and quality of pastures offered to horses in domestic contexts influence the amount of locomotion required for optimal foraging.

Although the forelegs alternate in leading during grazing, the time horses spend with the left

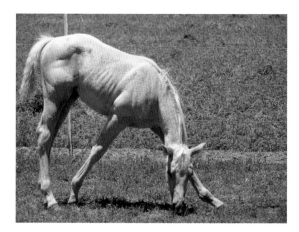

Figure 2.18 Even in the absence of lameness, some foals lock in a strong preference for an unbalanced grazing stance before weaning.

leg advanced is generally longer than that for the right (see Figure 2.18). This manifests as a significant directional bias to graze with the left foreleg in advance of the right (McGreevy and Rogers, 2005). If advancing a forelimb when grazing reflects greater mobility on that side of midline, then it is possible that the brains of left-preferent animals are right-hemisphere dominant. However, a counter argument is that the non-advanced limb is the more critical for survival because it supports more weight, reflects greater agility on the weight-bearing side of the animal and is arguably better positioned to launch the animal into a flight response and a more dominant left turn (owing to the abduction of the right foreleg in the stance phase; McLean and McLean, 2008). We are yet to study how this affects ridden work, such as canter leads and preferred side for lateral flexion.

Emotionality (or nervousness) in horses affects the frequency of eating and drinking, defecation, locomotion and contact with herd-mates (McCann *et al.*, 1988). As a consequence, the learning ability of an individual horse is influenced profoundly by emotionality (McGreevy and Thomson, 2006). Selection for heightened flight responses is more prevalent in racing breeds than in other horses, such as Warmbloods, draught horses and those used by riding schools. Escape tendencies, reactivity to people, behaviour after release and overall emotionality contribute to horses being

classified as highly nervous, nervous, normal or quiet.

Breed differences in the reactivity of horses and their tendency to be especially sensitive and thus easily sent into conflict are of great interest to those studying, working and competing with horses. Paedomorphosis, the retention of juvenile morphology at maturity, is important in generating evolutionary change and occurs in domestication through artificial selection. It may be that we have inadvertently selected for juvenile shapes and thus behavioural tendencies in some of our sport horses. When dogs are compared with their ancestral species the wolf, paedomorphosis manifests in the physical and behavioural traits of different breeds (Goodwin *et al.*, 1997). If this occurs in horses, it may explain physical and behavioural differences across the breeds and move beyond the current system of categorising horses as Hotbloods, Coldbloods and Warmbloods.

Ethological challenges

Like all sentient animals, the horse does whatever it can to reduce pain and discomfort. This underpins the basic responses of the ridden horse but equally explains the importance of pathologies in the emergence of behavioural responses that can cause problems. Physical causes of such behavioural responses should always be ruled out before any behavioural therapy is embraced. For example, undiagnosed pelvic or vertebral disorders can easily lead to poor performance in horses (Haussler *et al.*, 1999). The effect of disorders such as 'cold-back syndrome' and the relationship between dental problems and behaviour under-saddle also need to be more thoroughly explored (McGreevy, 2004).

Ethological challenges include interventions that generate both social and environmental stressors (see Figure 2.19). Although they may subsequently investigate them, horses are inherently cautious of new stimuli (neophobia). This is why jumping unfamiliar and unnatural obstacles initially presents an appreciable challenge to most horses. Examples of *social* challenges include leaving the social group, taking the lead in the company of established leaders, being forced to stay

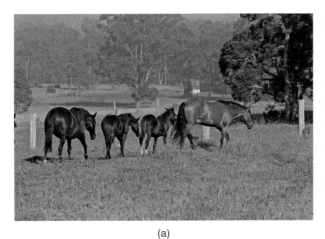
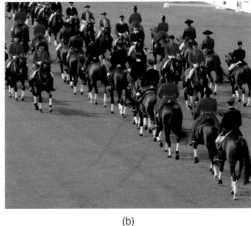

(a)   (b)

Figure 2.19   (a) Horses following one another. (b) Horses being ridden towards each other in a formal exercise (Photo courtesy of Julie Wilson).

at the rear, being close to aggressive conspecifics, walking abreast rather than trekking in a line, and ignoring displays by other horses. Enforced proximity to conspecifics can cause one horse to tread on another in ways that seldom occur in the free-ranging state. During steeple chasing, for example, when horses are clustered, vision is limited and the race becomes hazardous. Furthermore, as jockeys well know, when galloping horses are too closely spaced, they may be prompted by their conspecifics to jump when they are not close enough to the obstacle to clear it safely.

Even when riding alone, we may demand responses from the horse that naturally arise only in social contexts that are far removed from the manège. The elevated steps required in higher levels of dressage, for instance, may be appropriate when horses greet one another but may be ethologically discordant in the absence of a conspecific or a startling object.

Examples of *environmental* challenges include leaving the home range, deviating from an obvious track and traversing, rather than avoiding, obstacles. Other examples of the ways in which equitation provides environmental challenges to horses that run counter to their ethology appear in Table 2.2.

Riding brings both social and environmental challenges and is a useful example of the way we overcome and suppress horses' adaptive re-

sponses and thus ignore their preferences. For example, free-ranging horses rarely maintain a rounded posture while changing gait. The current debate surrounding hyperflexion (Rollkur; see Figure 2.20) highlights the extent to which riders can force a horse to maintain an abnormal posture and can sometimes gain a competitive advantage as a result (van Breda, 2006).

Responses to physical discomfort under-saddle generally have more to do with physiology than ethology. Here, the most obvious sources of *physical* discomfort are the bit, the rider's leg/spur, the whip, the 'carrot-stick' and the girth. This is important because there seems to be an implied assumption that the relationship between human and horse in-hand is identical to the relationship when mounted. It is by no means certain that horses connect pressure in the mouth with the rider. They have not evolved to expect that another animal can apply pressure to the inside of the buccal cavity via a piece of metal. This cognitive aspect may account for the apparent tolerance (or habituation) horses show when allowing heavy-handed riders to mount them time after time. It is therefore unnecessary and inappropriate to complicate a rider's interventions by giving them anthropomorphic labels, such as *asking* (e.g. asking the horse to lower his head), *encouraging* (e.g. using the inside leg to encourage forward movement) and *supporting* (e.g. applying

Table 2.2   Some examples of regular equitation that represent environmental challenges to horses by running counter to their ethology

In-hand	Under-saddle	Comfort
• Leading/following handlers • Lungeing • Entering small spaces, including trailers • Proximity to humans • Standing on moving platforms • Approaching erratically moving/sounding unfamiliar objects	• Walking, rather than running, through unfamiliar creekbeds • Overhanging elements • Approaching erratically moving/sounding unfamiliar objects • Maintaining speed while travelling from light to dark areas or across uneven terrain or downhill (head is usually lowered to assist detection of the safest path) • Maintaining a fixed postural outline while changing gait • Advancing when familiar conspecifics are emitting fearful signals • Walking backwards for more than a bodylength (i.e. entering any unfamiliar cul-de-sac that would require reversing)	• Not rolling when hot and standing in water • Walking on stony ground • Standing square for extended periods • The presence of a bit • Sweaty head covered with a bridle and back covered with a girth, saddle and saddle cloth

the outside rein to support the impulsion). It may be the intention to use words that are common in everyday usage and convey an attitude of co-operation rather than supremacy, but the abiding problem with the use of an anthropomorphic framework to explain rider–horse interactions is that it can disguise and justify abuse of horses that offer undesirable responses, even though these may have been accidentally induced/trained by humans. So, most horses benefit when science provides mechanistic explanations of equitation, even though some horsepeople argue that this is un-

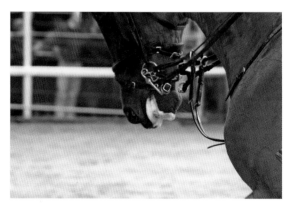

Figure 2.20   A horse being hyperflexed under-saddle.

dermining the bond they share with their horses (McGreevy, 2007).

Communicating ethologically

The complexities of the equine sociogram are explored elegantly elsewhere (Tyler, 1972; Houpt and Keiper, 1982; Keiper and Sambraus, 1986; McDonnell and Haviland, 1995; van Dierendonck *et al.*, 1995), but there remain a number of elements that are relevant to equitation. When riding in company, agonistic responses between horses that derive from unfamiliarity or previous aggressive encounters can be extremely dangerous. Riders can be seriously injured by kicking horses. Equally, sexual advances by stallions can injure riders of oestrous mares and, for that reason, owners of stallions and oestrous mares are encouraged to avoid taking them to shows and events. This may be part of the reason that the owners of competition mares look to hormonal treatments to suppress oestrous behaviour.

Aggression is not the only unwelcome influence from the equid ethogram in equitation. Social responses include the tendency to remain in the company of the herd. This provokes a suite of

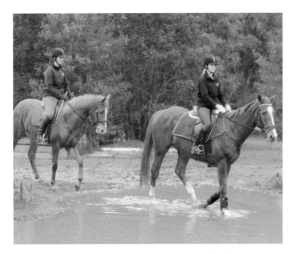

Figure 2.21   One horse following another's lead into water.

responses that can be described as separation anxiety (McGreevy and McLean, 2005). Horses may refuse to leave the stableyard, refuse to lead on the trail or over obstacles and bolt back to their group when turned for home. Instead of fighting these tendencies, it is preferable to focus on getting affected horses under stimulus control and to capitalise on the inclination to return to the herd (e.g. to train negotiating certain obstacles with the leadership of affiliated conspecifics; see Figure 2.21).

When free-ranging horses travel, they generally do so in company by trekking or, far less commonly, by being herded (McDonnell and Haviland, 1995). This explains why ridden horses travel well in single file. Experience shows that certain individuals prefer to take the lead but how this relates to social rank is far from clear. The racing industry could profitably invest in research that explores the social interactions between unfamiliar horses during a race, since this may partly explain why some individuals fail to reach the potential suggested by their cardiovascular attributes.

Applying elements of the horse's social repertoire in a bid to bond with them rarely has an impact on ridden work. Allogrooming may be an exception. Head-rubbing by horses on people (most often after the horse has developed a layer of sweat under its bridle) should not be reinforced because buckles on bridles can easily damage human skin. Horses quickly learn that head-rubbing on humans is fruitless if their handlers stand away when this behaviour is directed at them. Riders who wish to relieve the itchiness of sweat on their horses should remove the bridle and scratch the horse only when it keeps its head still. Stopping the scratching whenever the horse moves is a form of negative punishment (see Chapter 5, Learning II: Associative (attractive)). Equally, riders can scratch horses to reward them because when conducted in areas allogroomed by conspecifics, this has been shown to lower the horse's heart rate (Feh and de Mazières, 1993), an outcome indicative of calmness that in prey species is considered rewarding.

There is an appealing notion that we can apply equine social strategies to human–horse interactions, but data and scientific rigour are lacking in this domain. In the midst of social conflict among horses, it is often submission signals that switch off aggression (McGreevy, 2004) and determine the outcome. These signals may be very subtle: indeed so subtle that they are the subject of considerable debate among equine ethologists (Goodwin, 1999). Horses have rod-dominant photoreceptors arranged in a visual streak, giving tremendous peripheral vision, which contrasts with the cone-dominant trichromatic *area centralis* of humans (Evans and McGreevy, 2006). They are able to detect minute cues from animals (and not just horses) around them. It seems likely that most human signals are not necessarily interpreted as surrogate equine signals (Roberts and Browning, 1998). How crude are the signals from a human to an equine observer? With no tail, fixed ears, a short, inflexible neck and only two legs, we can hardly expect horses to regard us as equine. The chance that we can mimic equine signalling with any subtlety seems remote. Perhaps this is partly why humans rarely claim an ability to issue putative appeasement signals to horses and why agonistic advances from humans prevail. Humans who fall into the trap of assuming that they can communicate eloquently with horses may fail to recognise the aversiveness of some of their behaviour. Ultimately, however, any search for equine analogues of human interactions with a horse becomes virtually irrelevant when the human gets on the horse's back. This point is based simply on the observation that horses mount conspecifics far more occasionally and far more briefly, in play and sex, and, in feral horses, being mounted by another species is associated with predation. When we ride horses we should not expect all of the learned associations, affiliative and otherwise, based on the equid social ethogram to apply. That said, responses trained in-hand can reliably transfer to the ridden context.

Relating ethologically

There are great difficulties in determining social hierarchies among groups of horses. We can measure the relative ease with which one horse can displace another from resources but the outcomes of such interactions usually depend on the resource in question and, hence, reflect the current motivation of the individual to access or retain that resource (Weeks *et al.*, 2000). Even if we confine ourselves to a study of food-related displacements, motivation can change from one hour to the next. For example, a horse is less likely to defend a feed bucket after it has recently sated its appetite. Furthermore, hierarchies are often not simply linear because coalitions among horses within an established social group mean that the presence of key affiliates affects the ability of individuals to retain and access resources (McGreevy, 2004). Humans tend to walk away from feeding horses when they deliver food, with the exception of grass-kept horses, when routine hoof-care and grooming may take place as the horse feeds. However, food-related aggression towards people is atypical and most likely to be shown by stabled horses (see Figure 2.22). The extent to which horse–horse status translates to horse–human contexts seems minimal and is highly unlikely when humans behave in ways that are not analogous to elements of the equine social ethogram. It is also unlikely that horses see humans as horses (McGreevy and McLean, 2007; McGreevy *et al.*, 2009a). We do not and may never know precisely how horses perceive and interpret their world.

Despite this, most 'New-Age' training methods assume that the interactions between horses and humans are analogues of the social relationships existing between horses. Such methods claim that dominance, submission and leadership behaviours account for the quality of horse–human

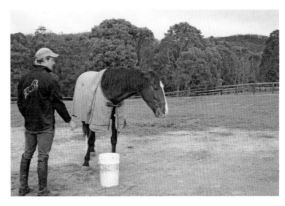

Figure 2.22   A horse showing signs of aggression towards a human at feeding time.

interactions and are apparently understood by the horse (Parelli, 1995; Roberts, 1997). At first glance, this may seem plausible, but equine scientists familiar with learning theory do not find this argument convincing. Horses do not do things for us because they sense strong human leadership. They learn to do things as a result of reinforcement of certain responses: because their human trainers have rewarded the correct responses.

As a trainer you need only to reinforce the correct response, clearly and consistently; you do not need to stand tall and puff your chest out. Your demeanour does not matter. What does matter is what behaviours you reinforce in the horse. For example, the horse that does not load into the float/trailer does not refuse to load because he does not trust or respect you or because he sees your leadership as weak. The horse refuses because his training to lead forward has not been sufficiently generalised to include leading into a trailer. The horse, therefore, remains more under the control of environmental cues than he is under the control of your signals in this context.

The horse's environment is full of competing stimuli, and in this case the contest for control is between the aversiveness of the trailer versus the conditioning of the lead forward signal. The horse that refuses to load into the trailer is clearly not under the control of the lead forward signals. Thoroughly attending to reversing this situation results in horses loading successfully because leading signals outcompete the trailer for salience. That said, it does not provide any justification for beating horses to drive them into a trailer, a practice that would be entirely counter-productive since most horses make an association between the trailer and the beating and learn to avoid all trailers.

Any consideration of human–horse interactions can be blurred by terms that only vaguely relate to equine ethology. From an objective point of view, we should also be cautious in ascribing terms such as 'trust' and 'respect' to horse–human interactions because these terms have little relevance in a scientific interpretation (see Figure 2.23). Such qualities (see Table 2.3) are impossible to identify or measure. We may very well sense that they exist, but if they cannot be clearly measured or defined, then their usefulness as components of systematic training will remain questionable. These topics are discussed in Chapter 8 (Training).

If, when handling horses on the ground, we are to correctly exploit the social organisation of horses, the distinction between alleged dominance characteristics and leadership is critical. It is important to recognise that in the equestrian

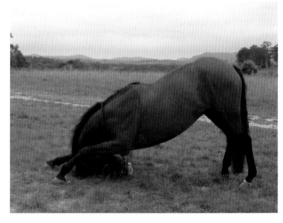

Figure 2.23   There is no convincing evidence that horses showing trained postural responses are offering either submission or respect.

context, when practitioners claim to be imposing their rank, this always involves the application and withdrawal of aversive stimuli and, therefore,

Table 2.3   Undesirable responses and elusive terms with plausible scientific interpretations

Term	Scientific interpretation	Likely extent of horse being under stimulus control of the rider	Likely extent of horse being under stimulus control of the environment
Honest	Compliant	+++	++
Genuine	Predictable	+++	++
Bomb-proof	Unreactive	++++	+
Thorough gentleman	Calm and compliant	+++	++
Perfect manners	Well trained	+++	+
Nice person	Well trained	+++	++
Forward going	Reactive	++	+++
Dirty (stop at a jump)	Unreliable go response	++	+++
Cheeky	Poorly trained	+	++++
Naughty	Poorly trained	+	++++
Sharp	Sensitive	++++	+
Prefers the company of other horses	Likely to stall when leaving conspecifics	+	++++
Not for a novice rider	Reactive, with a tendency to show flight responses and to be unresponsive to rein signals	++	+++
Keen	Tendency to show flight responses	++	+++
Bold	Tendency to traverse unfamiliar obstacles without stalling	++++	+
Lazy	Unresponsive to leg pressures	+	++++
Intelligent	Easily trained	Depends on the skill of the trainer	

cannot be considered outside the framework of learning theory (McGreevy, 2007). There is growing distaste among some authors (e.g. Goodwin, 1999) for the term 'alpha' since this implies non-negotiable and permanent status. This resistance is also found in dog-training circles, and has led to a preference for the notion of leadership.

The concept of humans as leaders of horses has subsequently gained currency in equestrian contexts, but this brings its own set of problems. It implies that all horses that 'respect' a human as leader and have subsequently bonded to him or her will follow that human to aversive places away from the sanctuary of conspecifics. Notwithstanding the rather blurred definition of leadership, there is no evidence in the scientific literature of such phenomena occurring. Furthermore, those who subscribe to the notion of leadership do not explain how leadership qualities can be developed. Rather, they describe operant techniques that condition some useful responses.

Unless they have been hand-reared or subjected to excessive early handling, horses will typically find conspecifics more salient than humans as leaders and, for that matter, companions. Analogues drawn between human–horse interactions and elements of the equine ethogram are tenuous. For example, it is suggested that simply being behind a horse and driving it forward (as in long-reining) is analogous to the herding behaviour of stallions (Zeitler-Feicht, 2004). This assumption is very difficult to test, but convincing evidence would include behavioural analogues in horses driven by humans of the responses herd members typically make when driven by a familiar stallion. Such findings are thwarted by the fact that, when long-reining horses, humans do not make snaking neck movements or bite threats. Equally, when horses direct horses, they never use pressure cues in the mouth. The analogues are elusive. Perhaps humans should simply accept that we are food-bearers and companions, and when we are not giving care and companionship, we are trainers. Conspecifics, including dams, can condition members of their social group (see Figure 2.24) and this activity may facilitate some later outcome, but it is unlikely that training is the intention. Although there is clearly some overlap between care-giving, companionship and training, it makes sense to compartmentalise them. To do so

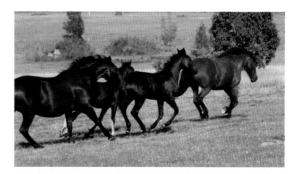

Figure 2.24 It is interesting to speculate on whether horses train one another.

helps us approach each set of activities with clear expectations of likely outcomes.

It has been suggested that humans can enter the social 'hierarchy' of groups of horses by mimicking their behaviour, most notably through their signals (Roberts, 1997; Sighieri *et al.*, 2003). This approach, based on the controversial premise that a herd is organised according to a social status established by means of ritualised conflict, has grown in popularity, but it lacks scientific rigour. Consider round-pen training, for example. The chief appeal of this approach lies in the notion that it is possible to manage unhandled horses without coercion by mimicking behaviours from the equid social ethogram. The merits of this type of hands-off training are purported to be that it is humane and carries with it little risk of learned helplessness. But round-pen training does involve coercion. For unhandled horses, being approached and touched by humans seems to lie on the same continuum of aversive interactions as being whipped: they are all interactions worth avoiding (McGreevy, 2004). Round-pen training may be ineffective insofar as achieving anything useful in human–horse interactions. Indeed, it has been proposed that horses might simply learn to avoid being chased (Krueger, 2007), in other words, negative reinforcement. In some circumstances (with fearful horses, for example), round-pen training can be inhumane. It can precipitate chronic stress if horses are conditioned into constant states of hyper-reactivity and, therefore, may increase behavioural wastage in the form of loss of usefulness and commercial value – a downward trend that can lead to euthanasia or the abattoir. Furthermore, rewards in round-pens often take the form of rubbing,

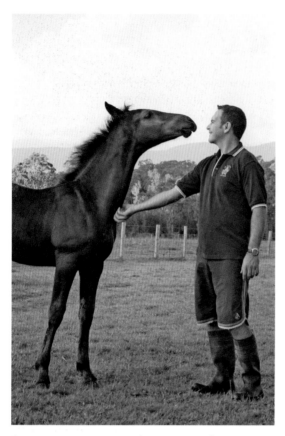

Figure 2.25   Humans groom horses in areas that are not groomed by other horses.

typically on the forehead. Although this intervention may indeed serve as an effective reward, it lacks ethological salience, given that allogrooming of the forehead by conspecifics is far rarer than wither-scratching. Interestingly, an investigation of responses to round-pen training states that grooming as a reward (see Figure 2.25), appeared to have no significant effect on the horse's tendency to follow trainers in the round-pen itself (Krueger, 2007). In other words, the following response was not placed under stimulus control (see Chapter 5, Learning II: Associative (attractive)).

An array of questions is launched by the philosophy of human-as-leader: What if, despite embracing the notion wholeheartedly, handlers cannot persuade their horses to comply? Does that mean the *horse* has better and more consistent leadership characteristics? If the horse fails to follow the handler into a trailer, does that simply

mean the human was perceived as a poor leader? What particular aspect of the human's leadership was lacking? How can this be studied scientifically? Are there negative welfare implications for the horse that does not recognise any human as leader? If a third party successfully leads the horse, using a correct application of negative or positive reinforcement, is he or she showing subliminal leadership?

One might expect horses that genuinely regard certain humans as leaders to seek out the company of the human leaders and forsake their conspecific affiliates. However, there is currently insufficient evidence that horses in a paddock approach humans for reasons other than mere curiosity or because they have been conditioned to do so. Indeed, considering that after 'successful' round-pen training, horses show no increase in their tendency to follow trainers outside of the round-pen, it leads us to question the utility of such a potentially detrimental technique.

If horses regard humans as other horses (which seems unlikely), or if they are deprived of equine company (which is a common mistake seen in rearing orphan or home-bred single, rather than stud-bred, multiple foals), they may engage with humans as play partners. Equine play involves biting, rearing, boxing and kicking (McDonnell and Haviland, 1995). It is never safe to encourage these responses in horses of any age or size.

Ethological solutions

Purely ethological solutions for horse-training are limited (McGreevy and McLean, 2006), confined as they are to the evolutionary adaptive behaviour of the animal that humans can capitalise upon or modify (social facilitation, stimulus enhancement and group behaviours such as trekking). However, horses did not evolve to carry people and so when we ride them, ethology has little further to offer. In contrast, learning theory provides greater possibilities to alter behaviour through the non-associative processes of habituation and sensitisation, and associative modalities, such as operant and classical conditioning.

It has been suggested that a trainer's interactions with horses should be based on three elements fundamental to the equilibrium of the herd:

flight, herd instinct and 'hierarchy' (Sighieri *et al.*, 2003). However, this approach overlooks the importance of foraging, coalitions, kinship and affiliation, as well as the reality of the effects of conditioning on all innate responses. Ethologically sound solutions should not depend on a notion of the horse's benevolence – that the horse is 'wanting to be with' or 'wanting to please' the trainer.

The importance of habituation, sensitisation, operant and classical conditioning should never be underestimated because they facilitate efficient learning and underpin training techniques. They are informed by learning theory and supported by ethology. All training systems use a blend of all of these processes, yet there are fundamental gaps in the understanding and acceptance of their place in equestrian coaching (Warren-Smith and McGreevy, 2006). Studying equine ethology demands consideration of how natural selection shaped horse behaviour and the learning capacity of the horse. Training philosophies that embrace learning theory can be ethological in the sense that they might take into account the types of stimuli horses are most likely to respond to and the types of reinforcers that are most rewarding (from our knowledge of ethology).

Instinctive responses predicted by ethology can facilitate horse-handling without the need for deliberate training. For example, allelomimetic behaviour (mimicry), stimulus-enhancement and social facilitation (McGreevy *et al.*, 2005) are all mechanisms for changing behaviour without associative conditioning. However, these are adaptive mechanisms that evolved for group cohesion, and they can and do act upon behaviours that are themselves subject to conditioning.

Ethologically based training solutions can capitalise on 'leadership' by conspecifics and possibly even the effects of psychopharmaceuticals (including synthetic pheromones; Falewee *et al.*, 2006). Labelling training systems as forms of ethology (e.g. for a short period in the UK, Natural Horsemanship was marketed under the brand 'Equine Ethology') denies the importance of learning theory and implies that we must 'speak the language of horse'. This may be a beguiling idea, but it is ultimately an illusion.

The illusions of horse-owners are generally harmless as long as they do not create unrealistic expectations. Learning theory can and should

be used to explain all training techniques, no matter how elaborately they are camouflaged. As noted previously, most round-pen techniques (e.g. Roberts, 1997) are based as much on negative reinforcement as the physical pressure/release systems used in the ridden horse (McGreevy and McLean, 2007). Similarly, advance-and-retreat techniques (e.g. Blackshaw *et al.*, 1983) are examples of negative reinforcement plus habituation in that the trainer's retreat is made just before the horse initiates a flight response.

Environmental enrichment

Social behaviour, dietary requirements, physiology, temperament and genetics all influence the way a confined animal behaves in its enclosure. Equally, the environment we provide for any domestic animal affects its behaviour and, therefore, its welfare. However, as the context and purpose of confinement change, so do our perceptions of what amounts to appropriate space and what that space must contain (Webster, 1994). Paddocks of adequate size reduce the amount of time spent standing passively (Jørgensen and Bøe, 2007). When stabling and isolation prevent horses from moving and playing, the motivation to perform these behaviours increases (Mal *et al.*, 1991; Houpt *et al.*, 2001; Christensen *et al.*, 2002; McGreevy, 2004; Chaya *et al.*, 2006). Clearly, this affects the work in-hand and under-saddle. Too much concentrated food and insufficient exercise can lead to hyper-reactivity (see Figure 2.26), and

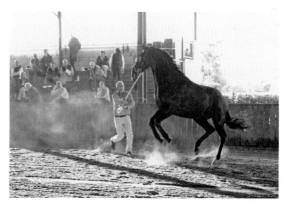

Figure 2.26 Behaviours described as exuberance can reflect previous confinement. (Photo courtesy of Sandy Hannan.)

even catastrophic muscular disorders, within a matter of 24 hours. So, all good horse-keepers appreciate the need to reduce food intake in anticipation of reduced exercise. Confinement to a stable becomes excessive if horses are maintained on full rations and not exercised at least once per day.

As horses spend most of their time not being ridden, their maintenance environment is a prime consideration in horse management. However, the behavioural relevance of this is frequently overlooked. There are a number of areas for consideration in improving a suboptimal environment. These include:

1. *Behavioural enrichment.* The main aim of this method of enrichment is to create an environment that mimics the horse's natural habitat and allows it to express its natural adaptive behaviours and so reduce frustration. Behavioural enrichment that requires an extremely diverse environment plus a large amount of space can be impractical, so the behavioural relevance of enrichment methods is paramount. Also, there must be limits on the extent to which full behavioural repertoires (within the equid ethogram) can be accommodated. We have to acknowledge that allowing a horse to 'express all its natural behaviours' is not entirely feasible. If it were, we would have to let them express their natural reproductive behaviour and fear. In the case of domestic horses, it is possible to argue that riding can offer a form of behavioural enrichment. Riding in environments that are more complex than a familiar arena, such as on reasonably familiar trails, may be akin to the treks free-ranging horses take within their home range. The risks of not doing so can result in horses for which riding outside the arena presents supernormal stimuli (Appleby, 1997) such that they become unsafe to ride. Riding out also appears to help horses to develop mental maps.

2. *Companions.* Like all social species, horses require companions (see Figure 2.27). However, many are housed individually, effectively preventing almost any social behaviour. This social isolation is likely to lead to frustration and suffering for the animals. Placing animals in groups is one of the most easily achieved forms of environmental enrichment but this is

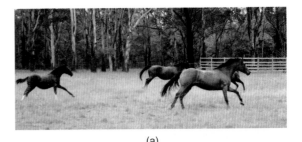

(a)

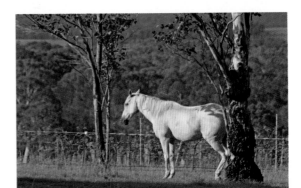

(b)

Figure 2.27   (a) A well-established social group provides important enrichment in domestic contexts. (b) Even at pasture, isolated horses may have compromised welfare.

often not implemented because of the prospect of fighting and injury at the time of mixing. It is not sufficient to assume that any horse will provide the right sort of company. Optimal stable management includes taking the time to establish which horses socialise appropriately as neighbours.

3. *Artificial appliances.* Various devices have been designed for confined animals. Although these may have little similarity to anything that horses are likely to encounter in their natural environment, nonetheless, they can provide suitable enrichment. Examples are plastic bottles suspended from the roof of the stable. Inexpensive items are preferred because they can lose their appeal completely as the horses become habituated to them. The less likely outcome is that these appliances can become the focus of abnormal behaviour patterns such as repetitive, invariant and apparently functionless interactions (i.e. stereotypies).

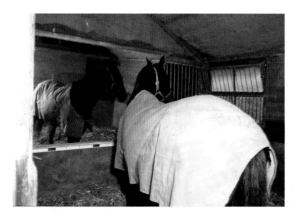

Figure 2.28 The value of ethologically relevant visual stimuli for stabled horses is becoming better understood.

While some yard managers insist that a quiet stable block is beneficial because it allows horses to rest, others play radios in a bid to keep horses mentally occupied. The efficacy of this approach remains unclear since studies have failed to show either an effect of music on ponies during isolation or any preference from one style of music over another (Houpt *et al.*, 2000). This contrasts with studies of dairy cattle, which have shown that classical music facilitated milk flow when compared with rock (Albright and Arave, 1997).

Cooper *et al.* (2000) showed the beneficial effects of providing a mirror for isolated horses, especially those that showed stereotypic weaving (see Figure 2.28). The apparent presence of a conspecific seems to be an effective stimulus for these horses since even a poster of a horse is sufficient to have a similar effect (Mills, 2005a).

4. *Foraging enrichment*. Concentrate feeds do not represent a natural diet for horses. The use of concentrated rations means that horses consume their daily ration very rapidly. This has at least two major disadvantages: it reduces the total oral activity per day and increases the risk of gastric ulceration. These consequences are probably linked in that reduced oral activity is thought to result in reduced saliva production and increased physiological stress responses, both of which compromise the stomach lining (Waters *et al.*, 2002). It seems likely that there is also a deleterious effect on

performance, but evidence of this is marginal to date. Stereotypies associated with low-forage diets may reduce the ability to learn, but it is not yet clear whether this has any effect on ridden work. One method of extending feeding time and mimicking trickle feeding is to feed concentrates in a way that makes the animal work for them (e.g. using the Equiball™ or Pasture Pal™; see Figure 2.29).

Increasing the variety of forage provided to stabled horses allows natural patch-foraging behaviour, and has been shown to reduce the performance of established stereotypies (Goodwin *et al.*, 2002). Thorne *et al.* (2005) report that offering multiple forages can help to normalise feeding behaviour. There is also evidence that offering multiple concentrate diets that vary only in flavour (viz., molasses, garlic, mint or herbs) can prompt stabled horses to show natural patch-foraging behaviour on concentrates (Goodwin *et al.*, 2005).

5. *Control of the environment*. The lack of control of the environment is often pinpointed as a cause of frustration and stress in confined animals. The absence of an ability to travel through time mentally may prevent horses from looking forward to better times ahead and ruminating on the past (McLean, 2003, 2004; Mendl and Paul, 2008). However, it does not mean that sub-optimal environments, including those of the past, do not affect welfare (Mendl and Paul, 2008). When the animal cannot control variables, such as feeding time or the lighting schedule, and when it cannot escape from events it finds unpleasant, it often behaves in ways that suggest frustration. Animals that have learned (as in so-called shuttle box experiments) that rewards and punishments are continually interchanged randomly tend to stop responding. They become withdrawn from their environment and exhibit what is termed learned helplessness. They have lost control of their environment. Learning that there is no escape from aversive stimuli differs from habituation (Hall *et al.*, 2007). Clearly, horses in training are vulnerable to this outcome because the pressures that underpin negative reinforcement may be excessive and sustained, even when horses have responded appropriately. When animals learn

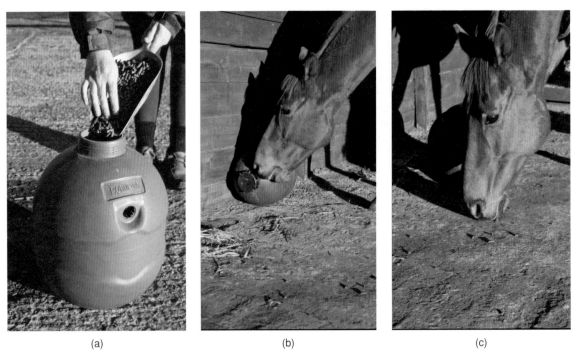

(a)   (b)   (c)

Figure 2.29 An Equiball™ feeding device is filled with pellets (a) before being left with the horse that rolls it around (b) to trigger the delivery of feed pellets (c).

that resistance is futile, they typically become apathetic (Webster, 1994). The lack of active behavioural responses in such animals increases the need for physiological measures that characterise the state of learned helplessness.

Giving horses control of their own environment can be a very successful method of enrichment. One application of such operant devices is in consumer-demand studies, where custom-built devices are operated by the horse (as the consumer) to grant it access to resources such as food, liberty and company. The work that horses put into using these devices reflects, at least in part, the value they place on each resource. Training horses to use switches of this sort can also allow them access to resources in commercial, rather than experimental, contexts. The results of trials of commercial systems that allow group-housed horses access to feeding stations have been reported (Gieling *et al.*, 2007) in descriptions of a one-size-fits-all stable-management system with automated feeding programs. This technology is still embryonic and the prospect of an error

leading to gastrointestinal disturbances is rather forbidding, but one day it may allow horses to be fed customised diets at times that suit their digestive physiology and current work commitments.

Ethologists are likely to contribute significantly to welfare by further explaining human impact on domestic horses while they work and rest. It is generally accepted that signals given to highly trained horses are elegant in their subtlety (Loch, 1977; Sivewright, 1984; McGreevy and McLean, 2007). The development of cognitive ethology and the application of learning theory to equitation may allow us to plot the emergence of the subtle signals given to horses as they progress through training and, thus, detect the transition between operant and classical conditioning.

Once we can distinguish between operant and classically conditioned cues, we will have all the mechanistic data that explain human–horse interactions in the context of the ridden horse. This will allow conceptual investigations of the unique characteristics of elite horses and riders (including talent, flair and intuition) that transcend scientific analysis. Although elite riders will always be those who learn the fastest and get the best from their horses with a minimum of apparent effort, the use of the mechanistic data from the studies of the horse–rider interface will be invaluable from an educational perspective, since it will allow novice riders to mimic elite riders and catalyse their ascendance from novice to advanced horses.

By measuring the pressures and weight distribution of riders and saddles on the horse's spine while in motion, we will also be able to relate lameness and performance problems to asymmetry (McGreevy and Rogers, 2005). An additional welfare benefit is that we will be able to measure the thresholds of tolerance of flexion and hyper-flexion in naïve horses and trained horses from a variety of disciplines. This will greatly inform the welfare debate surrounding Rollkur (McGreevy, 2007).

Ethology helps us to describe a ridden horse's responses as clearly as possible. This is the first step to measuring when they occur, what triggers them and what can be done to reduce their likelihood. The differences in the ethological and cognitive challenges of various forms of horse use appear in Chapter 9 (Horses in sport and work).

Conclusions

To apply learning theory correctly, we must identify the motivational state of the horse so that we can predict its responses and capture or redirect them as appropriate. Horsemanship depends on both detailed knowledge of functional patterns of equine behaviour and the flexibility to correctly apply learning theory. All good trainers display both attributes in a variable measure.

Take-home messages

- Equitation presents significant ethological challenges.
- Training must reflect the physical abilities and learning capacity of the horse.

- Any ability humans may have to relate to horses using equine communication cues is of no use once they mount to ride.
- A rider often runs into difficulties when he or she assumes that the horse knows what he or she wants to achieve.

Ethical considerations

- If laterality studies and temperament tests identify foals that are likely to prove difficult to train, how will this affect the commercial value of those foals and, ultimately, their welfare?
- Matching horses with humans raises ethical questions about whether certain humans should be allowed to ride horses with which they have a poor conceptual match.
- Biotechnologies (and perhaps cloning) may allow horses of extraordinary ability or tolerance to become more predictably available, meaning that humans do not have to modify or moderate their behaviour as much as they currently do.

Areas for further research

- Training and performance differences between crib-biters and weavers and other horses merit a thorough longitudinal investigation so that the long-term effects of stereotypy on learning can be evaluated.
- Temperament characteristics of elite horses should be measured and characterised more fully.
- Further exploration of temperament and laterality tests as predictors of reactivity and suitability for certain sports and work may reduce behavioural wastage.
- Future studies on social and observational learning that focus on the dam as tutor to her foal.
- Further study of the relationship between behaviour under-saddle and disorders such as 'cold-back syndrome' and dental problems will reduce the application of equine behaviour therapy to horses with clinical pathologies.

3 Anthropomorphism

Introduction

Assigning human characteristics to animals and other non-human agents (i.e. anthropomorphism) has been identified by many scholars (Hume, 1757; Darwin, 1872; Freud, 1930). Humans attribute human characteristics to a wide range of non-human agents, embracing such diverse notions as depicting God as having human-like features and crediting machines with feelings. The use of anthropomorphism is comfortable, on the one hand, as it may enhance the lives of people and the animals being anthropomorphised, yet detrimental on the other hand when the inverse process happens and people become dehumanised. Until fairly recently, anthropomorphism has been a common approach used to describe horse behaviour; it is unhelpful at best and may promote poor welfare at worst, particularly when it comes to describing problem behaviours as having some malevolent component. That said, the rejection of anthropomorphism certainly does not imply that horses have no emotions or feelings.

Non-human agents

Non-human agents can include a wide range of things: companion animals, natural phenomena such as the wind, and even mechanical devices. Debate still surrounds the validity of anthropomorphism in scientific discourse, but there is something inherently appealing in attributing human characteristics to non-human agents. When the computer crashes, we may playfully ascribe malevolent intentions to it, but when we do this with animals, it can colour our interactions with that animal. Perhaps because as humans we sense our isolation in terms of our language abilities and thought processes, we are desperate to find that, after all, we are not alone (McLean, 2003).

The cognitive boundaries between humans and animals are unclear; consequently, the boundaries of anthropomorphism are also unclear. We might say that a horse is naughty, but we must question whether our notion of human naughtiness can possibly apply to horses (see Figure 3.1). Perhaps the naughty horse is merely confused. The problem that then arises is what are we going to do about it? Do we have the right to punish the naughty horse? Clearly, there can be serious welfare problems in attributing human characteristics to horses because of the consequences for them. Horses are commonly described using terms such as brave, loyal, dependable, naughty, bad, nasty, malicious, bad-tempered, that he hates, loves, regrets, is compassionate and has a will to win, as well as benevolent with a will to please.

Horse-training and coaching literature abounds with anthropomorphic language where the horse is assumed to understand mental states. Even horse behaviour experts sometimes fall into this

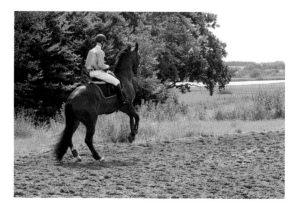

Figure 3.1 Horse misbehaviour – naughty or confused? Terms such as naughty inappropriately shift the blame from the rider to the horse. (Photo courtesy of Julie Taylor/EponaTV.)

trap. Cregier (1990), in the newsletter of the *Equine Behaviour Study Circle*, writes:

> Well-being also has a lot to do with a horse's name. 'A' has a name that draws spontaneous guffaws from all who are introduced to him, their perceptions of the horse are shaped by his name, their laughs diminish the horse. He shrinks further into himself. A horse should suggest his own name, a name that encourages intelligent questions about the horse's talents, personality, grace or origins. A horse's whole world can change when it is in a new place and given a new name that shows that it is cherished and admired for what it is. 'A's name must be changed and reflect the individual and proud animal that he will become.'

Of course, this article may be forgiven for its anthropomorphic transgressions as a result of its non-scientific pretension and being almost 20 years out of date. On the other hand, teleological explanations of purpose are more difficult to accept, especially from an author who claims horse behaviour expertise (although she is astute enough to point to the horse's confusion as being the key):

> Immortal's problem was that he was not only very sensitive (as Lusitanos tend to be), he was also very willing. He wanted to do his best to please, and while he understood exactly what was expected of him, he was fine. (Skipper, 1999)

Scientists neither confirm nor deny the existence of the equine mind, but hold that sensitivity and willingness are not measurable by any honest scientific means. As this is a second-hand account of someone else's horse, it is unclear whether this is what the author was told (and accepted) or, an interpretation of what was said. Skipper (1999) did not elaborate on what was meant by 'wanted . . . to please', although later mentioned how enjoyment of work is developed:

> It is true that, at the very outset of his education, the horse will generally not possess a great deal of inner motivation, except that he may enjoy exercise for its own sake. [. . .] However, he may not see the point of some fairly simple exercises we may ask him to do. When we set out to train a very green horse, there is no way we can explain to him that what we are asking of him is . . . for his own good. [. . .] The trainer . . . can only say something along the lines of, 'Because it will please me if you do.' (Skipper, 1999)

However, the mechanism or teleological implications of 'pleasing' are not addressed in the text. While there is an unnecessary assumption of cognitive capacities beyond behavioural reinforcement in explaining the acquisition of trained responses, it is clear that Skipper understands the importance of other motivating factors, which are discussed at length in her books. Unfortunately, this author seems to align her arguments with scientific principles when it suits her purpose but criticises scientific rigour when it runs counter to her anthropomorphic position.

Communication

Griffin (1992) believed that communicative gestures in animals convey conscious thoughts and subjective feelings from one animal to another. This, he claimed, is objective, verifiable evidence of the mental experiences of the animals themselves. Griffin also considered that versatile adaptability to novel situations is powerful evidence of conscious thinking in animals. Anthropomorphism is sometimes defended as legitimate within certain contexts, in that animals might, in fact, be able to think about certain things that are important to them (Fisher, 1990).

The recent spate of horse-whisperers represents a range of so-called Natural Horsemanship training techniques and an appealing message. Few horse-owners deny that harmony of horse and human is desirable, but many admit that it can be elusive. The appeal of direct communication between horses and humans is beguiling. Clever labeling of human–horse interactions may be designed primarily for educational purposes, but it can also make the interpretations of horse whisperers sound irrefutably plausible and humane. Unfortunately, such labels can be misleading, contradictory and constitute potential barriers to effective training. They can also lead to misunderstanding, conflict and reduced welfare for human and equine participants. For example, some practitioners insist that horses in round-pens signal to their human trainers as they would to high-ranking herdmates (see Figure 3.2), and that they are motivated to be with those humans simply because they 'respect' them. In contrast, it is possible that horses in round-pens are showing distance-reducing affiliative signals that are being misinterpreted (Goodwin, 1999). However, recent empirical studies suggest that the responses of horses to humans in confined areas, such as round-pens, are context-specific (Krueger, 2007) and may rely more on negative reinforcement than on innate equine social strategies (Warren-Smith and McGreevy, 2008b). These findings prompt us to question the interpretations of a horse's responses to round-pen

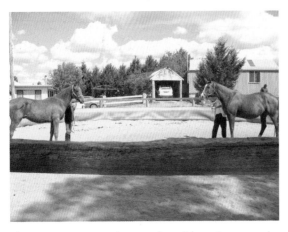

Figure 3.2 Recent evidence confirms that equine responses to round-pen training are not seen in intra-specific contexts. (Photo courtesy of Amanda Warren-Smith.)

interventions commonly offered by practitioners and to offer more scientific, measurable interpretations in horse handling and training.

Anthropocentrism

The doctrine of the human-centred universe is pivotal to the anthropomorphic mindset and makes a number of assumptions. One of the most detrimental is assuming that the horse *knows* and, if this is so, he must *know* the difference between right and wrong, so punishing him when his response is incorrect is an appropriate human intervention. Teleological explanations attribute purpose to an organism's behaviour and can also lead to assumptions that are difficult to prove, or are perhaps simply convenient oversimplifications. For example, 'my horse behaved badly because he was paying me back for my being late to feed him last night'; or he is 'thinking of ways to get out of work'. Attributing human thought processes to animals may be the most inappropriate way of describing cognitive processes. For instance, when the horse is given a spell after a period of work, one hears that it 'gives him time to think about what he has learned'. The unique effect of human language on human thought processes provides reason for caution in attributing the same processes to other species. For this reason, the term higher-order linguistic thought (HOLT) was coined and considered to be a uniquely human capability (Rolls, 2000).

It is often suggested that one of the main reasons horses comply with riders' requests is their willingness to please (Warren-Smith and McGreevy, 2008a). Although appealing to some horse-owners, the chief problem with this approach revolves around the higher cognitive skills required for this to come about. Also, it is questionable whether horses are motivated to please other horses, let alone humans, or indeed, that human expressions of pleasure can even be correctly interpreted by horses. Why should a horse wish to bring pleasure to its rider by jumping a fence when its species-specific response is simply to avoid it?

Beyond mere compliance lies the implicit assumption that horses may actively cooperate with riders to achieve shared goals (e.g. in play; Goodwin and Hughes, 2005). True cooperation

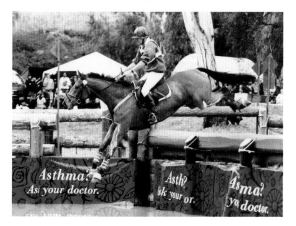

Figure 3.3   The horse is not likely to share the same goals as humans.

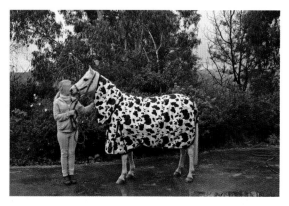

Figure 3.4   The pet horse: a projected image of ourselves?

would demand very complex cognitive skills, as the horse would have to know the outcome and want it for some reason (see Figure 3.3). For example, to be considered 'cooperative' a racehorse would have to know that it is racing, presumably over a certain distance, and recognise the critical importance and benefits of being in the lead when running past the finishing post. One of the dangers in adopting a teleological and anthropomorphic framework to explain horse motivation is that a rider may assume that a horse knows what the rider wants. This can lead the rider to give unclear cues and become angry and perhaps feel disappointed when these fail to produce the desired outcome.

How did anthropomorphism come about?

Anthropomorphism has an appeal to many observers of animal behaviour, especially novices, because it by-passes dry descriptors. Epley *et al.* (2007) suggest that at least two dimensions of similarity need to be present for anthropomorphism to occur: similarity in morphology and similarity in motion. Children as young as 9 months seem able to attribute intentions to an action when performed by a human-like hand but not when performed by a wooden rod (Woodward, 1999). Furthermore, if robots are given human-like faces and bodies, they are anthropomorphised more readily, and when products are designed with human features they are more successful in the marketplace (Epley *et al.*, 2007).

Anthropomorphic behaviours include regarding the pet as a family member or best friend, assigning a human role, such as baby, to the pet, taking on a specific maternal or paternal role (Greenebaum, 2004), and even dressing the pet in human clothing and celebrating its birthdays (Archer, 1997). These human behaviours are increasing at a surprising rate. Data from a US pet hospital (Gardyn, 2002) revealed that between 1995 and 2001 there was a 28% increase in pet owners describing themselves as the father or mother of their pets. Commercial interests have been quick to capitalise on this behaviour so that pet owners can now send their pets to daycare, weight-loss holidays and spas, massage and homeopathic therapy, as well as taking them to cafés and restaurants and taking them on holidays (Duvall-Antonacopoulos and Pychyl, 2008). The vast array of colours and styles of horse rugs/covers and equipment available is testimony to the horse-owners' participation in this response (see Figure 3.4).

What purpose does anthropomorphism serve?

Epley *et al.* (2007) proposed that anthropomorphism satisfies a desire to feel efficacious in one's environment and to increase a sense of social connection – it should increase as a function of these two motivational states. They suggested that anthropomorphism has an important function in humans in reducing uncertainty and increasing understanding of one's environment and the tendency positively correlates with loneliness. In such states of isolation, a lonely person is likely to see a pet as thoughtful and consecrated but less likely to see it as vengeful or deceitful (Epley *et al.*, 2007). Their research also reports that developmental influences such as the quality of social relationships and feelings of attachment to animals or detachment from other humans also increase the likelihood of anthropomorphism. So, it seems that anthropomorphism serves to increase predictability and, therefore, controllability in an uncertain world, which would have made it attractive to our ancestors since time immemorial. Surveys by Beck and Madresh (2008) revealed that relationships between humans and their pets were more secure than human–human relationships on every measure. In addition, relationships with pets affect other aspects of the pet-owner's life, perhaps by buffering the experience of negative human social interactions.

Using a scale for anthropomorphism designed by Albert and Bulcroft (1988), studies by Duvall-Antonacopoulos and Pychyl (2008) revealed that on a scale of increased anthropomorphism:

- women scored higher than men;
- unmarried people scored higher than people in married or de facto relationships;
- people without children at home scored higher than those with children at home;
- people without university degrees scored higher than those with degrees;
- people with less family support scored higher than those with greater family support.

Anthropomorphism can, thus, be seen as an adaptive human behaviour. Surprisingly, however, the studies showed a small but significant positive correlation between a person's stress level and the tendency to anthropomorphise pets.

The dangers of anthropomorphism

Fisher (1990) has argued that the mistakes or fallacies of anthropomorphism are neither well-defined nor fallacious. He claims that the charge

of anthropomorphism oversimplifies a complex issue and, worse, it inhibits examination of vital issues in an empirical sense. Human language provides unclear boundaries of anthropomorphic possibilities. For example, a racehorse might be trying hard to be in front of other horses, thus allowing it to win the race, but it probably has no idea of the consequences of winning. It is even more inappropriate to describe it as courageous. Fisher distinguishes between making descriptive mistakes where we misinterpret behaviour (such as a stallion's bared teeth being mistaken for smiling and affection) or anthropomorphism as a result of inaccuracy (what might not be anthropomorphism when describing a chimpanzee's behaviour could well be when describing a worm's). Thus, caution is required in laying charges of anthropomorphism. Fisher concludes that critics of anthropomorphic thinking require a plausible argument that ascribing human thinking to non-human agents is fallacious. He concedes that the general response of humans to animals is also based on an innate but crude cognitive emotional framework within which there is no clear differentiation between ourselves and other animals.

Fisher's caution regarding the fundamentalist scientific approach in describing animal behaviour is encapsulated in the term mechanomorphism (Caporael, 1986), the doctrine that the universe is fully explicable in mechanistic, reductionist terms. It implies that living beings can be described in purely mechanistic and, by implication, inappropriately simplistic terms.

Dennett (1996), however, cautions us against assuming without proof that animals have insight into their innate behaviours. To do so 'is to ignore the null hypothesis in an unacceptable way – if we are asking a scientific question'. Scientifically, such a view is unnecessarily complex and it is incorrect to assume without proof that animals have 'a stream of reflective consciousness something like our own' that accompanies apparently clever activities (Dennett, 1996).

Anthropomorphism remains an important cautionary beacon for horse-trainers. For example, Midkiff (1996) illustrated the benevolent and anthropomorphic viewpoint: 'One of the most compelling reasons women love horses is the promise and reality of unconditional love.' However, anthropomorphism also allows for the malevolent notion. For example, Schramm (1986), writing on the subject of difficult horses, describes some as 'depraved'. McBane (1987) quotes an experienced groom as saying that some people are born bad and the same is true for horses. Such anthropomorphism provides a great danger in diagnosing and treating behaviour problems and training issues in general that may compromise the welfare of the horse. It can encourage punishments that bear little or no relation to the original (incorrect) response.

When humans have expectations that animals 'understand' what is required, they are likely to give inappropriate signals to the animals, such as delayed, inconsistent or meaningless reinforcements, resulting in deleterious behavioural changes. These changes are manifest in conflict behaviours, such as redirected, ambivalent and displacement behaviours, stereotypies and injurious behaviours (Wiepkema, 1987). Concepts such as respect and submission can have negative welfare consequences for horses when applied within the context of unwelcome or problematic behaviour. In the minds of some, the terms respect and submission may justify delayed punishment ('He knows what he did wrong!'), poor timing of signals and reinforcement ('He knows what I am asking for!'). However, the chief problem of describing horse behaviour other than in subjective terms is that there has been no consistent scientific descriptive terminology even among horse enthusiasts (Mills, 1998).

Empathy is the ability to simultaneously experience another being's emotional state. It is a characteristic of human thought processes that, as a result of the discovery of mirror neurons in monkeys (Rizzolatti *et al.*, 1996), we now extend to include other primates. This mirror neuron system is central to the ability of humans to empathise with other humans and possibly other animals about their emotional states. However, if empathy results in projection of our own personality onto the object of our empathy, it may be the first step to misunderstandings between man and horse because it deprives the horse of its own 'horsonality'. A truly empathetic approach involves understanding the horse's nature as far as possible, and may actually describe what is known as 'feel', 'horse sense' and having a 'way with horses'.

Communication between humans and horses

Using principles of symbolic interaction, Brandt (2004) claimed that humans and horses have created a language system with rules of 'grammar' that allow effective communication through body-to-body contact. Mead (1934) considered that animals were more impulsive because they do not have language. Maybe this is true but we have to be careful how we define language. Stone (2001) uses Shapiro's idea (1990) that 'kinesthetic empathy' communication between horses and humans is an embodied experience, but is this really language? Language is defined as a systematic (i.e. ordered, planned) means of communicating by the use of sounds or conventional symbols. Human listeners treat words and phrases that describe objects as implying the speaker's disposition and propensity to act towards those objects or events in certain ways (Pinker, 1994); in other words, as implying something about the speaker's mental state. While non-human listeners acquire a raft of information from the communications of others, there is little evidence to suggest that anything is conveyed about the speaker's mental state. For example, consider the behaviour of a subordinate horse when threatened by a more dominant individual. The subordinate's submissive behaviour thwarts further attack, which causes a change of behaviour in the dominant horse. One might conclude that the subordinate horse has recognised a change in the *attitude* of the dominant horse, or that the dominant horse is now seeking to lower the fear of the subordinate horse. It is just as likely that the subordinate is simply acting on the basis of a genetic predisposition that has been modified by learning. The difference between the two scenarios may seem minimal but the latter does not require an unnecessarily complex theory of mind or purposive intention (teleology); in other words, it does not require one animal to *understand* and infer the mental state of the other.

What about racehorses?

Surely, when racehorses make a supreme effort, they do so in order to get or stay ahead of the others. Or, do they? In Chapter 11 (Biomechanics),

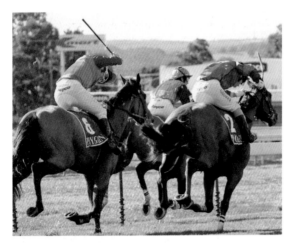

Figure 3.5 The factors that determine whether a horse will overtake others and win a race are more likely a result of conditioning than a desire to win in order to please humans. (Photo courtesy of Sandra Jorgensen.)

we will look at the powerful influence of social facilitation. This influence appears to be principally what causes racehorses to run (see Figure 3.5). It may well be that some horses *do* want to be in front, and there could be many reasons for that (to avoid being crowded is one possibility). There is also the possibility that galloping fast in company may satisfy an internal drive that is rewarding in itself. Some people insist that dominant horses make the best racehorses, but there is little evidence that this is actually the case. Sport horses do not – and cannot – share our ambitions with regard to those sports. True cooperation would demand very complex cognitive skills, as the horse would have to know the outcome and want it for some reason.

Training and handling

In the broadest sense, approaches to training and handling horses have been assigned to two categories: a so-called cooperative approach based upon the belief that horses want to please their riders, handlers and owners, and an alternative approach based on human dominance and equine submission (Goodwin, 1999; van Dierendonck and Goodwin, 2005). This categorisation may seem to explain responses by the trained horse but over-

looks the possibility that most naïve horses respond to humans as they would to conspecifics or predators and that, in moving away posturally or bodily, they avoid physical and psychological pressure (McGreevy and McLean, 2005). So, we might refer to counter-predator responses as core elements of the *predator model* and responses based on the equid social ethogram (Goodwin, 2002) as core elements of the *conspecific model*. It is unclear whether these two possible models must necessarily be mutually exclusive.

There are several limitations to this binary interpretive framework. While it is convenient to identify the ethological relevance of a response, and tempting to assign an appropriate affective state to horses as they show them, the cognitive pitfalls are considerable. For example, it engenders the idea that horses use a functional classification (i.e. that anything to be avoided is a predator). There are interpretive problems with a functional species-based classificatory perceptual system in contrast to one based on more general stimulus qualities, which we know underpin many perpetual processes (e.g. stimulus configuration, and other simpler properties such as perceived velocity and size, which influence the response elicited).

McGreevy *et al.* (2009a) tested the validity of the conspecific model, since that is the model for which ethological data are most readily available. In their analysis, they accept that it may be that the predator and conspecific models apply in series, such that if the actions of the human do not continue to elicit counter-predator responses, then this deficit may stimulate an array of conspecific responses. Notwithstanding the above-mentioned arguments against such interpretive labels, this approach may be plausible, given that horses show some pre-adaptation for domestication by forming and maintaining inter-specific associations in the same way that zebra and wildebeest do (Estes, 1991). Perhaps this manifests as an ability to interpret agonistic behaviours in both their own and the accompanying species. Thus, the predator model may reflect a set of default responses but is succeeded by the conspecific model. However, as McGreevy *et al.* (2009a) emphasise, there may also be an important departure from either of these ethological models when horses are ridden.

The distinction between intra-specific and counter-predator responses is inherently blurred since some counter-predator responses, such as biting and kicking, may be used in agonistic responses to other horses. Regardless of the respective order or exclusivity of the two prevailing models, the waters are muddied by claims that horses operating under the conspecific model *trust* trainers and *accept* them as dominant members of the dyad (as discussed by Waran *et al.*, 2002). This might be referred to as the sympathetic model and features in Natural (sympathetic) Horsemanship. Of course, these approaches are currently beyond the reach of scientific enquiry since emotional qualities, such as trust, are difficult to define and measure. That said, there is some evidence that relative social rank affects the way observer horses may learn from potential demonstrator horses (Krueger and Heinze, 2008).

In support of the conspecific model over the predator model, there are some highly specific behaviours that horses do to other horses and which they may show to humans but never to predators. Examples include foal snapping, head lowering (Goodwin, 1999), mutual grooming, vocalisation and oestrus display. When horses exhibit these behaviours to humans, it seems unlikely that they perceive us as predators at that time. Compelling scientific evidence in support of the conspecific model comes from studies showing that stroking or vigorous grooming of the withers or back by humans can have effects similar to allogrooming by horses (Feh and de Mazières, 1993). In addition, many naïve horses attempt to reciprocate wither grooming by humans (McGreevy, 2004). However, there will always be *some* difference when humans are substituted for a horse in horse–horse interactions, such as not using teeth in mutual grooming, human ears will always be immobile and we will never have tails to swish. Feh and de Mazières (1993) showed that heart rates fall in horses groomed at the withers. It seems likely that this is a difficult region to autogroom, being situated so far from the hindfeet and so close to the head, the body parts used for autogrooming. It may also be that grooming the forehead and the pectoral region has a similar effect on cardiac responses even though it is far less common to see allogrooming of these sites. Thus, we contend that the biological correspondence, proximate benefits and context specificity of such interactions between horses and humans merit consideration.

The emergence of the equid ethogram (McDonnell and Haviland, 1995; McDonnell and Poulin, 2001; McDonnell, 2003) allowed McGreevy *et al.* (2009a) to consider the breadth of horse–horse (social) interactions that may have analogues in human–horse interactions. They explored the impact and relevance of plausible analogues of the equid social ethogram that may appear in human–horse interactions in common equestrian and stable-management techniques, especially as they relate to riding, driving, round-pen training, lungeing and leading as well as handling in the stable and paddock. In summary, McGreevy *et al.* (2009a) argue that it is more accurate to replace predator, conspecific and sympathetic models with *avoidance* and *approach models*, the latter being sub-divided into approach for investigation and subsequent approach for affiliation.

Analysis of the equid ethogram

The tables below offer an exploration and analysis of elements of the equid social ethogram that may be analogous to interactions with humans in the domestic context. Activities for which a naturally occurring analogue exists appear in Table 3.1, which is sub-divided into activities for which naturally occurring analogues exist in both directions: human–horse and horse–human (Table 3.1a) and activities for which a naturally occurring analogue exists in only the horse–human direction (Table 3.1b). For clarity, we distinguish between horse–human and human–horse interactions, the latter and more common of these being where the human initiates the interaction. We have clustered these analogues together in Table 3.1a to highlight where characteristics such as 'attractiveness of outcome for the initiator' differ depending on the direction of the interaction.

In our analysis of the equid ethogram, we have assumed that horse–human interactions are motivated by proximate outcomes rather than a learned goal. Thus, in our tables, horses that threaten humans do so to move the humans away, even though it is possible that some horses learn to be aggressive and threatening for different ultimate goals (e.g. these responses may have been inadvertently reinforced by poor timing of food offers at feeding time). Such outcomes are not

Table 3.1a Activities for which naturally occurring analogues exist in both directions: human–horse and horse–human

Horse–horse interaction (McDonnell, 2003)	Human–horse interactions	Horse–human interactions	Biological correspondence	Stability/Context dependence	Attractiveness of the proximate outcome for the horse	Extent to which the horse may have control over the interaction
Alert	Staring at horse while standing within its visual field	=[a]	+/?	+	–	+
Approach	Walking/running directly up to horse	=	++	+	–/?	+
Avoidance/retreat	Withdrawal (e.g. during round-pen training or simply moving away from horse)		+	+	+	–
		Horse avoiding being caught	++	+	+	++
Balk[b]	Stopping suddenly while walking		–	–	–	–
		Horse ceasing forward movement while being led	++	++	++	++
Bite threat	Rapid turning of the head towards horse		++	+	–	–
		Horse threatening to bite handler	++	+	+	++
Boxing	Hitting a horse with fists, hands or whips		+/?	–	–	–
		Horse rearing and paddling forelegs at handler	++	+	+	++
Chase	Running after horse to catch it or harry it away from given spot[c]		+/?	+	–	–
		Horse chasing human out of the stable, paddock or round-pen	+	–	+	++
Grasp	Neck twitch or so-called gaucho twitch		+/?	+	–	–
		Horse grasping handler	++	+	?	++

Behaviour	Description				
Head bump	Head- (or possibly hand-) to-head contact with horse's head or neck	−	−/?	?	−
	Head-to-head contact with human	+	?	+	+
Head on neck, back or rump	Head- (or possibly hand-) to-head contact with horse's neck, back or rump	−	−/?	?	−
	Head-to-neck, back or rump contact with human	+	?	+	+
Head-bowing =	Horse bowing towards handler	++	+	?	++
Herding and driving	Moving horse(s) from behind with mildly aversive stimuli	++	+	−	+/?
Interference[d]	Human in paddock or stable with more than one horse, attempt to 'split up' fight	+/?	−	+	++
	Mare protecting foal	+	+/?	−	−
Kick	Some humans do kick horses[e]	++	+	++	+
	Horse kicking handler	++	+	−	−
Kick threat	Threaten to whip or sound the whip[e]	+/?	+	+	++
	Horse threatening to kick handler	++	+	−	−
Lunge	Moving rapidly towards horse	+/?	+	+	++
	Lungeing towards handler	+	+	−	−
Mutual grooming	Grooming/scratching a horse's lower neck/withers	+	+	+	+
=		+	+	+	+
	Nuzzling	+	?	+	+
Mounting	Mounting-to-ride?	−	−	+/−	−
	Attempting to mount human	?	−	−	−

(Continued)

Table 3.1a (*Continued*)

Horse–horse interaction (McDonnell, 2003)	Human–horse interactions	Horse–human interactions	Biological correspondence	Stability/Context dependence	Attractiveness of the proximate outcome for the horse	Extent to which the horse may have control over the interaction
Nip	Brief pinching of skin (often lip) as punisher		—	—	—	—
		Horse nipping handler	++	+	+	++
Olfactory investigation	Nose-to-nose exchanges as advocated by some trainers		+/?	+	?	+
		Responses to novel human-borne odours	+	+	?	++
Parallel prance	Leading in-hand at the trot (as in in-hand showing)		+/?	+	?	+
		Prancing alongside handler	+/?	+	?	+
Push	Moving horse with pressure on shoulders or flanks		++	+	—	+
		Barging	++	+	+	+
Stomp	Stamping foot near horse		+/?	+/?	?	—
		Stomping at handler	+/?	+	+	+
Trekking[f]	Leading a horse without rein pressure		+/?	+	—	+
		Following a horse (e.g. in long-reining)	?	+	—	—

[a] = denotes the existence of a corresponding activity in the opposite direction to the usual.

[b] Abrupt halt or reversal of direction with movement of the head and neck in a rapid sweeping dorsolateral motion away from an apparent threat while the hindlegs remain stationary. The forelegs lift off the ground.

[c] Loose jumping sometimes involves this interaction.

[d] One or more horses may simultaneously interfere with an ongoing agonistic encounter between conspecifics. Disruption of combat occurs by moving between the fighting individuals, pushing, attacking or simply approaching the combatants.

[e] Hitting, using a whip, is a closer analogue of a kick than a bite, since it causes sharp pain and is the result of a movement that extends towards the target but does not involve teeth.

[f] Two or more animals moving together, typically following one another.

Table 3.1b Activities for which a naturally occurring analogue exists in only one direction: horse–human

Horse–horse interaction	Horse–human interactions	Biological correspondence	Stability/context dependence	Attractiveness of the proximate outcome for the horse	Extent to which the horse may have control over the interaction
Arched neck threat	Flexed necks are favoured in dressage competitions	-/?	-	-	-/?
Bite[a]	Horse biting handler	++	+	+	++
Circling[b]	Horse being lunged or worked in a round-pen	+/?	+	-/+	-
Dancing[b]	Horse attacks human Circus/Pignonesque tricks	-/?	-	-	-
Ears laid back/pinned	Ear threat towards human	+	+	++	++
Erection	Erection while being groomed, shod or otherwise handled	+/?	+	?	++
Flehmen	Responses to novel human-borne odours	+	+	?	++
Head threat[c]	Horse threatening handler	+	+	++	++
Neck wrestling[d]	Same as dancing (above)	+/?	+	+	+
Pawing	Pawing in presence of handler	+/?	+	?	+
Posturing[e]	Posturing towards handler	+/?	+	?	+
Rearing	Rearing towards handler	+	+	+	++
Rump presentation	Presenting rump towards handler	+/?	+	?	+
Snapping[f]	Foal or young horse snapping towards human	+/?	+	+	+
Receptive and non-receptive female responses	Mare displaying to human	+/?	+	?	+

[a] Arguably, bite has analogues in pinching and whip use.
[b] Two stallions rear, interlock the forelegs and shuffle the hindlegs while biting or threatening to bite each other's head and neck.
[c] Head lowered with the ears pinned, neck stretched or extended towards the target and lips often pursed.
[d] Sparring with the head and neck that may involve one or both protagonists dropping to one or both knees or raising the forelegs.
[e] Posturing describes a suite of pre-fight behaviours that includes head-bowing, olfactory investigation, stomping, prancing, rubbing and pushing, all with neck arching and some stiffening of the entire body.
[f] Moving the lower jaw up and down in a chewing or sucking motion, with the mouth open and lips drawn back.

Table 3.2 Elements of the equid ethogram that do not appear in horse–human dyads (horse–horse activities, but not horse–human or human–horse)

> Maternal licking (although sponging may equate).
>
> Suckling (although equivalent may appear as hand-stripping prior to bottle feeding).
>
> Blocking (defined in ethogram as foal stopping in front of and perpendicular to mare).
>
> Mutual insect control (although a human may swat flies away from horse, and may also be a target of tail swishing from horses, these two activities rarely occur simultaneously, so it seems inappropriate to call it 'mutual').

considered within a framework because we are seeking to focus entirely on the most ethologically plausible proximate functions of responses. Solitary activities are not listed because they lack relevance to this argument.

Elements of the ethogram that do not arise in horse–human dyads (interventions humans never undertake with horses) appear in Table 3.2. These include maternal licking, suckling and mutual fly-swatting. Activities for which no naturally occurring analogue exists (interactions horses never engage in with each other) appear in Table 3.3.

What is really going on?

Table 3.1 shows how common analogues of horse–horse interactions may be adaptive and appropriate in interactions between horses and humans. Table 3.2 reminds us that some elements of the equid ethogram cannot translate to horse–human interactions, and Table 3.3 highlights interactions for which horses may not offer an intra-specific social response. Taken together, the tables strongly suggest that interactions between humans and gentled, unridden horses are informed more by a notional conspecific model than those by a notional predator model. However, even the correspondent behaviours in Table 3.1a may lose relevance for horse members of a dyad because they are of inappropriate duration, context, consistency, contiguity or contingency. For example, a human grooming a horse may persist in this activity for much longer than any conspecific would. That said, the duration of events may be of less consequence than we might imagine because we have no evidence that horses are able to project into the future (McLean, 2004) and, so, cannot know that an activity is going to carry on; instead, they focus on the present and relate the present set of stimuli to innate

Table 3.3 Activities for which no naturally occurring analogues exist (things horses never do to each other, i.e. no biological correspondence)

Human–horse interaction	Attractiveness of outcome for horse	Extent of horse's control
Picking feet up, hoof trimming and shoeing	+	+
Leading into trailer or box	+/−	+/−
Trailer loading without leading	+/−	+
Feeding by hand or from bucket	++	+
Invasive veterinary work (e.g. injecting and suturing)	−	−
Grooming inguinal, ventral and perineal regions	+/−	+/−
Pulling hairs from the mane and tail	−	+/−
Spraying against flies	+/−	−
Clipping	+/−	−
Branding	−	−
Driving in close proximity to other horses (e.g. driving horses side-by-side demands tolerance of breached individual space)	+/−	+/−
Mounting-to-ride	+/−	+/−

Other things we make or train horses to do:
Bow, hyperextension, capriole, jump over another horse, walk on hindlegs, tolerate predator on back
Vaulting, towing, jumping, racing, driving, showing/parading, treadmill training
Semen collection

responses. If no resources are present, pushing a horse out of one's way may lack any ethological relevance. Meanwhile, consistency may be lacking when humans chase horses and yet expect them to approach in a round-pen. Contiguity and contingency describe the links between cues and responses. An example of these being interrupted arises when a human rejects a horse's attempts to reciprocate allogrooming.

Perhaps the most profound intervention we undertake with horses is requiring them to tolerate potential predators (humans) on their backs. It is significant that, within the social ethogram, mounting-to-ride could be the only activity for which a naturally occurring analogue exists in only one direction: human–horse. Horses mount horses primarily in juvenile play and subsequently during courtship and copulation. However, it is likely that a human mounting-to-ride is not perceived by the horse as sexual, otherwise mares would respond as they would to a stallion mounting, either rejecting or acquiescing. The duration of human presence on a horse's back during foundation training is also far longer than any intra-specific mounting activity. Furthermore, one would see a distinct sex difference in horses during foundation training, so perhaps mounting-to-ride belongs in Table 3.3 as an activity for which no naturally occurring analogue exists. If this is the case, it implies that there are no intra-specific interactions in the equid social ethogram that we do to horses but they do not do to us.

The tables above suggest that we are far more likely to be able to use relevant analogues of horse–horse interactions when handling horses and training them in-hand than when riding them. Riders are obliged to apply learning theory and use novel inter-specific signals. The tables also emphasise that the proximate benefits for horses of most interactions decline as their control over the interactions decreases. For most ridden training and competition, the horse has negligible autonomy. This and the fundamental role of negative reinforcement in training and riding a horse underpin rider safety. Nevertheless, time spent training horses in-hand seems to pay dividends even in the ridden horse (McGreevy and McLean, 2005). Perhaps it is effective in habituating horses to humans. Inter-specific communication may help them overcome fear and, therefore, reduce their tendency to use counter-predator responses. It is important that the translation of trained responses from in-hand to under-saddle cues is better understood. It may simply be that an unconfused horse in-hand is a better prospect for training than a confused one. In any case, such a line of enquiry may allow us to describe and even measure the bonds that form between horses and their trainers.

Horsemanship and horse sense

How do we define good horsemanship? Generally, the word implies practices and skills without regard to learning theory. Its traditional focus has been on handling and husbandry that encompassed knowledge of nutrition, conformation, reproduction, farriery and veterinary skills. Because of their love of traditional horselore, horse-trainers have been predictably slow in adopting new approaches (Warren-Smith and McGreevy, 2008a). They contrast poorly with dog-trainers in this regard (see Figure 3.6). There is an unfortunate expression: 'You can always tell a horseman; but you can't tell a horseman anything.' This implies that horsefolk are immune to new information but, in fairness, they could not expect to find the same trove of applicable psychology-based training principles that dog-trainers have. As previously discussed, horse-training cannot easily be reward-based. And since we cannot ride rats, the study of training by negative reinforcement is still in its infancy.

Horsemanship tends to reflect detailed knowledge of functional patterns of behaviour typical to the species (Rees, 1997), and is more or less aligned with the correct application of learning theory, even if practitioners do not appreciate the significance of the science in their art. It covers a multitude of skills, including stable-management, horse-keeping and horse-training, but has recently been re-packaged by proponents of so-called horse whispering and Natural Horsemanship. All are underpinned by that highly valuable commodity: horse sense. Horse sense is poorly defined but generally refers to the inherent way of being that some people have around horses. Their timing, sensitivity and resolve to pursue a training opportunity allow them to get the best out of their horses.

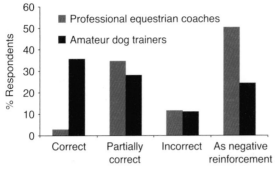

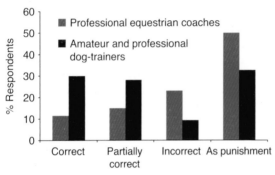

Figure 3.6   Results of a survey of Australian equestrian coaches (professional, *n* = 830) and dog-trainers (amateur and professional, *n* = 430), showing the distribution of correct, partially correct and incorrect explanations of key terms in learning theory. **Note.** The poor performance of equestrian coaches shown in this table does not necessarily mean that they were less effective as coaches than dog-trainers, but it does imply that they apply less scholarship to learning theory and developments in training protocols.

Horses also train us, or at least the training process trains humans, to modify their training behaviour (e.g. offering the correct response results in the trainer releasing the pressure or using a lighter cue next time). Sensitivity to such cues from horses is a critical element in good horsemanship. Excellent horse handlers often struggle to describe what it is they do that makes horses respond well to them. From first principles this must involve timing and consistency. But, even with the best timing and consistency, some people fail to achieve calmness in horses and, given that calmness is a precursor to optimal training, these practitioners can never excel in training. There is anecdotal evidence that horses can perceive a lack of relaxation in their handlers, and this may manifest as decreased compliance (Chamove *et al.*, 2002). There are also early, unreviewed reports of horses' heart rhythms responding to the emotional state of nearby humans (Gehrke, 2007). It is worth noting that there is a persistent belief that a special connection exists between women and horses (Midkiff, 2001) and that this allows them to train with less force than men use. Technological advances (such as those that measure rein and leg pressures) should help to establish the validity of such claims.

New age approaches

For centuries, shamans, medicine men (see Figure 3.7) and gypsies would travel from village to village plying their skills. The reason their practices were often called 'whispering' relates to the calmness of horses and the lack of noise brackets, including verbal commands that generally accompanied training. The mystique these people built around themselves and the secrecy with which they guarded their methods meant that best practice in horse-training was not widely dispersed. In a sense, these gurus relied on other people's mediocrity as horse-trainers and handlers.

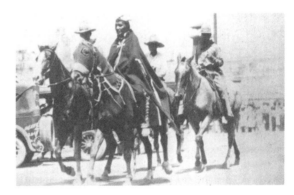

Figure 3.7   A horse tamed in 1 hour using the Indian blanket act is featured in this photograph of a 1922 parade. Outriders were used as extra insurance against an accident, although the Medicine Man insisted that they were not necessary. (Photo by George Dawson.) The use of equipment, such as blankets, in horse-taming techniques may distract from the importance of pressure/release, timing and consistency. (With permission from Jeff Edwards, Wild Horse Research Farm, Porterville, CA 93257.)

Using the same skills as shamans of old, modern horse-whisperers have had a renaissance, sparked in part by the Nicholas Evans book and the Robert Redford movie. But rather than adhering to codes of secrecy and practising quietly in stables behind closed doors, latter-day practitioners have started to promote their techniques and even to franchise them.

While the use of multimedia has made distance education and the marketing of horsemanship styles possible, it has also inspired an encouraging increase in the focus on horse welfare as a priority. Natural Horsemanship and so-called 'horse whispering' have emerged as a form of horsemanship that is underpinned by tremendous tact and subtlety. However, there is one fundamental problem: the notion that philosophies rather than mechanisms matter to the horse. This allows good technique to be eclipsed by a certain mental state in the handler. The terms energy, leadership and domination are as prevalent in these circles as love, harmony and willingness to please are among committed social scientists.

The widespread adoption of Natural Horsemanship, despite its lack of reference to learning theory, is seen by many as being preferable to traditional practices, probably because the media has chosen to focus on rough techniques throughout the world that are sometimes used on horses as foundation training. This generalisation overlooks the way in which many traditional practices are conducted in a humane way, and many foals and youngsters are gentled.

The reality is that Natural Horsemanship and allied techniques such as Join-up also rely on negative reinforcement (McGreevy and McLean, 2007). Yet again, pressure is applied to prompt a response and its release rewards the horse and makes the animal more likely to offer that response in future. The chief difference is that the pressure applied can be so subtle as to be imperceptible. Sometimes it involves only slight movements towards the horse. This is largely why early practitioners were assumed to be only 'whispering' to the horses. This has been positive for horses since it has renewed an interest within more traditional circles for lightness of touch and has also, in an unlikely sidestep, spawned an emerging line of scientific inquiry into horse-training, now called Equitation Science (McGreevy, 2007).

Towards a more scientific approach

As scientists, we may be able to measure and define the personality traits of more successful and empathetic equestrian personnel. At the same time, it would be helpful to log the behaviour of these humans. If they apply stimuli with more consistency than other riders, this quality may be more critical than the effect of any empathy they may have with their horses on the ground. This, in itself, raises the matter of how accurately we can measure empathy from humans to horses. It may be useful to measure a human's apparent attractiveness (see Figure 3.8) to both naïve and experienced horses after contact that provided no edible inducements or negative reinforcement for remaining close. However, the hunt for this sort of measure may be flawed if it is based on the assumption that horses want to remain with one conspecific to the exclusion of all others.

It is also worth considering how horses with multiple riders establish any significant relationship. Some argue that military riding techniques, many of which still prevail, were developed to obviate such relationships and allow any rider to get the best out of any horse (McLean and McGreevy, 2004). Cues need to be broadly consistent among riders so that horses do not need to learn a new set of cues for each. The same goes for service dogs, as the person who trains them may not be the person who eventually works with them. However, even with the best military regimentation, humans are

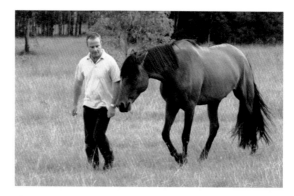

Figure 3.8 Many training methodologies feature the horse seeking to follow a human. This behaviour is a result of the innate tendency of a social animal to follow conspecifics.

not all the same and so human culture, habits or idiosyncrasies introduce additional layers of complexity. For example, males are more likely than females to be punitive (Brown, 1984). Furthermore, it is not clear how easily individual humans can be recognised by horses. Clothing, scents and even hair colour can change from one day to the next. Given that they are very responsive to whole-body signals, horses may use stance and movement patterns to distinguish among individuals.

During equitation, tactile contact between horse and human lasts much longer than contact between conspecifics ever does. And as far as attempted predation is concerned, the duration of contact is again extended. Perhaps, during foundation training (breaking in), horses simply learn that humans are ineffective predators. Naïve horses are usually frightened of being handled by humans but are seldom actively aggressive, preferring to avoid contact (McGreevy, 2004). This is the usual response of a prey species and, indeed, is central to early round-pen training. Horses that have learned that being ridden does not lead to extreme discomfort rapidly learn to tolerate it and then may even begin to associate it with positive outcomes (e.g. as a prelude to meeting other horses or as an opportunity to explore).

The responses of ridden horses deserve special attention since they can most directly affect the usefulness, commercial value and, indirectly therefore, the welfare of the horse. They also have a direct effect on the safety of the rider. It may be that at their most dangerous (e.g. when bolting and bucking), ridden horses have simply reverted to avoidance responses. This, in itself, is interesting because it suggests that no matter how ethologically parallel in-hand work may be, a ridden horse can revert to these counter-predator responses. This seems to emphasise that under-saddle work is not within the horse's ethogram.

One model for all situations is unlikely to hold true in all contexts. Even if horses deploy responses that align with the approach model more than the avoidance model, it would be imprudent to imagine that these responses are stable or unvarying. For example, when a pony is groomed every day it may make associations with humans that relate to the approach model but may react completely differently (e.g. with a flight response) when clipped once a year. We have to accept

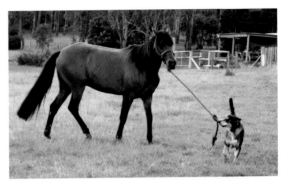

Figure 3.9 Conditioning rather than leadership qualities provides a more plausible explanation of leading behaviours. A horse will lead forward from pressure even from a well-trained dog.

that the behavioural flexibility of the horse has contributed a great deal to its success as a domesticated animal, so it is important to note the influence and indeed the inevitability of experience. The behavioural flexibility of horses is fundamental to their utility in the domestic context (see Figure 3.9). It allows them to respond to negative reinforcement more than most domestic species and also explains why they are subject to tremendous abuse by clumsy and ignorant handlers (McGreevy, 2004). In addition, horses and asses habituate to stimuli far more readily than zebras, a feature that undoubtedly enhanced our ability to use them safely.

Learning in domestic contexts may result in horses undertaking many activities that bear no semblance to naturally occurring responses. For example, we make or train horses to bow, hyperextend, capriole, walk on hindlegs, tow objects, race, and jump obstacles that would normally be avoided.

Husbandry practices can influence the way horses respond to humans. For example, a horse's social environment is more likely to affect the way it reacts to humans in its home environment than in a novel environment (Søndergaard and Halekoh, 2003). Similarly, it is important to acknowledge that predictions about the nature of relationships cannot be made with confidence for all horses and all humans. Differences arise as a result of a human's demeanour (which may be characterised by the quiet but purposeful manner of those with an inherent 'horse sense' or otherwise), their attitude towards horses (Chamove *et al.*, 2002) and the horse's experience.

Table 3.1 includes 'Parallel prance', one example of moving together, but the full equid social ethogram has other examples of moving or standing in *groups* (e.g. stampede and huddle). So, beyond dyadic interactions, it is worth considering two synchronised activities not explicitly mentioned in the current tables: 'standing/lying together' and 'moving together in a coordinated way' (not leading, driving or following). As noted by Wasilewski (2005), social grooming may be associated with initiating bonds, whereas resting in close proximity may strengthen newly formed ones. The way in which we *move* in relation to horses may be just as important in shaping their responses and 'attitudes' to us as what we *do* to them. This aspect of horsemanship is often less obvious and may be harder to describe and measure than the interactions themselves, but it should not be overlooked.

It may be that deliberately evoking approach in a horse can accelerate a reduction in anti-predator responses. So, for example, stimulating the mutual grooming response in foals at a stage where they would not tolerate general handling/touching is an effective way to lessen the drive to flee from the handler, allowing subsequent desensitisation to touching to proceed more rapidly than if the handler attempted first to habituate the foal to being touched (e.g. on the face). It is worth exploring whether this difference is merely due to the fact that the foal is positively reinforced for allogrooming the human or whether an additional factor comes into play when the touch elicits the desire to reciprocate the action *as if the human were a conspecific*. Foals make excellent subjects for this sort of enquiry since they are behaviourally naïve, and they should be used to test the possibility that allowing the horse to reciprocate in full by grooming the human reduces avoidance faster than simply grooming, but not allowing any reciprocal contact.

It may also be that when horses interact with humans under the approach model, analogues of a matriarchal society prevail (Goodwin, 2002). Jones (1983) showed that girls care more than boys about their horses. But does this mean that a pony prefers being cuddled or groomed by a girl to being fed by a boy? There are anecdotal reports to suggest that horses can detect sex differences in

humans and empirical evidence that dogs respond differently to male and female humans (Wells and Hepper, 1999). It is unclear to what extent horses relate such perceived differences in humans to their innate responses to male and female horses. Given that male humans are more likely to be a source of aversive stimuli, it may well be salient for horses to learn the cues that help them distinguish between men and women.

Apart from body proportions and locomotory style, the voice is the only constant that distinguishes one handler from another. Since, along with timing, good training relies on consistency (McGreevy and Boakes, 2007), it is surprising that the use of the voice is forbidden or discouraged in many equestrian codes and equitation manuals. It is worth exploring the relevance of human vocalisations to equine listeners (as has been published in studies of vocal cues to dogs; Fukuzawa *et al.*, 2005; Mills, 2005). As they busy themselves around horses on the ground, humans frequently chat to human and equine companions and sometimes just to themselves. On the whole, horses must learn to discriminate between background conversation and commands intended for them. Equally, horses sometimes vocalise to us as if we were conspecifics (e.g. mares may nicker to humans as if to a foal, and stallions sometimes direct courtship nickers to familiar handlers). However, although foals can sometimes be triggered to vocalise by human whistling imitations of their high-pitched wavering call (Francis Burton, unpublished data), to our ears human vocalisations scarcely ever sound like those of horses. It seems likely that the vocalisation humans use to call horses in a field, to drive them away from inappropriate locations or to prompt them to make upward or downward transitions under-saddle are all conditioned cues. These are meaningless to naïve horses and must acquire relevance by classical conditioning. So, certain vocalisations may appear to have a direct effect in some situations because they are, often subconsciously, coupled with and, therefore, become classically associated with 'body language' that bears the equivalent message. For example, shouting at a horse to go away is likely to be accompanied by a threatening stance and jerky movements; invitations to approach may be conveyed more by the relaxed, unthreatening posture than by the gentle voice.

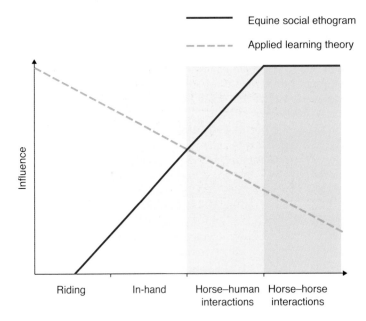

Figure 3.10   The relative influence of learning theory and ethology changes with context.

The relative importance of applied learning theory and the equid social ethogram depends on the context. In the ridden horse, learning theory is of more importance than the social ethogram (see Figure 3.10).

Conclusion

Equine scientists assert that learning theory is at the core of training (Mills, 1998) and re-training (McLean and McGreevy, 2004), but the application of a mechanistic view is to regard the human as just another part of the horse's environment. Every response in the ridden horse can be explained by the use of punishers and reinforcers, both primary and secondary. Mechanistic analyses are decried by some horse-lovers as being Cartesian and unenlightened because they appear to deny that horses have minds (Skipper, 1999). Presently, scientists can neither confirm nor deny the existence of the equine mind, love and respect, but accept that these qualities are not currently within the realm of an honest scientific approach.

Behaviourism is espoused in round-pen training that hinges on the handler advancing and retreating as a means of negatively reinforcing the horse's approach or response or immobility (Blackshaw et al., 1983). No need for interpretation of the relationship seems necessary if there is a simple association between cause and effect (Warren-Smith et al., 2005b).

Given the importance of timing and consistency in animal-training, the value of bonding with horses as pseudo-conspecifics may have been overstated by popular practitioners. Ultimately, we humans seek to refine our horsemanship for either competitive success or empathy or both. It may be that the useful, competitive horse simply has to respond consistently and appropriately to stimuli. Meanwhile, companion horses can behave with the autonomy that prevails in a free-ranging herd. In some contexts, horses may regard us as neither predators nor conspecifics, but perhaps more closely akin to objects in their environment. This may occur, for example, when we dispense food treats or when we exert mysterious forces on them via ropes.

Given the tremendous breadth of horse–horse interactions, it is striking how few interactions are required to train complex responses in horses. Perhaps equestrians will become increasingly subtle and sophisticated in their use of the analogues from the equid social ethogram we have described here. However, we hope that the continuing debate over the extent to which horses respond to them as stimuli or recognise them as attempts to communicate will now have a consistently scientific focus.

Take-home messages

- When applied to descriptions of horse behaviour, anthropomorphism is an unhelpful and unreliable tool at best and may promote poor welfare at worst.
- Training of horses in round-pens relies on negative reinforcement rather than human mimicry of equine social communication.
- There is no evidence that horses comply with human requests because of a 'willingness to please' or a desire to complete a shared goal.
- On the ground, some specific horse–horse interactions appear to have a corresponding horse–human interaction. However, this does not hold true when the horse is ridden.

4 Learning I: Non-associative

Introduction

In earlier chapters we examined the terms and mindsets that divert us from an objective appreciation of equitation. These were contrasted with mankind's current knowledge about the mental and physical capabilities of the horse as they relate to equitation. Despite the lack of an evidence-based framework, we have used horses successfully in war, agriculture, transport, sport, recreation, leisure and companionship roles. Now, we must look at learning itself. In this chapter, we will consider the general phenomenon of learning and the different forms it takes.

Learning

One definition of learning is: A process in which an individual's experience results in a relatively permanent change in behaviour. As a process, learning is not directly measurable; what *can* be measured is what has been *remembered* as a result of learning (i.e. when the association is remembered). Humans generally make better subjects for learning studies than non-human animals because language facilitates communication. Human learning can be tested by recall, where the subject might recite what has been learned; or by recognition, where the subject recognises the correct answer from an array. Recognition is an easier task because the situation provides stimuli that trigger the memory of the correct answer. When we test an animal, such as a horse, in a maze (see Figure 4.1), it cannot provide us with a map of its path, so we have to rely on observing its behaviour as it traverses the maze. If the horse fails in the maze, we have no way of knowing whether its failure was a failing of learning or of recall or even a manipulation of the motivation for the end-goal in the maze. So there *are* limitations in measuring learning.

Until the 1970s, animal-learning studies were dominated by the contributions of experimental psychologists. Behaviourism, founded by J. B. Watson, firmly established the laboratory rat and the pigeon as the standard species for learning studies. From this foundation sprang new schools of learning dominated by psychologists C. L. Hull, E. C. Tolman and B. F. Skinner, which focused on constructing a system of behavioural laws. These laws were intended to predict conditions under which learning will occur. Their approach to understanding learning in animals was entirely mechanistic. Following the work of these behaviourists, particularly Skinner, animals not only in laboratories but also in zoos, aquaria and circuses were trained using their theories and exhibited performing routines featuring increasingly complex trained behaviours. However, the major weakness of the early animal-learning studies was

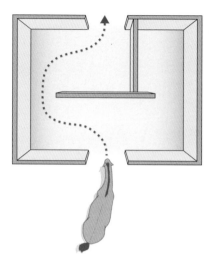

Figure 4.1   An example of a maze. Simple experiments, such as maze learning, allow us to compare cognitive processes (e.g. recall) between species. (Reproduced from *Equine Behavior*, copyright Elsevier 2004.)

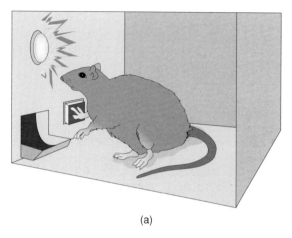

(a)

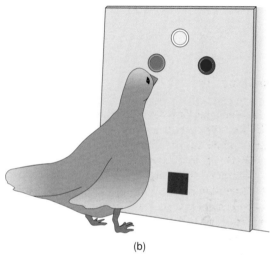

(b)

Figure 4.2   An illustration of a rat (a) and a pigeon (b) in Skinner boxes. The contribution of the behaviourists resulted in a wealth of knowledge derived from experiments largely conducted on two easy-to-keep species: the rat and the pigeon. Skinnerian principles have emerged largely from studies of just two operant models: rats pressing levers and pigeons pecking keys. (Redrawn with permission from Sandro Centini.)

their excessive focus on these two species, the rat and the pigeon (see Figure 4.2). Despite this, when we consider how dissimilar phylogenetically these two species are, any evidence of parallels in learning infers that such abilities could also be expected in other mammals and birds.

After the 1970s, behaviourism fell out of favour for a couple of decades as a result of its purported rigidity as well as sociocultural factors of the era (Skinner, 1971). The behaviour of animals was seen to be more complex than behaviourist models implied. The predominance of behaviourist theory was replaced with cognitive psychology. Behaviour was no longer seen simply as a product of reinforcement or punishment, but as a result of more complex agents. Rejecting behaviourism had both positive and negative implications for our understanding of learning. On the one hand, the rejection of simplistic approaches was an important step forward, but on the other, it resulted in studies of associative learning coming to a virtual standstill for some time. More recently, cognitive ethology has emerged, which is a multidisciplinary blend of behaviourism, cognitive psychology, neurophysiology, cognition and ethology. Shettleworth (2001) pointed out that a multidisciplinary approach is essential for real progress to be made in understanding the animal mind.

Some schools of thought in psychology share a central theme that learning follows some general laws that apply unequivocally in all situations. However, reviews by Seligman (1970) and Manning (1972) suggest that this assumption was too simplistic. Nevertheless, it is helpful to distinguish various categories of learning while keeping in mind that those categories may be arbitrary and seamless. The chief merit of such categories lies in their capacity to illuminate our understanding of learning processes. To this end, it is helpful to distinguish between two basic categories: non-associative learning and associative learning.

Non-associative learning

Whereas associative learning describes the formation of a relationship between at least two stimuli, non-associative learning, by contrast, occurs when exposure to a single stimulus results in either habituation or sensitisation. Both are fundamental to effective horse-training and are interconnected at almost every stage of training. Despite this, there has been little published research on non-associative learning abilities in the horse (Nicol, 2002) until the recent work of Christensen (2007) and Christensen *et al.* (2006).

The evolution of habituation and sensitisation

Habituation and sensitisation are adaptive responses that enable organisms to function effectively in their environments. Both involve animals learning not to respond to one type of stimulus without associating it with any other stimulus (Kandel, 2006). It should be remembered, however, that aside from learning, behaviour can also change because of motivational factors, physiological variables, sensory adaptation or fatigue (McGreevy and Boakes, 2007). In general, habituation manifests as a decrease in the size of an innate response to a stimulus after exposure to it (see Figure 4.3). In contrast to habituation, sensitisation involves an increase in the size of a response to a salient stimulus.

Central to evolutionary theory is the necessity for animals to exploit their environments optimally and in particular their various umwelts. Energetic efficiency is therefore of crucial importance, and it is not difficult to imagine the critical importance of habituation and sensitisation in the evolutionary process. In short, it is a waste of precious energy to react to stimuli that prove innocuous and, on the other hand, it may be critical to become sensitised to stimuli that predict predation, pain or injury.

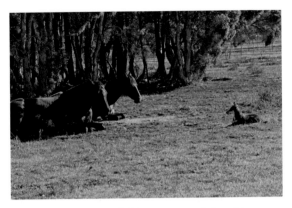

Figure 4.3 Horses can habituate to potential predators.

Habituation

Habituation is the simplest and oldest form of learning: even invertebrate animals such as earthworms habituate to stimuli. Typically, a worm in a Petri dish reacts aversively when the dish is tapped, but after a few repetitions of tapping, the response wanes. Similarly, horses that live beside railway lines or airports may initially show a strong reaction, but this soon fades and trains or planes no longer elicit any response.

The speed and likelihood of habituation are dependent on the nature of the stimulus, the rate of stimulus presentation and the regularity with which it is presented (McGreevy, 2004). It is important when habituating an animal to a stimulus to continue presenting the stimulus regularly, well past the point of initial habituation. Ceasing the stimulus early can cause the fearful behaviour to return quite suddenly, in a process called spontaneous recovery (Marks, 1977). Even when the habituation is reliable, a prolonged absence of the stimulus can eventually cause the original response to return.

Habituation is easily confused with extinction. Habituation occurs when the unconditioned stimulus (UCS) is repeatedly presented until the associated unconditioned response (UCR) fails to appear. On the other hand, extinction (see Chapter 5, Learning II: Associative (attractive)) results when the conditioned stimulus (CS) fails to predict the associated UCS, so that the CS no longer elicits the conditioned response (CR). Thus, horses that have habituated to a human sending them away in a round-pen can spontaneously become fearful of humans at some later point. Again, this is spontaneous recovery and can occur not only with habituated responses but also with extinguished CRs (Lindsay, 2000). A horse can fail to respond to a trained cue and then spontaneously recover its original responses.

Habituation in human–horse interactions

As discussed in Chapter 2 (Cognitive ethology), habituation is fundamental in many human–horse interactions and especially in horse-training. The selective processes of domestication have considerably increased the likelihood of habituation in the horse (McGreevy and McLean, 2007). It is plausible that those horses whose habituation was absent or slow during interactions with humans in former times would have been rejected in favour of those that habituated more easily. The wild horses that habituated quickly may even have been selected preferentially simply because they were the easiest to catch. By contrast, associative learning processes would seem equally salient in the domestic as in the natural state.

Habituation is readily seen in horses in situations both with and without direct human intervention. For example, horses generally habituate to all innocuous features of their local environments. If they are regularly exposed to them, horses soon become accustomed to children rushing by on bicycles, and even animals that they typically seem to find aversive, such as dogs, pigs, donkeys, camels, elephants, emus and kangaroos. When horses habituate to these stimuli in the absence of human intervention, they generally do so *gradually*.

In horse-training, habituation (desensitisation) is mostly employed while the animal is *restrained* to some extent. Restraint may be through stabling, yarding, tethering or restricting locomotion via in-hand or under-saddle signals that have been installed by negative reinforcement (the removal of pressure at the onset of the desired response). Under certain conditions, preventing animals from escaping aversive stimuli has been shown to facilitate habituation to fearful stimuli (Baum, 1970; McLean and McLean, 2008; see Figure 4.4). Be-

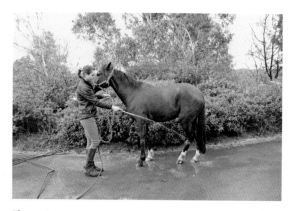

Figure 4.4   During aversive encounters, trainers commonly utilise the advantage of immobility, using the stop response to expedite habituation. (Photo courtesy of Amelia Martin.)

cause high levels of fear have an inhibitory effect on learning (see Chapter 13, Fight and flight responses and manifestations) and the emergence of the phenomenon of flooding at some point in the elevation of fear levels, preventing such flight response should be carefully managed. Flooding is the forced exposure to noxious situations or objects for an extended length of time without an opportunity to escape. In contrast, exposing the ridden, held or tethered horse to low-threshold aversive stimuli with gradual increases in intensity avoids the likelihood of flooding, with habituation being established at each stage (Lindsay, 2000).

Habituation/flooding as part of horse-training

The young horse learns to habituate to various equestrian paraphernalia, including the bit in its mouth (part of what is known as mouthing, described in Chapter 7, Applying learning theory) and other aspects of the bridle, head-collar and horse boots (see Figure 4.5). To a limited extent, the horse may have habituated to these while at liberty, for example, turned out into a round-yard or small enclosure. On the other hand, restraint, and therefore low-intensity flooding, is frequently used when it comes to habituation to the saddle, saddle blankets, numnahs, covers, rugs and girth pressure. The girth constricting the thorax possibly represents the greatest challenge

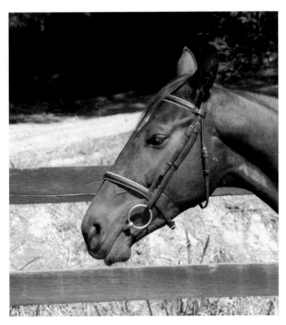

Figure 4.5 During foundation training, horses are expected to habituate to the bridle and the bit.

are known as girth-shy. There are also claims that girth hypersensitivity is due to birth trauma. However, as yet there are no evidence-based data (double-blind trials and age-matched controls) to support this interesting possibility.

The horse also habituates to the presence of a human on its back. For example, during foundation training, the horse may be habituated to having a person above him (e.g. on a fence beside the horse), and instead of completely mounting the horse, the rider may break this down into small stages, gradually getting higher and higher onto the horse's back. In some methods such as the Jeffery method, the rider may stretch the habituation procedure out further and progress to lying along the horse, placing each leg on the horse's sides and then sitting up very gradually (Wright, 1973; see Figure 4.7). A typical habituation procedure would entail the rider repeatedly putting weight on one stirrup, then when the horse shows adequate habituation, quietly standing on that

to habituation in horse-training. Even with the use of gradual habituation and apparatus such as elastic girths, many horses may continue to respond with persistent hyper-reactivity when first girthed, and this reaction may reflect variations in thoracic sensitivity (McLean, 2003; see Figure 4.6). Horses exhibiting such behaviours

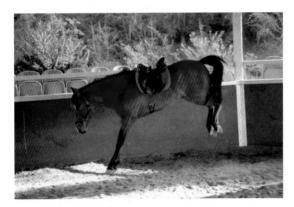

Figure 4.6 The constant pressure provided by the girth is the most difficult stimulus for some horses to habituate to. There are few comparable human-horse interactions that entail habituation to inescapable discomfort. (Photo courtesy of Christine Hauschildt.)

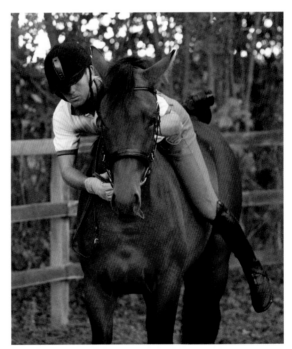

Figure 4.7 Mounting the horse bareback during foundation training is employed in various methods. This has a number of advantages in habituating the horse to human body contact and separates it from the sometimes troubling girth/saddle experience with human astride.

stirrup and holding the pommel (top front) of the saddle. Next, the rider swings his or her leg to the other side of the horse and when the horse has habituated to this activity, the rider may place his or her right foot in the stirrup and gradually begin sitting upright. At each of these stages, habituation has occurred when the horse no longer attempts to escape the primarily aversive stimuli and shows relaxation (McGreevy and McLean, 2007).

During subsequent training, horses in all equestrian codes are required to habituate to visual, auditory and olfactory stimuli. Most ridden horses encounter traffic, other animal species, objects that are blown past in the wind, and other changes within their environments. Stimuli that present significant habituation challenges to horses are novel, large, sudden, erratic or advancing stimuli (see Chapter 6, Learning III: Associative (aversive)). In some breed societies, such as the Verband Hannoverscher Warmblutzüchter (the Society of Hanoverian Warmblood Breeders), horses are scored and ranked for their ability to habituate and these attributes are broadly referred to as temperament and, to some extent, rideability.

Habituation is important for all trained horses and especially so for police horses as well as those trained for film and exhibition work. These horses are trained to ignore almost any novel visual, auditory, tactile and even olfactory stimuli. During training, these stimuli are gradually brought closer to the horse and as a result, they become more threatening. At some point, they compete with the rider's signals and may outcompete them. This competition for salience is implicit in the overshadowing phenomenon. In such a situation, in which the rider or handler finds his or her signals overshadowed by external stimuli, he or she may attempt to reverse the process and increase the salience of his or her signals by increasing the pressure of the reins or legs. The seamless nature of learning processes is again revealed in such events. There are many examples where habituation results from overshadowing, when trainers attempt to desensitise horses to aversive stimuli and events by increasing the intensity of the rider's or handler's signals to overshadow the relatively weaker but formerly aversive stimuli. Overshadowing offers a promising method of desensitisation for modifying fearful responses to stimuli

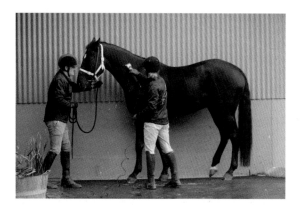

Figure 4.8   Overshadowing aversive stimuli, such as noisy clippers, provides a rapid method of habituation and desensitisation.

(such as clippers and needles), or in treating shying (McLean, 2008; McLean and McLean, 2008; see Figure 4.8).

From the standpoint of training, habituation can be thought of as anathema to operant conditioning. In all forms of equitation, the horse learns to respond to signals provided by the bit in its mouth and signals from the rider's legs (McLean, 2003). This is learned through the operant process of negative reinforcement (see Chapter 6, Learning III: Associative (aversive)) in which the removal of the aversive stimulus is reinforcing. Hence, in most equestrian codes, the bit and the rider's legs are not neutral signals. In other words, the horse must not habituate completely to these signals; if it does, conflict behaviours and distress may ensue. The terms *hard mouthed* or *dead sided* are used to describe horses that have, to some extent, habituated to the bit and rider's legs and possibly spurs. Habituation is a more plausible explanation than 'laziness' for sluggish or inadequate responses to the rider's acceleration signals (McGreevy, 2004). Being a discriminative grazer, the horse has a very sensitive mouth and can discern a fly landing on its thorax, so there can be little doubt about the physical sensitivity of this species.

Clinical experience suggests that habituation of the mouth results in more expressions of conflict (such as rearing, shying and hyper-reactivity) than habituation of the sides (McLean and McLean, 2008; see Figure 4.9). Because the problem is a result of human intervention rather than non-compliance of the horse, it has been suggested that

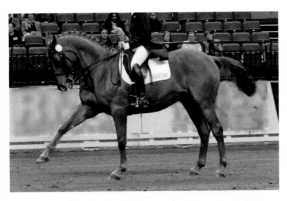

Figure 4.9 A horse can habituate to various stimuli, but owing to the great sensitivity of its mouth, it is difficult to habituate a horse to strong inescapable mouth pain without it developing conflict behaviours and, in the worst-case scenario, learned helplessness. (Photo courtesy of Minna Tallberg.)

the term habituation should be used in such cases (McGreevy and McLean, 2005). This is an example of the way in which the language of learning theory can make training more logical and accessible.

Repeated habituation to painful stimuli increases the likelihood of learned helplessness. For example, when riders resort to using ever-more severe bits on horses that fail to slow appropriately, a process of progressive habituation may set in as the horse deadens to lower/lighter pressures. While habituation to relatively innocuous stimuli may not affect the animal's wellbeing, there is a point on the pain continuum where habituation may escalate into learned helplessness—this term, which describes an animal's apparent habituation to painful stimuli, is discussed in Chapter 6 (Learning III: Associative (aversive)). Similarly, when riders resort to using spurs because the horse fails to learn to respond to the lighter leg signals, habituation and the possibility of a degree of learned helplessness may ensue. When a rider applies two or more signals at one time, such as the opposing signals of go and stop (legs and reins), habituation of one or both may occur. Overshadowing may occur such that the horse habituates to only one signal or indeed both signals (McLean and McGreevy, 2004). Again, learned helplessness may result from such a situation.

Contact

While optimal training requires that reins and leg signals should not become neutral, one exception to that rule occurs in the sport of dressage (including its offshoots, eventing and show-jumping). Here, some amount of bit and leg pressure *is* neutral. This, together with the seat, is known as *contact* (Decarpentry, 1949; German National Equestrian Federation, 1997; Hinnemann and van Baalen, 2003). Rider skill is critical here since the benefits of continuous contact, which relate to delivering subtle signals, may be outweighed by excessive, relentless tension and random hand movements. Current dressage practice requires that for all locomotion, including intra-gait and inter-gait transitions, the reins must be straight and the rider's legs must be in direct contact with the horse's thorax (German National Equestrian Federation, 1997). Data suggest that rein pressure during contact lies typically (but perhaps not optimally!) between 30 and 60 N (Preuschoft *et al.*, 1999; Clayton *et al.*, 2003; Warren-Smith *et al.*, 2007a). The Newton (N) is the international unit to measure force. One Newton is about 0.224 809 pounds of force (lbf) or about 0.101 972 kilogram of force (kgf). Using kitchen-bench science, the effort required to hold 3 kg of sugar in each hand provides an indication of how much force is required to apply 60 N of rein pressure to a horse's mouth.

While previous studies have recorded rein pressures (e.g. Preuschoft *et al.*, 1999; Clayton *et al.*, 2003) found a range of pressures up to 60 N, on the other hand, Warren-Smith *et al.* (2007a) found that when specific cues were given to the horse via the reins, the range of pressures employed was much lower (less than 30 N). This, in itself, highlights the need for further research to be conducted on the pressures applied to horses and, importantly, the subsequent education of riders and trainers so that horses are not subjected to unnecessarily strong pressures.

Habituation in behaviour modification: desensitisation

Habituation, generally in the form of desensitisation, is commonly utilised by horse-trainers to detrain fearful responses. Horses that require

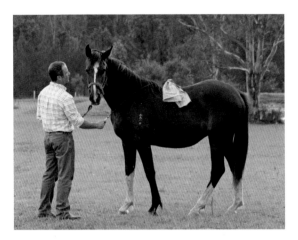

Figure 4.10 'Bagging down' is a term used by horse-trainers in some countries to describe a handler repeatedly flailing a bag or a towel on a horse's body until habituation occurs. (Photo courtesy of David Faloun.)

desensitisation typically have intensely fearful reactions to certain stimuli. Successful desensitisation requires that flooding be avoided, and that the horse be gradually exposed to lower thresholds of fear that gradually increases in stages, with habituation required at each stage until the flight response fully subsides (Marks, 1977; McLean and McLean, 2008).

In some methods of foundation training, the flooding process of 'bagging-down' (or 'sacking-out') is employed (see Figure 4.10). In this process, the horse is restrained while a person flails a towel or sack over much of its body until it ceases to attempt to escape. Restraint (and so reduction of the flight response) in this case may involve hobbling (see Chapter 10, Apparatus). Hobbling can entail securing the distal part of the forelimb to the proximal part by fully closing the knee joint. For hindlegs, it involves hoisting and securing the limb towards the ventral thorax. It may also involve tying one leg to another (an anterior pair, a posterior pair or an ipsilateral pair) or even securing three legs together.

In the USA, wild mustangs have been corralled into raceways culminating in a crate. When a horse enters the crate, the entrance is closed with only the horse's head protruding. The crate is then filled with wheat and the mustang is subjected to a flooding procedure. While descriptions of this method suggest some amount of habituation has

occurred (Grandin, 2007), they tend, anthropocentrically, to describe the encasement as comforting (they cite the tenuous analogue of autistic humans apparently deriving comfort from broadly applied pressure). The most simple and plausible explanation is, again, that the legs are restrained and habituation or flooding is occurring. Learned helplessness may also be implicated. This procedure is similar to the treatment of young elephants in some parts of Asia. An elephant is tethered tightly to a post (Nepal) or contained tightly in a pen (Thailand and elsewhere) and the animal may be subjected to flooding with painful stimuli.

Desensitising hypersensitive body regions

A biological characteristic of all species is that all traits show some variation, which is central to natural selection. The variation in sensitivity and subsequent learned reactivity of various parts of animals may have selective advantages in survival because protection of vital body parts may result from subsequently learned reactivity. Hypersensitivity to tactile stimuli may be generalised across the whole body. We see that, alongside head-shyness, horses may show hypersensitivity around the thorax, flanks and legs. When contact with specific body sites results in hyper-reactive withdrawal responses, there is usually an epicentre of heightened reactivity surrounded by a less reactive area (see Figure 4.11). Reactivity positively correlates with proximity to that epicentre. For example, in most cases of head-shyness, the horse's ears represent the epicentre of reactivity.

Many trainers, particularly those skilled in behaviour modification, recognise the importance of maintaining the stimulus until some habituation has occurred. Let us consider the example of head-shyness further. Head-shyness is a reaction with a significant learned component (the reaction can become stronger) even though it is likely that there is also a genetic predisposition for such behaviour. The development of this reactivity is easy to imagine. The human unwittingly touches the young horse on or near the ear, which is immediately and rapidly withdrawn. This withdrawal response becomes faster and is reinforced by the removal of the human's hands (negative

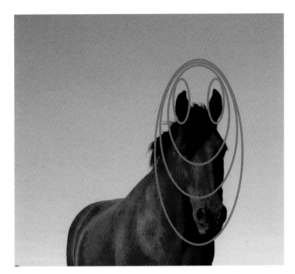

Figure 4.11   Head-shy horses tend to show increasing sensitivity towards an epicentre of the ears or a single ear.

reinforcement). So, the response becomes amplified and the withdrawal response becomes increasingly violent. The human hand touching even a formerly neutral site on the animal's head now elicits a violent withdrawal response. The horse is now sensitised to the tactile stimulus of being touched on the ear. If the handler had not removed his or her hand in the first place, then habituation might have occurred. The sensitisation of the horse to the human hand occurs as a result of the immediate removal of the hand. It is easy to see how neatly sensitisation processes dovetail with negative reinforcement. Resolution of head-shyness is discussed in Chapter 7, Applying learning theory.

Sensitisation

When an animal is sensitive to a stimulus, there is an increase in its associated response after repeated presentations of that stimulus, so the stimulus becomes noxious. When an intense sample of the stimulus is presented and the animal's escape is thwarted, it may become increasingly sensitive to the stimulus. The animal is then said to be sensitised to that stimulus (McLean and McGreevy, 2004).

Sensitisation results in the opposite effect to habituation. For example, after a person is startled by a gun going off, even an unexpected touch on

the shoulder will probably be more alarming than usual. Although it is generally regarded as a non-associative learning process, there are some examples of sensitisation described later that involve associated stimuli. This again shows the seamless and interactive nature of natural phenomena, and how they resist discrete labelling.

Unlike habituation, sensitisation evolved to ensure that animals paid attention to a variety of stimuli, even previously inoffensive ones, because of potentially dangerous consequences (Kandel, 2006). Some of these consequences reflect innate predispositions while others emerge from direct aversive experience, such as injury. Sensitisation may last from just a few minutes to the longer term, depending on the characteristics of the sensitising stimuli. Established learned responses can subsequently be enhanced by sensitisation or inhibited by habituation.

Sensitisation plays a significant role in the ontogeny of behaviour problems, for example, escape learning. A sudden aversive event can sensitise a horse to a previously innocuous stimulus. For example, electric fences sensitise a horse to ordinary wire (see Figure 4.12). The faster the horse can escape the now-aversive stimuli, the more likely the escape reaction becomes. If a horse is hurt or frightened inside a trailer, it learns to rush out of the trailer very fast. While shying frequently involves aversive classical conditioning (see Chapter 6, Learning III: Associative (aversive)), it can also arise when a previously innocuous stimulus becomes sensitised. A rabbit that suddenly scuttles from the bushes beside a letterbox can, if the horse's reaction is strong enough, sensitise the horse to the letterbox. In Hong Kong, a sound is emitted from the apparatus of the starting gates just before they open. The racehorses sprint out and that escape sensitises them to the preceding sound.

Sometimes horses seem dull to signals, but in horse-training, the problem is not a lack of sensitivity or intelligence but of responding: the horse has learned to respond only to strong signals as a result of poor application of either pressure or timing, or both. Because training requires full expression of all components of the operant contingency (see Chapter 5, Learning II: Associative (attractive), and Chapter 6, Learning III: Associative (aversive)) timing is imperative. With poor timing,

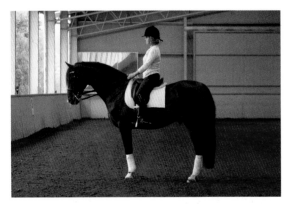

Figure 4.13 Halts that are square in the forelegs from light rein signals signify sensitisation to the signals of the light reins. This suggests relaxation and looseness of the forelegs, which are the goals of correct training.

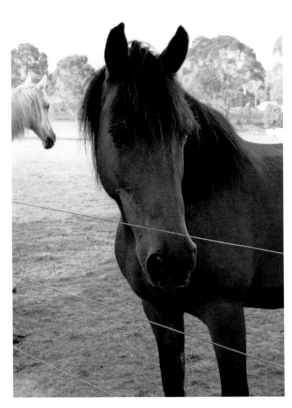

Figure 4.12 If a stimulus is highly aversive, such as an electric shock, the horse may become sensitised to previously innocuous stimuli, such as an ordinary wire.

horses can become dull to the rider's or handler's signals. Prior to foundation training, horses may offer no response to the rider's light signals from the reins and legs, so training involves the sensitisation of the horse to these signals. If the rider's timing is suboptimal, some horses may become dull to the signals as training and riding proceed. Typically, it is the more sensitive horses, those prone to hyper-reactivity, that become dull to the stop response of the bit, and it is the less sensitive horses that are prone to become dull to the rider's go signals. In both cases, the response must be re-trained: generally, sensitive horses require sensitisation of the stop signal while less sensitive ones are more likely to require sensitisation of the go signal. Here, it becomes clear that isolating sensitisation from negative reinforcement is problematic.

Sensitisation of the stop signal demands the same process as the initial training of the stop signal (see Figure 4.13). It involves increasing the intensity of the discriminative stimulus (the light stop signal) until a sufficient response occurs, in which case the stimulus is immediately withdrawn. Sensitising the go signal follows the same format: increasing the intensity of the go signal until the response occurs and then immediately releasing.

Sensitisation can also occur if a stimulus of low salience is associated contiguously (i.e. temporally connected) with a more intense stimulus (Lindsay, 2000). In other words, sensitisation can involve a paired association. For example, the whip is sometimes used in association with leg signals to train the go response, particularly in situations where that response begins to show habituation. Sometimes the addition of the whip initially helps the rider's leg signal through a process of classical conditioning. However, the response may soon show habituation to the paired association. To sensitise the horse to the light leg signal, there are two possibilities that have a place in operant conditioning. The first involves applying the light leg signal and contiguously increasing the intensity of the whip-tap until the horse shows sensitisation to the antecedent leg signal (German National Equestrian Federation, 1997). The second technique, developed by the Finnish trainer Kyra Kyrklund, is to train the horse to respond to the

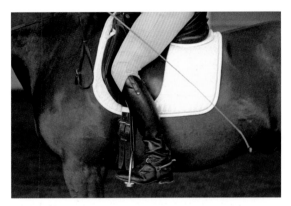

Figure 4.14 If the whip is to be used to fortify the 'go' response of the rider's legs, it is useful to train the horse to go forward from a light tapping motion of the whip. The whip should not be used to punish and should never be delivered in a strong one-off application because this can result in the horse becoming afraid of it.

whip-tap alone until the horse goes forward from one or two taps (see Figure 4.14). In this method, the whip-taps are increased in frequency until the horse goes forward (as described in Chapter 8, Training). When the horse is sensitised to the whip-taps, it will consequently show sensitisation to light leg signals (Kyrklund, 1998; McLean and McLean, 2008). These processes can be used to sensitise horses both in-hand and under-saddle to the relevant signals.

Imprinting

Imprinting is a form of learning in neonate animals at a highly sensitive period in their development, when they are receiving their very first stimulation from the outside world. It is considered to be a separate category of learning. The first to make systematic observations of this phenomenon was Spalding (1873), who reported that shortly after hatching, young chicks followed any moving object. However, it was Lorenz (1937) who made the topic popular among behavioural scientists. He described imprinting as a unique process in precocial birds characterised by a sensitive period outside which the process was less likely to occur. During the sensitive period, 2- to 3-day-old hatchlings would imprint on a 'mother figure'. Typically, of course, this would be their real mother, but Lorenz recognised that they would follow almost *any* moving object during their growth

period. The tendency to follow any moving object made imprinting a popular practical ethology topic in universities throughout the world. Ethology students imprinted chicks onto all sorts of moving inanimate objects such as themselves or moving balloons. Lorenz described imprinting as a rigid phenomenon that was irreversible and determined future mating partners. Indeed, birds hatched by other species have been shown to court and attempt to mate with the foster species.

With regard to horses and other mammals, the questions are: does imprinting occur; does it have the same characteristics as in precocial birds; and is it of any use in training and management? The term imprinting was first used to describe the behaviour of young foals by Miller (1991). Miller suggests that the sensitive period for foals is within the first 48 hours of life when the 'following response' is learned. At this time, the foal apparently learns to follow its mother, which is usually the nearest large moving creature in its world (McLean and McGreevy, 2004; see Figure 4.15).

Imprinting is facilitated largely by the sense of sight, but sound and olfaction are also involved. Miller not only described imprinting as a process in foals but also introduced the prospect of *imprint training* as a viable methodology for training newborn foals that is said to reduce the prevalence of aversive reactions, defensive aggression as well as sensitise the foal for pressure release (Miller, 1991, 2001). Miller's observations about the phenomenon of imprinting are noteworthy, because unlike pups and kittens, horses are precocial and are mobile soon after birth. If Miller's claims are

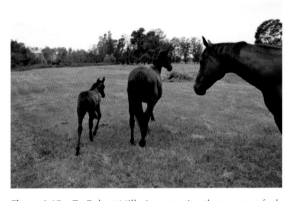

Figure 4.15 Dr Robert Miller's contention that a young foal can imprint onto humans is based on his interpretation of its neonatal tendency to follow its mother.

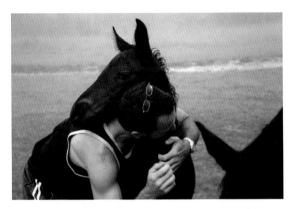

Figure 4.16   Imprint training includes desensitising the newborn foal to human touch.

correct, it makes sense to spend time imprint training foals rather than training larger, stronger and more dangerous youngsters.

The process of imprint training recommended by Miller is lengthy, requiring habituation of the foal to common stimuli as well as sensitisation to other pertinent stimuli (see Figure 4.16). Miller advocates multiple interventions with the foal that he calls 'stimulations'. He prescribes between 30–50 stimulations of each body region. Imprint training begins with severing the newborn's umbilical cord and drying the foal. On the first day, the process of habituation begins with holding the foal securely before it stands, and continue holding it until it relaxes and ceases to resist. Then, it is rubbed all over its body until it again shows relaxation. This is repeated, beginning with the ears (including ear canals), face, upper lip, mouth, tongue and nostrils, followed by the eyes, neck, thorax, back, legs, feet, rump, tail, perineum and external genitalia.

The next steps are more controversial because of the apparent flooding with novel aversive stimuli. They involve the introduction of artificial devices, such as clippers and a rectal thermometer, as well as mock rectal examinations. Following this, further habituation to unusual stimuli occurs. The handler rubs a piece of crackling plastic over the foal's entire body until 'panic subsides'. Gunfire, hissing sprayers, whistles, loud music, flapping flags and swinging ropes are also included in the imprinting program. Next on the agenda is habituation of the girth region. The handler's arms surround the foal, compressing rhythmically until habituation has occurred.

Following habituation, sensitisation to pressures for leading via the head-collar is carried out. This is not exclusively part of so-called imprint training; rather, it is the first step in negative reinforcement. Training the foal to lead at any early age would seem a sensible protocol that facilitates and helps ensure safety in any veterinary intervention before foundation training.

In recent years, as a result of the increase in popularity of imprint training, imprinting has attracted much attention from scientists owing to the possible implication of flooding and learned helplessness in techniques that involve restraint and aversive stimuli. A considerable amount of research has suggested limitations to Miller's schema. The critical period during which foals can be imprinted is not clearly defined. Mal and McCall (1996) concluded that handling throughout the first 42 days of life improved performance in a halter-training task compared with handling from 43 to 84 days of age. They concurred with Miller about the likely existence of a critical period, but their study suggested that this period is more likely to be within the first 42 days of life.

Heird *et al.* (1986b) reported that when foals were moderately handled from weaning until 18 months of age, they showed enhanced problem-solving abilities. Extensively handled horses were slower to learn the correct route in a maze than minimally handled horses, but faster than unhandled horses. It is possible that progress through the maze was thwarted by fear and that the aversiveness of confinement was greatest in the unhabituated, unhandled foals. Meanwhile, extensively handled horses, having been trained to wait for cues, may have been somehow made more dependent on human signals to advance through the maze. Heird *et al.* (1986b) also reported that horses that were continuously handled as weanlings and yearlings were less emotional, showed a higher maze-learning performance and were more trainable for riding than were horses receiving less early handling. This evidence supports handling protocols that reduce flight response through habituation and flooding, approaches that do not necessitate imprint training per se.

Most scientific evidence suggests that imprint training does not correspond to any natural analogue and that the foals frequently resist strongly and endure high levels of stress while undergoing imprint training (Diehl *et al.*, 2002; Sigurjonsdottir and Gunnarsson, 2002). It is not clear whether this early stress can be justified in terms of later benefits (Hausberger *et al.*, 2007b). Williams *et al.* (2002, 2003) reported that when foals were handled at birth and/or 12, 24 and 48 hours after birth, there was no beneficial effect on their later behaviour when tested at 1, 2 and 3 months of age (Williams *et al.*, 2002) or at 6 months of age (Williams *et al.*, 2003).

Distinguishing among the benefits of habituation, any equine analogue of filial imprinting (as described in birds) and the more radical elements recommended by Miller is far from simple. So, it is not surprising that some studies have shown some positive effects of imprint training. For example, foals handled early tend to approach familiar humans (Simpson, 2002) and accept feet handling (Spier *et al.*, 2004) more readily than unhandled ones. That said, acceptance of aversive stimuli was not facilitated by imprint training. Fitting halters or clipping was just as traumatic for handled foals as for unhandled foals at 3 or 4 months of age (Simpson, 2002; Williams *et al.*, 2002; Spier *et al.*, 2004). Significantly, imprinted foals without regular handling were as difficult to approach as controls (Sigurjonsdottir and Gunnarsson, 2002).

Some of the studies on imprint training have been summarised by Houpt (2007) as shown in Table 4.1.

Research on the effects of handling after the putative sensitive period also suggests only transient benefits (Lansade *et al.*, 2005). While Mal *et al.* (1994) showed no beneficial effects when foals were handled during the first 7 days, later research showed that when handled in the same way (stroking, haltering, picking up feet) at 14 days of age, the foals at 3 months were more tractable than non-handled foals. However, when tested at 6 months of age, there were fewer differences between the handled and unhandled foals, and by 1 year of age there were no differences at all (Lansade *et al.*, 2004).

Heird *et al.* (1986b) and Lansade *et al.* (2004) reported higher trainability and easier handling, respectively, of foals handled regularly from weaning. Similarly, Hausberger *et al.* (2007b) suggested that the beneficial effects of early handling rely on regular repetitions of handling. Handling foals 5 days per week (tasks included catching, leading, picking up feet, grooming and being approached by an unfamiliar human) until they are 2 years of age results in improved manageability at 12, 18 and 24 months compared with unhandled foals (Jezierski *et al.*, 1999). However, the optimal time for handling seems to be at weaning and this should be followed up with regular handling. This would reduce the chance of interfering with the mare–foal bond, which must present a significant risk in imprint training.

Hausberger *et al.* (2007b) concluded that there is no clear evidence in foals for the existence of a sensitive period in development, which may facilitate the establishment of a foal–human bond. It is appropriate to reflect on the direct benefits for the foals themselves of being near humans. What's in it for them? Especially prior to weaning, they seem to find being scratched highly reinforcing but Søndergaard and Halekoh (2003) proposed

Table 4.1   Results of imprint training

Imprint age	Repetitions	Test	Age of	References
14 days	Until 24 weeks	Hoof[a], lead[a], approach[a]	6, 12, 18, 24 months	Jezierski *et al.* (1999)
24 hours	Daily for 42 days	Halter, lead[a]	85 days	Mal and McCall (1996)
6 hours	Daily for 14 days	Halter[a], hoof, lead[b]	16 days, 3 months, 6 months, 1 year	Lansade *et al.* (2005)
10 minutes	24 hours	Restrain, halter, worm, vaccinate, hoof[a]	90 days	Spier *et al.* (2004)
Birth	Daily for 7 days	Approach responses to stimuli	120 days	Mal *et al.* (1994)
2–8 hours	Daily for 5 days	Approach stimuli[a]	4 months	Simpson (2002)
45 minutes	12, 24, 28 hours	Approach stimuli	1–3 months	Williams *et al.* (2002)

Source: Adapted from Houpt (2007), with permission from Elsevier.
[a]Significantly better than non-handled.
[b]Three-month results.

that unhandled 2-year-olds become as familiar as handled animals, probably because humans bring food. As Hausberger *et al.* (2007b) point out, the affiliative qualities of human–horse interactions may be more important than when the interactions occur.

The reactions of the mare during handling have an impact on the foal's behaviour. Sigurjonsdottir and Gunnarsson (2002) found a positive correlation between the mare's nervousness and the imprinted foal's resistance to capture, haltering and leading at the age of 4 months. In short, they showed that the calmer the mare, the easier the foal was to handle. This finding could simply reflect the inheritance of flightiness or social learning. Henry *et al.* (2005, 2006) showed that forcible handling of foals (e.g. where they have been coercively brought to the mare's teat) tended to result in reluctance to make contact with humans later on. On the contrary, a passive human presence tended to induce less flight response than in controls, although the effects were short-lived.

More direct activities such as brushing and hand-feeding of the mare in the presence of the foal have been shown to have a positive effect that may last for some time (Henry *et al.*, 2005). Foals handled in this way have been shown to be more easily approached in the paddock and stroked by a familiar or unfamiliar human 1 year later, without any handling in the interim. This contrasted with controls that showed greater resistance to capture and to the presence of humans. Hausberger *et al.* (2007b) concluded that establishing a positive human–dam relationship may therefore be an important key to durably enhance the manageability

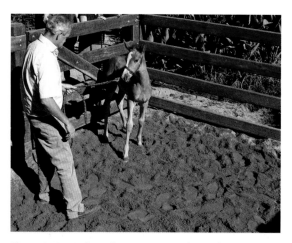

Figure 4.18 Perhaps the greatest contribution from Dr Miller is the assurance that as a precocial neonate, some training, such as lead training, can begin early in the foal's life. This can help ensure safety when veterinary attention is required.

of foals. Of equal importance is establishing clear and consistent interactions with the foals themselves, and as far as training is concerned, to use techniques that fully align with learning theory and, in particular, to time pressure release accurately (see Figures 4.17 and 4.18).

Take-home messages

- Non-associative learning occurs when exposure to a single stimulus results in either habituation or sensitisation. Both are fundamental to effective horse-training and are interconnected at almost every stage of training.
- Habituation as a result of poor application of pressure or timing or both is a more plausible explanation than 'laziness' for sluggish or inadequate responses to the acceleration cues.
- When a rider applies two or more signals simultaneously, such as the reins and the legs, habituation of one or both may occur. This is undesirable for both rider safety and horse welfare.

Areas for future research

There is a need for further research to be conducted on the pressures applied to horses via bit, legs, seat and spur and, importantly, the subsequent education of riders and trainers so that horses are not subjected to unnecessary pressures.

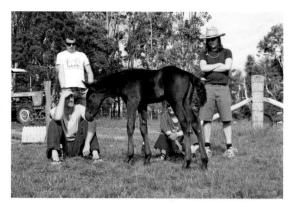

Figure 4.17 It is important to reflect on the effect of the foal's first experiences with humans.

5 Learning II: Associative (Attractive)

Introduction

Animals learn to tailor their responses to environmental changes in order to survive. The way they learn about feeding is a fundamental example. From the first minutes of life, a foal learns the cues that help it find milk. Its performance in acquiring the teat rapidly improves as long as it is rewarded by milk in its mouth. By learning to avoid pain and discomfort, an animal can make its life more pleasant. Even invertebrates, such as flies and slugs, show advanced forms of learning when avoiding unpleasant stimuli. When animals cannot evade pain or aversive stimuli, they become distressed. We manipulate animals' experience to train them, so there is a huge onus on trainers to keep any distress involved to an absolute minimum.

As the term suggests, associative learning involves an animal experiencing events or stimuli in close association in either time or space. There are two types of associative learning (or conditioning): operant (or instrumental) and classical (or Pavlovian). Broadly speaking, in the context of horse-training, links between two or more signals result from classical conditioning, while links between signals and outcomes develop because of operant conditioning.

Operant conditioning

An operant response is a voluntary activity that brings about a reward or allows an animal to avoid an aversive outcome, such as punishment. In operant conditioning, the animal must operate within its environment to get what it wants. The learned link between the particular behavioural response and the reward is what learning theorists call a contingency. This sort of learning underpins most horse-training. The horse has to offer a particular response to get the reward. To some extent, the horse has to choose whether to respond appropriately or not, so operant conditioning increases the horse's control of its environment.

To study the principles of operant conditioning, a US scientist, Edward Thorndike (1911), focused on the behavioural responses of cats in so-called puzzle boxes. The cats were left in a box without food and water (Figure 5.1). They wanted to leave but had to undergo trial-and-error learning to escape. The box had within it a lever that, when pulled, released the catch and allowed the cat out. Let us break this down into its constituent elements: to solve this problem, the cat had to see the lever (*the cue*) and pull it (*the operant response*) to obtain liberty (*the reward*). As we will discover, every operant response has these three

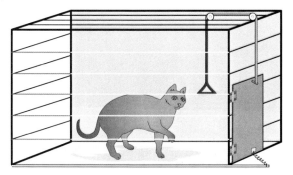

Figure 5.1 A cat in a puzzle box has to trial the use of a lever (make an instrumental change) to access its reward (liberty). (Redrawn with permission from Sandro Centini.)

core elements. They are referred to as the operant contingency. Consider a horse that has sensed its rider's leg pressing against its side (*the cue*). The horse moves laterally leg-yielding (*the operant response*) and, if the rider behaves appropriately, is relieved of the irritant pressure on its side (*the reward*). Thorndike referred to this kind of learning as 'trial-and-error learning with accidental success'. At the time it was widely believed that animals must understand a problem to solve it. Thorndike's investigations blazed the trail for animal learning studies in operant conditioning and provided a model that is of tremendous use when we think about any horse faced with a challenge during training. This label has largely been replaced by the terms instrumental learning and operant conditioning.

Operant or instrumental conditioning consists of presenting or omitting some reward or punishment when the animal makes a specific response (Kratzer *et al.*, 1977). The effect of the reward is to strengthen the likelihood of a correct response being offered again. This strengthening is called reinforcement. The term reinforcement refers to the process in which a reinforcer follows a particular behaviour so that the frequency (or probability) of that behaviour increases. The relationship between the first event and the second makes an association possible; the links between the two are called stimulus–response–reinforcement chains.

In general, the kind of learning produced by a response–reinforcer relationship – or *contingency* – is now called *instrumental conditioning* since it applies to any procedure in which a response is 'instrumental' in obtaining a reinforcer. In the 1930s,

Skinner studied the effects of response–reinforcer relationships on the behaviour of rats and developed a novel research tool that permitted a major leap forward in the study of instrumental conditioning. His experimental chamber, the now-famous Skinner box, had three main components: something the animal could operate, a *manipulandum* (usually a lever); a means of delivering reinforcers in the form of small food pellets; and a stimulus source such as a light or loudspeaker that could be used to signal to the animal a particular response–reinforcer relationship. Using a Skinner box, the experimenter did not have to intervene each time the animal received a reinforcement. Skinner called the response–reinforcer relationships he studied in this chamber *operant conditioning* (Skinner, 1938), since the behaviour 'operates' on – or makes changes to – the animal's environment. So, operant conditioning is a type of instrumental conditioning.

Operant conditioning in the horse has been studied under two sets of experimental circumstances: 'discrete' trials and 'free operant' trials. 'Discrete' trials involve exposing the horse to the learning task, requiring it to make a response and then withdrawing it from the situation. For example, a horse may be led into a simple T-maze and then has to choose one of two directions, left or right. In contrast, a 'free operant' involves allowing the horse to operate freely in its environment. For example, it may be led to a paddock and released to do whatever it likes, and then trained by reinforcement of whatever responses it happens to offer. Horses such as those that open their stable doors or dunk their own hay are good examples of free-operant conditioning: they work within their environment to acquire a reward.

It is not difficult to see that learning about the environment and how to make rewards appear will enhance a horse's umwelt. But, if the contingencies are unreliable and the horse's expectations are not met, we see signs of conflict reminiscent of experimental neurosis. Several studies suggest that lack of control over aversive events can bring about major behavioural and physiological changes (Wiepkema, 1987). For example, after being exposed to uncontrollable electric shocks, rats have increased gastric ulceration, increased defecation rates and are more susceptible to certain cancers when compared with individuals that retain control over comparable shocks (Moberg and Mench, 2000). Furthermore, training animals to expect enrichments that are associated with specific cues can increase their anticipation and play (Dudink *et al.*, 2006).

A trained response can tell us a great deal about not just the trainer but also the animal. If all the training is the same and there are differences in the performance of the response from one animal to the next, we can be fairly confident that the motivation of the animal is the chief cause of the difference. This is exciting because we can use this principle to let animals tell us what they want. Operant devices can be used to determine the preference animals have for certain environmental variables. As noted in Chapter 2, horses can easily be trained to use operant devices in consumer-demand studies. Some have been trained to break photoelectric beams to turn on lighting in their accommodation and, using this device, have demonstrated a preference for an illuminated environment (Houpt and Houpt, 1988). Others have been trained to nuzzle buttons to access resources (Figure 5.2).

Training generally means drawing out desirable behaviours and suppressing undesirable innate behaviours. In training horses we must exploit their need as prey animals to avoid discomfort and, indeed, threats of discomfort. Generally, we apply pressure to attain the desired response and remove it when we get the response we want. As we will see, delaying the removal of pressure is appropriate only when we are pushing the horse to try harder; in other words, when we are

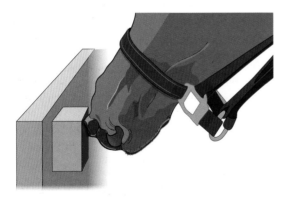

Figure 5.2 A horse using an operant device to turn on a light.

shaping an improved response (see shaping in Chapter 7, Applying learning theory, and Chapter 8, Training).

The aim of training is to install signals that elicit predictable behaviour patterns. For a response to be regarded as being under *stimulus control*, it must satisfy two requirements. First, it must be offered reliably after every presentation of the stimulus (cue) and, second, it must be offered after the cue. At this point, the cue is known as the discriminative stimulus.

There are two main ways to train a discrimination using positive reinforcement: *simultaneous discrimination* and *successive discrimination*. In *simultaneous discrimination* training, the horse is presented with two or more stimuli at the same time and is rewarded only if it responds to the correct stimulus. In contrast, in *successive discrimination* training, the differing stimuli are presented to the horse at different times.

The trained horse's task includes being able to discriminate not only between general grooming pressures and the trained signals, but also between one trained signal and the next. Isolating horses from their trainers, when trained responses are not required, can be an effective means of reducing *generalisation*, that is, horses offering a trained response to a cue similar to the cue used in training. Such isolation can ensure consistency in the effectiveness of pressure cues.

A similar approach to discrimination training is called *fading*. This is intended to ensure that few, if any, responses are made to any stimulus other than the discriminative stimulus. If successful, it leads to *errorless learning*. The aim is to reduce the number of errors a horse makes. There are two basic sequential steps in fading: the first step is to train the horse to respond to the discriminative stimulus (critical cues) rather than other stimuli; the second step is to gradually introduce the similar stimulus, or stimuli, that the animal is being trained *not* to respond to. The emphasis here is on gradual introduction. The duration and intensity of similar stimuli must be very gradually faded into the animal's perception. An example occurs in police horse-training where the horse is trained to attend to the rider's signals, not stimuli coming from people on foot. Once basic distracting stimuli on the ground have been successfully faded, they are gradually magnified.

Training horses, whether under-saddle or in-hand, stabled or in the paddock, basic, advanced or remedial, involves operant principles. Before giving a reward, the trainer must wait until the animal produces the desired activity. Rewarding the desired behaviour relates to the law of effect, which states that whatever behaviour immediately precedes reinforcement will be strengthened. When the association between pressure, response and timely release becomes highly predictable, a habit emerges. If a habit does not develop, the horse may have learned that it cannot offer any response that reliably causes the pressure to be released. Unfortunately, there are many horses in all spheres of ridden and draft work that have developed such apathy and lack of responsiveness. They are often unfairly labelled dull or stubborn (see Chapter 12, Unorthodox techniques).

The changing role of the horse in developed countries, at least, demands a greater emphasis on humane treatment and more research into horse education. In this context, prevention is better than cure, so correct foundation training of naïve horses is generally preferable to re-training animals with inappropriate experience. There is certainly less detraining (unlearning) to do and one of the ways in which this manifests is with less frustration. All animals that have learned to expect relief from pressure by adopting a certain unwanted response will eventually stop when the rewards are removed. However, most will show *more* of the response before it disappears completely.

If an animal is exposed several times to a conditioned stimulus before structured conditioning commences (i.e. before reinforcement), its acquisition of a conditioned response to that stimulus will be retarded. An example is a horse that is habituated to sustained pressure on its sides before being trained to produce a locomotory response. The horse has simply learned to ignore the pressure because it has no important consequences.

All therapeutic behaviour modification programs identify the motivation, remove the rewarding aspects of the unwelcome behaviour and reinforce a more appropriate alternative. If the strategy does not work, the most common explanations are either that training has been insufficient to establish the new associations or that the reinforcement for the new response is insuf-ficient to overcome gratification from the existing behaviour.

Classical conditioning

Classical conditioning is the acquisition of a response to a new stimulus by association with an old stimulus. From the outset, it requires a stimulus that evokes an innate or learned physiological or behavioural response. Also labelled Pavlovian conditioning, it has its origins in the studies of gastric physiology conducted by Ivan Pavlov, who spotted his experimental dogs salivating when they heard his technician tinkling a bell as he approached the kennels to feed them. Determined to establish how accurately dogs could develop these associations, Pavlov replaced the sound of the bell with more easily varied sounds made by a buzzer and then a metronome. To measure the rate of saliva production, Pavlov surgically implanted a tube into the dogs' cheeks and used saliva flow and volume as a measure of the association between the novel cues and the food.

Pavlov linked a novel stimulus (the buzzer) to a physiological stimulus (food in the mouth) and response (salivation; see Figure 5.3). The dogs quickly began to salivate in response to the buzzer, a new stimulus that had previously been irrelevant or neutral. The labels Pavlov created for the elements in this process are still used today. Before the learning experience, only meat powder, the *unconditioned stimulus* (US), produced salivation as an *unconditioned response* (UR). After learning, the buzzer became a *conditioned stimulus* (CS) and the salivation response to the conditioned stimulus became the *conditioned response* (CR, also known as the learned response).

The sound of a buzzer was consistently followed by the delivery of food to the mouth, regardless of what the dog might have done when it heard the buzzer. This is of critical importance in understanding the difference between classical and operant conditioning. Classical conditioning enables the animal to associate events over which it has no control. This increases the *predictability* of an environment. (In operant conditioning, the animal operates within its environment to get a reward or avoid punishment and so makes the environment more controllable.) The more

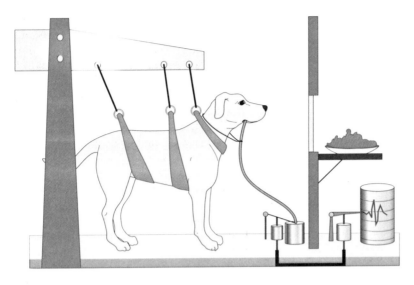

Figure 5.3 Pavlov's apparatus for collecting saliva as a measure of the association between food and various novel stimuli.

frequent and consistent the pairing of the neutral stimulus and the unconditioned stimulus is, the more rapidly the association develops. In some cases, usually involving the most critical pain or pleasure, the association is formed with a single experience (Lieberman, 1993).

There are numerous examples of classical conditioning in the horse world. Most stud managers will agree that stallions become aroused when they hear the sound of a particular bridle if it is the one used to control them in the breeding barn. Racetrack grooms use classical conditioning when they whistle each time they see their charges urinating (see Figure 5.4). Once the association between the whistling and urination is made, the

horses urinate on cue for post-race urine tests (see also Chapter 7, Applying learning theory).

Some horse-trainers use it to pair verbal praise (which, of course, means nothing to a naïve horse) with an inherently rewarding outcome such as food. The strength of associations that are built in this way can be assessed by the extent to which horses will work for these learned rewards. If the associations between primary and secondary rewards are too loose, the quality of the animal's performance will decline, because of a process called extinction. Pavlov found that if a CS, such as the sound of a metronome, were paired with food as a US, it would continue to make the dog salivate just as long as the CS continued to be followed by the

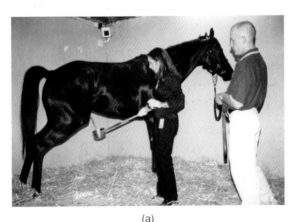

(a)

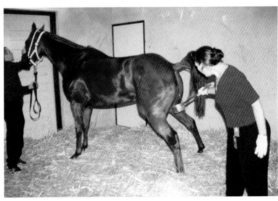

(b)

Figure 5.4 Post-race urine samples being taken on cue from a gelding (a) and a mare (b).

arrival of food. If the buzzer was sounded again and again but food no longer arrived, then *extinction* resulted in the disappearance of salivation to the tone. Extinction can apply to all examples of classical conditioning.

Riders use classical conditioning when they replace hand or leg pressure cues with previously neutral signals such as changes in their position or movement of their seat. It is difficult to train a horse to stop from the seat alone. Instead, you must train a stop response with an unconditioned stimulus from the rein and then link it with a specific cue from your seat (CS, e.g. bracing against the action). Trail-riding operators sometimes do the same with a whistle (CS) that is linked to bilateral rein signals (US) as a means of stopping horses in an emergency should novice riders lose control. The training of responses to a piece of string around a horse's neck is largely the product of a similar approach (Figure 5.5). The critical skill in training a classical conditioned association is to ensure that the links are made frequently because the associations will not last indefinitely. In building associations, it is important to present the CS before or at the same time as the US. Presenting the CS after the US leads to no association, quite simply because this order of events cannot increase the predictability of an environment.

A particularly useful variant of classical conditioning is called *counter-conditioning*, a procedure that changes an aversive or noxious stimulus into one that is positive for the animal. The first known example comes from Pavlov's lab. He used a mild electric shock, which initially elicited signs of pain, as a conditioned stimulus. After the shock had been paired repeatedly with food, it began to elicit salivation and there was no sign that it was still painful. Counter-conditioning can be very useful in animal behaviour therapy and in getting animals to accept painful therapeutic interventions. An example is when clippers (an aversive outcome that elicits fearful responses in many horses) are associated with feeding (an attractive outcome for all horses).

An important feature of classical conditioning is that it is selective and is dependent on the relative closeness of competing stimuli. So, as one particular stimulus, such as the noise from a clicker, becomes strongly associated with some important event, such as food, we see a weakening of the associations between other stimuli and food.

An example of this selectiveness and the effect of competing stimuli is *overshadowing*. A trainer may intend that the horse learns to associate a certain word with food or with an appropriate response. However, if the trainer always makes

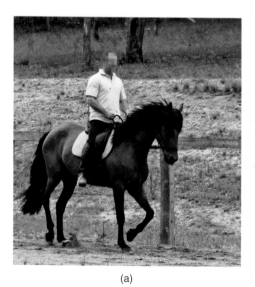
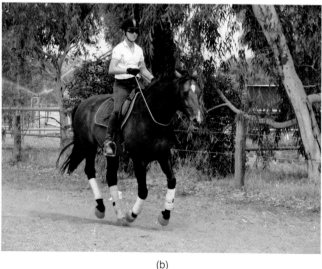

(a)   (b)

Figure 5.5 Horses being ridden without a bit (a) and without a bridle (b). (Photos courtesy of Pierre Malou and Portland Jones.)

an unintended hand gesture or body movement when uttering that certain word, the visual cue from the hand or body may become the effective conditioned stimulus instead. In this case, the body language signals have overshadowed the spoken signal or command. Consequently, they need either to become the cue in the trainer's mind or to be watered down by making them more variable. We will see more examples of overshadowing in Chapter 8 (Training).

Selective learning is seen in a process called *blocking*. If a stimulus is established as a consistent and reliable signal for a reinforcer, learning about a second stimulus that accompanies the first, is retarded or blocked. So, if a hand signal on its own has already become a strong conditioned stimulus, the later addition of a verbal command, even if issued at the same time as the hand signal, is likely to remain ineffective. If your aim is to train with clarity and consistency, avoid blocking and overshadowing because they impede training programs. Fundamentally, good trainers are careful to make sure that only the intended stimulus can serve as a signal to the horse.

Another important characteristic of classical conditioning is that associations between two events are more rapidly acquired if the events are *novel*. If a horse is exposed to a conditioned stimulus on a number of occasions before the conditioning procedure commences (i.e. before it is paired with the US), the conditioned response to that stimulus will be acquired more slowly. It is as if the animal has simply learned to ignore the stimulus because it has no important consequences. When pre-exposure to a stimulus produces retardation of learning, it is called *latent inhibition*. An example from a stable-yard might be the relative sluggishness with which a stallion would learn to get aroused by a head-collar, if he had been led around by that piece of equipment for years and then it was only used to lead him to the breeding barn. Similarly, a horse that has continually been told he is a 'Good boy' with no salient consequences (such as the release of pressure or arrival of food) will take longer to learn this as a secondary reinforcer, when associated with primary reinforcers, than an entirely naïve stablemate.

So, we can see that poor timing and inconsistent signalling can produce only weak, and sometimes even the wrong, associations. Good trainers

have excellent timing and consistency, often without having to think about it.

Like all good scientists, Pavlov kept a notebook and it is from this source that one of his most telling observations emerged. He noted that his dogs would race ahead of their handlers and jump onto the table in the experimental area. Instead of waiting for any stimuli (either unconditioned or conditioned) that made their mouths water, the dogs would actively try to place themselves into situations and perform activities that led to rewards. This resulted from trial-and-error learning and foreshadowed the other important category of associative learning: operant conditioning.

Reinforcement and punishment

Reinforcement, whether it is positive or negative, will always make a response more likely in future. Conversely, positive or negative punishment will generally make a response less likely in future (Table 5.1). Both punishment and negative reinforcement are central to operant conditioning because they can be applied as consequences of behaviour. Many trainers who claim not to use negative reinforcement are simply confused by its unpleasant connotations (Warren-Smith and McGreevy, 2008a). In the scientific study of cognition and ethology, negative is used in the arithmetic sense referring to the subtraction or removal of something from the animal's world, while positive refers to an addition. Negative reinforcement differs from positive reinforcement not least

Table 5.1 Punishment versus reinforcement – effect of the treatment (with examples)

Reinforcement	Punishment
Response becomes more likely in future	Response becomes less likely in future
Positive reinforcement (titbit reinforces begging)	Positive punishment (applying tension on the rein increases discomfort in the mouth)
Negative reinforcement (easing tension on the rein reduces discomfort)	Negative punishment (the complete removal of food extinguishes mugging)

because of the point at which stimulus control is achieved. When using positive reinforcement, trainers may wait until the shaped behaviour is offered before expecting it to come under stimulus control, whereas with negative reinforcement they are obliged to begin each pressure with a light version of the signal to prevent distress arising from the pressure and thus rapidly focus the horse on the light signal.

Using attractive stimuli

A reinforcer is any event that increases the frequency of the particular behaviour that it follows. Whether some event is called a reinforcer is related purely to the effect it has. So, the value of a reinforcer can be measured only in terms of the degree to which it makes the behaviour more likely in future. If a trainer's saying 'good boy' in response to a horse's leg-yielding has no effect on the horse's future behaviour then, according to this definition, reinforcement has not occurred. The trainer's words have had a neutral effect. A scratch on the head may be less reinforcing than a scratch at the withers, but a good trainer watches the animal to see how it responds not just to these comparable interventions but also to whether they genuinely make the preceding behaviour more likely.

Therefore, *many* different contextual features associated with both stimuli and reinforcers can be integrated to maximise differentiation and thus enhance performance (Nicol, 2002). Palatable foods are generally more reinforcing if they are not normally part of the horse's diet. However, this is less likely in naïve horses because of neophobia (literally, fear of the new). Horses that have been exposed to highly valued foods and do not receive them as part of a daily ration may perform with a higher level of consistency for such reinforcers. They recognise these foods as highly palatable and seem more motivated to work for them because they receive them infrequently. Clearly, this has a bearing on the rewards used in training since it explains why some horses appear to become rapidly sated (over-faced) with one type of food reward.

A horse's ability to discriminate between colours improves if the reward outcome differs. For example, in a discrimination task, if the colour of a central panel signals that either a left or a right lever response was correct, horses perform best when different reinforcers (food pellets for one lever, chopped carrot for the other) are linked with each lever, than when reinforcers were randomly assigned or identical (Miyashita *et al.*, 2000). This suggests that the cues for one reward are learned by classical conditioning so the horses would probably show a preference for one reward over the other and this preference would eventually affect their motivation to choose both panels equally.

Significantly, horses work to avoid aversive stimuli, even when this interferes with their access to positive reinforcement (Nicol, 2002). Acquiring food is generally rewarding but when the mouth that chews it contains a bit, enjoyment may be compromised by discomfort from the metal. In practical terms, this adds to the problem of blending negative and positive reinforcement (Warren-Smith and McGreevy, 2007c).

A significant problem when trying to use food reinforcers is the difficulty in delivering food immediately after the ridden horse offers a desirable response. Leaning out of the saddle after every good response is likely to train horses to slow down and halt, since this is the response they make immediately before we can easily flex forward from the saddle. So, devices that instantly deliver rewards to the mouth allow the time between performance of the desired behaviour and its reinforcement to be minimised, effectively enhancing the speed of learning. In trials with positive reinforcement alone, some horses took longer than control horses to complete a maze; this apparent stalling may reflect the nature of innate foraging strategies in horses in that they have not evolved to keep moving when feeding (McGreevy, unpublished data). So-called reward devices or sugar-bits, which deliver food rewards (such as molasses or carrot juice) orally, via a remotely controlled hollow bit, have been used successfully in experimental situations used in combination with bit pressures (Warren-Smith and McGreevy, 2007c).

Reinforcers can be either primary or secondary. Primary reinforcers are any resources that animals have evolved to seek. When the animal needs them, acquiring them is rewarding. In contrast, when the animal has just satisfied its need for them (i.e. it is sated), such resources are no longer rewarding. If the animal's motivation can be correctly predicted, food, water, sex, play, liberty, sanctuary and companionship can all be used as primary reinforcers. Secondary reinforcers are stimuli that are not intrinsically rewarding but that have become linked (by classical conditioning) with some kind of primary reinforcer. These associations make great sense in evolutionary terms since an auditory, olfactory or visual cue that has become reliably linked with a primary reinforcer will hold an animal's interest much longer than a neutral stimulus.

It is worth considering the innate value of things we class as rewards. Horses are often praised with tactile stimuli, chiefly with a scratch at the withers or a pat on the neck. Horses have evolved to find grooming one another (allogrooming) rewarding. So, a scratch on the appropriate part of the withers is a primary reinforcer. By comparison, the far more common practice of patting horses on the neck, if too forceful, can even be aversive. Patting is reinforcing only if the owner has coupled the pat with something inherently pleasant (McGreevy, 2004). Horses have not evolved to be motivated to offer certain responses for pats on their necks, so patting, if it is going to be used at all, must be conditioned as a secondary reinforcer. We have seen already how two stimuli can become linked as a result of classical conditioning. An interesting example is the way in which the bridle used for restraint during mating, the environs of the breeding barn, and the dummy used for semen collection can all become arousing for breeding stallions because they become reliable predictors of sex. The inadvertent emergence of similar links can easily arise during feeding time. Horses have not evolved to eat discrete meals and, so, the appearance of concentrated food in bulk causes inordinate excitement, especially for horses that do not have foraging opportunities between meals. This means that the sight of feed buckets, the sound of feed buckets and even the arrival of humans who frequently supply feed may all become secondary reinforcers. It is important that personnel who work around horses are aware of this possibility because they may inadvertently reinforce inappropriate behaviours such as pawing and aggression at the time of feeding. Feeding horses immediately after inappropriate responses is inadvisable but so is rattling buckets and then feeding. Clearly, feeding cannot be achieved without some

noise, so the best advice for owners of horses that get boisterously over-excited at feeding times is to feed plenty of roughage (so that horses are not frustrated by periods without food) and to stagger feeds throughout the day so that noise and the sound of feed buckets (being used to deliver food to *other* horses) become less likely to predict the delivery of food. In this way, any inadvertently rewarded responses will become extinguished. There are many ways in which we inadvertently reinforce our horse's responses. Just because we are not intending to train a response does not mean that the horse will not be learning something. Horses are learning all the time since they make no distinction between associations built through regular handling, regular riding, training and competition.

Given what we know about the horse's ability to discriminate between cues that are linked to a given reward (Miyashita *et al.*, 2000), in the most elegant case, a specific secondary reinforcer tells the animal that it will reliably encounter or receive a certain primary reinforcer. In this way, a trainer can mark excellent responses with a secondary reinforcer that delivers the resource for which the horse is most highly motivated.

Horse-trainers rarely need to question whether a technique is based on classical or instrumental conditioning, but it pays to look at possible interactions between the two types. Declines in performance of trained behaviour can sometimes result from competition between classically and instrumentally conditioned responses. They arise when unwanted responses that would be innate responses towards resources in more natural settings are offered in response to learned cues. A useful example is seen when a horse feeding from a bucket begins pawing at the ground; pawing is thought to be an innate activity horses use to expose forage covered by snow and so is a natural response to slightly frustrating feeding in a domestic context. This reversion to innate responses is known as *instinctive drift* (Breland and Breland, 1962).

Trick-trainers risk instinctive drift when they build a chain of instrumental responses that produces the reinforcer. For example, they may train a horse to pick up a hat, carry the hat and then relinquish it into the correct receptacle (e.g. the trainer's hand) to receive food. As performance improves, an increasingly consistent relationship develops between a stimulus, the hat, and the food; the hat becomes a conditioned stimulus that reliably signals the arrival of food (the unconditioned stimulus). This CS–US relationship produces classical conditioning, and so the hat acquires the properties of a surrogate food item and the horse will tend to hold onto it rather than let it drop. Responding to the hat as a food object, therefore, competes with the operant response of releasing it, so that this trained response is performed more slowly and less reliably.

Reinforcement schedules

Until a given response behaviour is under stimulus control, the trainer must be consistent in applying cues and providing rewards. If consistent reinforcement is not provided for correct responses, the horse's behaviour becomes unpredictable. Once a response is consistently elicited as a conditioned response, it can be made more resistant to extinction by means of a variable reward schedule. The desired behaviour can then be rewarded unpredictably. Horses respond to different *fixed-ratio* positive reinforcement schedules, in which partial reinforcement is delivered on the basis of the number of correct responses made, and *fixed-interval* positive reinforcement schedules, in which reinforcement becomes available again only after some specified time has elapsed (Myers and Mesker, 1960). This aligns them with other animals trained using positive reinforcement. When shaping novel responses, practitioners find that continuous reinforcement schedules rapidly increase the response rate (McCall and Burgin, 2002). However, once the response has been shaped and is under stimulus control, intermittent reinforcement can be used (with a resultant increase in its resistance to extinction).

Horses cannot be expected to learn well if reinforcement is delayed, because the delay prevents them from relating the reinforcement to the behaviour. Previous work has shown that horses have short-term spatial recall of less than 10 seconds in a delayed-response task (McLean, 2004). It is also necessary to obtain the same results in multiple locations for the behaviour to become generalised and not context-specific (some training systems refer to this quality as 'proof'; e.g. McLean and McLean, 2008).

The predominance of negative reinforcement in the training of horses means that much of what we know about positive reinforcement cannot automatically be applied to the ridden context. Trainers cannot choose to reinforce sometimes and not others (as in a variable reward schedule) since maintaining pressure leads to habituation. If, in a negative reinforcement system, riders delay reinforcement (release of pressure), they should do so only when shaping an alternative response. The horse subjected to sustained pressure may try harder to offer a response that solves its current problem but the rider has to know what he is waiting for in terms of an improved response since failing to reward the improvement will again lead to habituation. It pays to consider why this practical skill is so hard to teach to riders. There is evidence that judges (and therefore, presumably, coaches) fail to detect lightness in observed riders (de Cartier d'Yves and Ödberg, 2005). This means that they are likely to fail to spot removal of pressure and so are currently poorly placed to comment on the rider's most critical means of reinforcement.

Shaping behaviour

Shaping is the principle of reinforcing successive improvements that are approximations of the final response. Trainers seeking to reinforce particular responses can either wait for the behaviour to occur spontaneously – it can be readily reinforced if the behaviour occurs frequently – or they can shape the behaviour pattern. Using this technique, trainers can move from a point where it is impossible to reinforce a desired response (because that response never occurs), to one where basic attempts are offered, to one where the response is offered with increasing reliability. A common characteristic among good trainers is their ability to recognise an opportunity to reinforce improved 'approximations'. While less effective trainers complain that their animals fail to understand what is being asked of them and feel that the animals have peaked in their training, superior trainers have the skill and patience to capitalise on each tiny improvement as the only way of moving towards the final response.

Crucially, shaping relies on reserving the reinforcement so that the animal has to keep trialling new responses or responses that are developments on those that have previously been reinforced. For example, when training a horse to approach a target (in so-called target training), rewards are given chiefly when the horse travels closer to the target or does so faster than on previous occasions. While shaping a new response or, for that matter, modifying an existing one, it is important to reward target responses immediately. To delay in delivering reinforcement is to allow intervening responses to be linked with the reward.

Clicker training

If every delivery of a reward depends on the close presence of a human, its effect can quickly become context-specific to human proximity, so that a horse fails to perform the behaviour at any distance from its trainer. The cue of a human is an important contingency for these animals. Clickers that can be used to reinforce at a distance really come into their own here. These devices are currently the most popular example of a secondary reinforcer; they are being used by thousands of trainers worldwide (McCall and Burgin, 2002).

Clickers developed in the field of marine-mammal-training, a context in which restraint of the animals during training is impractical and in which the application of pressure for negative reinforcement or punishment is virtually impossible. By creating a classically conditioned association between the particular sound and the arrival of a primary reinforcer (most commonly a food reward), the trainer can *bridge* the gap between the moment an animal performs a response correctly and it receiving the reward. Essentially, the clicker comes to mean, 'Yes, that's good – a reward is coming.' When a clicker is first used, the correct association is established by making the sound just before giving a highly valued reward. Repetition of the pairing between the two stimuli assures the animal of the signal's reliability.

Some trainers deplore the use of food in training since they see it as a cause of biting. This may be true in horses and ponies that have been allowed to 'mug' their owners for food. Good clicker trainers never feed unless they have made a clicker

noise so their subjects expect food only on cue. These trainers also feed only at some distance from the receptacle containing the store of food (usually from a pocket or pouch on a belt). This breaks any direct connection between the food and its source and restricts the horse from helping himself. Moreover, consistency in this practice places the feeding response itself under stimulus control and extinguishes begging or nuzzling responses, which are never reinforced (and if they have been previously reinforced by another trainer, they are rapidly extinguished). Mugging can also be thwarted by reinforcing the horse for looking away. The clicker noise occurs when the horse offers the correct response and this should, in turn, make the food appear. It is certainly unwise to use food to lure horses during training since this makes desirable responses contingent on the presence of food (no food, no deal).

After establishing desirable responses through negative reinforcement, trainers can use clicker training to help maintain the acquisition of the light signal. The benefits of positive reinforcement as applied in clicker training are largely to do with the ephemeral nature of light pressure signals and the likelihood that it may be more humane than traditional negative reinforcement training. With clicker training, 'what you click is what you get', so if your observations and timing are not perfect you will inadvertently shape some responses you do not want. Subsequent adjustments that remove this reinforcement mean that these inadvertently shaped responses are extinguished. So, while poor timing can make clicker training ineffective, the same trainer error in traditional negative reinforcement training could amount to abuse (see Chapter 6, Learning III: Associative (aversive)).

Commercial clicker devices make a sharp and distinctive noise. The brevity and clarity of the click facilitates precise capture (reinforcement) of transient responses, such as the horse bringing forward its ears. Also, being pocket-sized or attachable to keyrings, clickers are very convenient, but they are not an obligatory item for so-called clicker training. An important caveat on the topic of clicker training is that its focus on the clicker sometimes obscures the fundamental message: that any secondary reinforcer, when developed appropriately, can be a powerful training tool. Virtually, any discrete auditory stimulus can be linked to a primary reinforcer to become a secondary reinforcer.

Some horses are fearful of the click per se and are, therefore, candidates for such alternative secondary reinforcers. Indeed, as long as they cannot be confused with words that appear in common parlance, any consistent vocalisation by a trainer (so-called clicker words) will be effective. 'Yes!' or 'Good boy!' are examples, but it is worth emphasising that the reinforcing value of any noise is a function of the degree to which it is associated with a primary reinforcer. Trainers who click (or say 'Good boy!') without delivering a primary reinforcer just afterwards are diluting the impact of the secondary reinforcer. This explains why horses show a rapid decline in interest in responding for the secondary reinforcer only, and the temporal link between the primary and secondary reinforcers is also critical (McCall and Burgin, 2002). Thus, the fundamental rules of learning theory apply, and trainers who maintain the horse's motivation for the primary reinforcer and build the firmest association between the primary and secondary reinforcers can most effectively shape desirable responses.

Secondary reinforcers are most effectively established when presented before or up until the presentation of a primary reinforcer. Simultaneous presentation of a reward and a novel secondary stimulus is less effective because the primary reinforcer will block or overshadow the new stimulus. Presentation of the secondary stimulus after the primary reinforcer is entirely unproductive, because although an association may exist between the two, it will not help the animal to predict the arrival of a reward.

The use of secondary reinforcement seems to increase a horse's interest in performing novel tasks (Myers and Mesker, 1960) and this creativity in the horse's approach to problem-solving accounts for the growing appeal of clicker training in behaviour-modification programs and some higher movements (such as piaffe; see Figure 5.6b and c), especially where traditional remedial approaches have failed (see Chapter 12, Unorthodox techniques and Chapter 14, Ethical equitation). Furthermore, the principles of clicker training can be very helpful in shaping and modifying unwanted responses. By deconstructing a series of undesirable responses that arise in a given context, we can counter-condition fear responses (see Figure 5.7). For example, by training a trailer-shy horse to approach a target and then moving the target towards a ground-based aversive stimulus (such as a tarpaulin; see Figure 5.6a), we can shape approaching hazards and then ultimately the trailer without using any pressure.

When selecting primary reinforcers, experienced trainers observe the horse's responses to determine the reinforcing value of a novel reward. Many horses respond well to carrots as the primary reinforcer in a clicker-training protocol, but more so if carrots are not routinely offered in regular meals. The relationship between motivation and the reinforcing value of any food should be considered here. The speed or strength of learning increases with the value of the reinforcer. This explains why horses will learn to run faster to the sound of a rattling bucket (a secondary reinforcer associated with concentrate foods) than they will to the rustling of a hay-net (a secondary reinforcer associated with hay).

Generally speaking, the larger the reinforcer, the greater is its effect on behaviour. This may suggest that big is always better, but the effectiveness of a reinforcer may decline when many reinforcers need to be given within a short period. An obvious example of such a satiation effect is the use of a food reward to a hungry animal that will soon lose its appetite for frequent large rewards. So, many trainers use small rewards within a session and then end when the horse completes a 'high note' – that is, performs particularly well – at which point it is given a large reward, a 'jackpot'. Learning theory suggests that jackpots should be used sparingly, since once the horse starts to expect large reinforcers in a given context, small reinforcers may start to lose their effectiveness. Therefore, it is advisable to start training with large rewards and short sessions and progressively move towards smaller rewards given in longer sessions. Sometimes horses get overexcited by large rewards so they should not be allowed to see jackpots before they are given (e.g. conceal rewards in a pouch).

Contiguity

The principle of temporal contiguity states that events that occur closely in time become associated. As we will see in the next chapter, the longer the delay between a warning sound and the

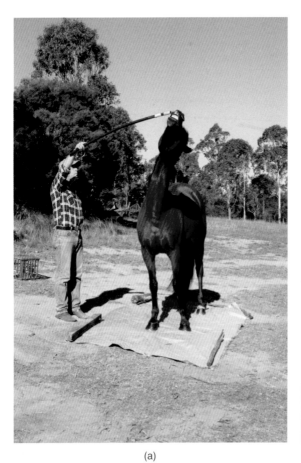

(a)

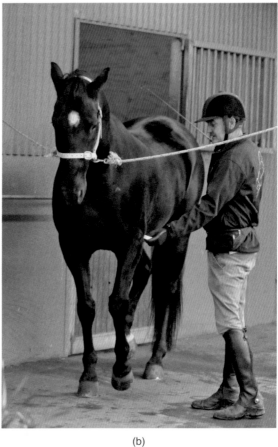

(b)

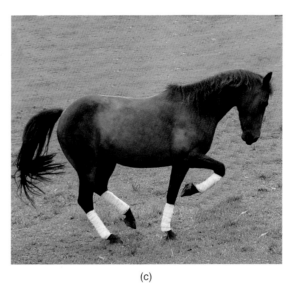

(c)

Figure 5.6 (a) A horse stretching (i.e. making an operant response) towards a target, as a part of being trained to traverse a ground-based obstacle. (b) A horse in early training of piaffe being reinforced using positive reinforcement. (c) A horse trained to piaffe at liberty using positive reinforcement. (Photo (c) courtesy of Georgia Bruce.)

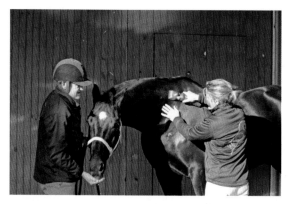

Figure 5.7   Horse being clipped in the presence of food – an example of counter-conditioning.

arrival of an aversive outcome, the weaker will be the horse's fear response to the sound. Similarly, giving a carrot to a horse 2 minutes after a pat on its neck will not make the pat reinforcing. The carrot would have to arrive within seconds of the pat if reinforcement is to occur. The interval between stimuli is usually, but not always, the most important criterion for the establishment of an association. Events distanced by time can still become associated as long as there is a high predictive link between them. The best example of this is food-aversion learning, which helps animals avoid food items that have previously made them ill. Novel flavours are more likely to be associated with later sickness and, therefore, horses may be alert to this possibility when they consume novel foods. Operant conditioning has been used to indicate the behavioural effects of drugs. So, for example, a horse trained to press a lever can be monitored before and after the administration of a pharmaceutical test. Since the reward for pressing is usually food, a decrease in the rate of demand suggests that the drug has either depressant or anorexic effects. Food-aversion learning has also been used by scientists interested in the consequences of proprietary drugs on horse welfare. The aversive effect of drugs can be calibrated by the degree to which a food associated with it is subsequently avoided.

Combining positive and negative reinforcement

Most research involving positive reinforcement with horses has been conducted on non-equitation related activities such as mazes (e.g. Haag *et al.*,

1980; McCall *et al.*, 1981; Heird *et al.*, 1986a; Marinier and Alexander, 1994) and so, while they may yield valuable results, they are not always directly transferable to traditional equitation (Dougherty and Lewis, 1991). Only a limited number of studies have reported using both positive and negative reinforcement for comparison. Haag *et al.* (1980) found a significant correlation with the learning ability of a group of ponies in both a shock-avoidance trial and a single-choice maze. Visser *et al.* (2003) used an avoidance test that involved puffs of air being given for the wrong choice and measured learning performance by percentage of correct responses, and in a reward test, measured performance by latency to obtain the reward; some horses did not respond to the aversive stimulus.

Employing a remotely operated pump that delivered a small food reward into the horse's mouth via a hollow bit (see Figure 5.8), Warren-Smith and McGreevy (2007) assessed the effectiveness of a blend of both positive and negative reinforcement in shaping responses to a halt stimulus. They found that, although it did not increase the speed of learning, horses subjected to this blend nodded their heads and mouthed the bits less and were more likely to lick their lips than those reinforced with negative reinforcement only. It will be interesting to see how research in this domain develops.

Long-term potentiation

As learning proceeds, memories encoded in short-term memory begin to become established as more durable long-term memories. This is known as long-term potentiation. Implicit in this transition is the neurotransmitter serotonin, and experimental studies have shown that five spaced deliveries of serotonin over a period of 1.5 hours have produced long-term changes lasting several days. Studies both in animals and with cells in vitro indicate that long-term memory is an extension of short-term memory. As short-term memory develops into long-term memory, they are seen to share many physical similarities, such as broadening of the action potential, an increase in excitability and enhanced release of transmitters of sensory neurons. Long-term memory, however, is also characterised by synthesis of new

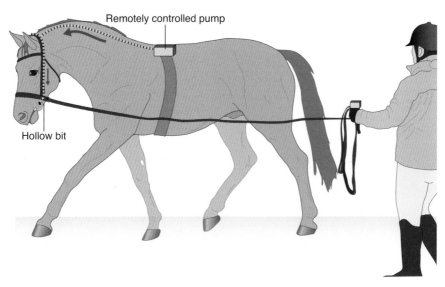

Figure 5.8   Remotely controlled reward devices (delivering positive reinforcement) can be used in combination with bit pressure (negative reinforcement).

protein molecules (Castellucci *et al.*, 1989) as well as further structural changes (Bailey and Chen, 1983). The persistence of structural changes correlates with the behavioural duration of the memory (Bailey and Chen, 1989). This more elaborate memory structure confers stronger resistance to forgetting, which characterises long-term memory (Kandel, 2006). For example, long-term memory is more resistant to various chemicals and traumas than short-term memory.

Take-home messages

- Just because a horse can be trained to offer a particular response, we should not assume it enjoys giving that response. After all, dogs can be trained to salivate in response to electric shocks.
- Horses are learning all the time since they make no distinction between associations built through regular handling, regular riding, training and competition.
- Effective trainers are clear and consistent in their signals and the way in which they set up challenges for animals to solve (i.e. the way in which they pose questions).
- Effective training relies on timing and consistency.
- Detraining can take the form of inconsistency and variable timing.

Ethical considerations

- The reliance on pressure and release in horse-riding distinguishes it from training in most other species. Animal welfare considerations put the onus on trainers to use minimal pressure and release it immediately.
- Should novice riders (including children) be taught the principles of cause-and-effect with positive reinforcement before being permitted to ride, balance and use negative reinforcement?
- The governing bodies of horse sports should encourage research into the most humane application of pressure and alternative means of communicating with horses and reinforcement during training.
- Ethical investigations into the use of positive and negative reinforcement should compare and contrast the motivations of hunger and pressure removal.

Areas and anticipated limitations for further research

- There are many questions remaining about positive reinforcement as it can be administered to horses. Results to date are in no way the full story.
- Can we discover ways to deliver 'jackpots' (a primary reward that is substantially bigger than usual and comes as a surprise) to ridden horses?

6 Learning III: Associative (Aversive)

Introduction

While the previous chapter focussed on training with attractive stimuli, aversive events are far more critical with the ridden horse. This chapter explores the use in horse-training of aversive stimuli, most of which are tactile. The trainer is well placed to deliver tactile stimuli, because the ridden or led horse is in direct physical contact with him or her. Aversive stimuli underpin the horse's learning of responses evoked by the rider's legs, reins and lead-reins, as well as whips, spurs and possibly seat and weight signals. No matter how much we are able to positively reinforce velocity and directional mobility responses, any tactile signals that elicit them are necessarily aversive, at least initially. Moreover, the acute sensitivity of horses to cutaneous irritations is well known, so the fundamental challenge in the initial training of horses is that they must respond calmly yet sometimes powerfully to aversive stimuli.

Equestrian technology has undergone very few quantum leaps. The chief milestones have been the bridle, the curb bit, the stirrups and the (saddle's) tree. Although horse-riding may have benefited from adjustable trees, air-filled panels and spring-loaded stirrups, it is essentially a low-tech activity. Despite the contribution of some innovative technologies, a successful partnership between horse and rider still relies predominantly on the skills of the rider. It is the development of such skills that have enabled humans to manipulate and control the behaviour of the horse. It is, thus, helpful to consider how humans learned to modify the behaviour of other animals in general and, from that point, how basic horse-training know-how developed. Undoubtedly, humans learned some basics from handling their own children or even captive members of enemy groups. Perhaps the first training interactions between humans and other species began inadvertently when food was thrown to scavenging animals. Humans would undoubtedly have noticed that, as animals ventured ever closer, the arrival of food made their tentative but significant steps forward more likely. It would also have been clear that any sudden, threatening moves by humans would cause the animals to scurry away (see Figure 6.1), becoming more wary and more distant. What these people were seeing were the effects of reward and punishment, always uneasy partners in learning.

The use of aversive stimuli to control horses has a long history. There is archaeological evidence of restraint artefacts from around the end of the third millennium BC (Levine, 2005). Xenophon, writing more than two millennia ago in his treatise *Hippike*, wrote extensively about the varied uses of aversive stimuli to control horses.

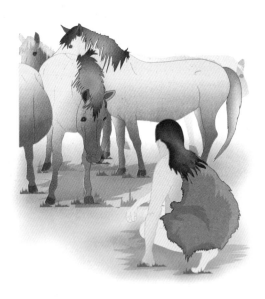

Figure 6.1   In ancient times, it is likely that humans learned to adapt their body posture to facilitate making contact with the horse in order to capture it.

Experimentally, our understanding of aversive learning is comparatively recent. The famous Ivan Pavlov mostly used food in his learning experiments, but a Russian contemporary, Vladimir Bechterev, also experimented on dogs using electricity. He showed, perhaps unsurprisingly, that if a conditioned stimulus (CS) such as a buzzer was repeatedly presented just before a dog's hind paw was shocked, the dog very quickly learned to lift its leg in response to the buzzer alone. Bechterev's experiments provided the first objective study of aversive learning in animals. Animals generally find an electric shock so aversive that they resist habituation to it, even at mild levels.

Stimuli that are generally aversive for horses

Many events are aversive for horses; for example, a sudden noise, the sudden appearance of a stimulus, large and/or moving objects and unfamiliar animals, including even their close relative, the donkey. Horsepeople typically claim that the more unusual looking a species appears to the horse (compared with those to which it has previously habituated) the more aversive it is. For example, the novel sight of ostriches and emus is particularly alarming to most horses. As prey animals, horses may even become sensitised to aversive events and this can occur after surprisingly few exposures (McGreevy and Boakes, 2007).

While being ridden, novel fear-eliciting stimuli may be encountered by the horse. Furthermore, they can even become aroused and subsequently fearful as a result of rider anticipation. For example, when riders were told to expect a fear-eliciting stimulus to appear suddenly, their horses' heart rates rose, indicating that they were mirroring their rider's increased arousal (Von Borstel et al., 2007).

Characteristically, horses maintain general surveillance and visually inspect novel objects that may constitute a threat. Hunting strategies including stealthy stalking and ambush are employed by carnivores that prey successfully on large social herbivores, so it is not surprising that horses rely heavily on their visual abilities to avoid predation. It warrants reflection that when ridden, the horse's head is in front of the rider, so the animal is possibly at its most aroused, flighty, wary and dangerous when it is under-saddle, particularly when it detects visual threats.

It is the magnitude, novelty, proximity or sudden occurrence of visual, tactile and auditory stimuli that make them aversive to the horse (see Figure 6.2). With visual stimuli, movement is particularly important. Objects are especially alarming if they appear suddenly, move erratically (and are, therefore, hard to identify, even if familiar), or if they are advancing (towards the horse). It seems that novel objects are dismissed as potential threats if they are moving away from the horse. This feature of equine responses to novelty can be utilised in training. For example, in police-horse-training, it is possible to reinforce appropriate behaviours by causing novel objects (such as large, fear-eliciting, stability balls) to retreat.

Although horses have limited ability to focus on objects that are close to them, they have good distance vision and a very extensive visual field (Harman et al., 1999). This is important as it allows them to scan the horizon for potential threats. However, they rarely need to see close up with high acuity and because the eye's proximity to objects is generally limited by the length of the

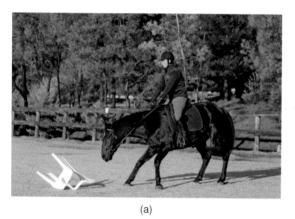
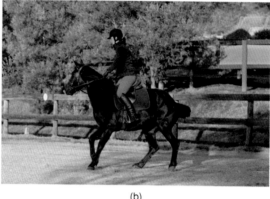

(a)   (b)

Figure 6.2   Even an up-turned chair can be perceived as a novel object worthy of fear (a) and horses may learn to shy away suddenly from stimuli they perceive as aversive (b).

nose (Wouters and De Moor, 1979), objects very close up are felt via the skin and vibrissae of the muzzle. Within the retina of the horse there is an area of maximal sensitivity (similar to the fovea of the human eye) termed the visual streak and it is only in this area that the horse has any real visual acuity (Ehrenhofer *et al.*, 2002). In the more peripheral areas of the retina, the structure suggests that the horse is particularly sensitive to subtle changes in light and stimulus motion (Ehrenhofer *et al.*, 2002).

The way the horse sees determines how it will react to different stimuli and head movements may be the result of the horse trying to see an object more clearly. The horse may either raise or lower its head to focus the image on the visual streak, or cock its head sideways to see an object more clearly. Movement of the head may bring into focus images that originally fell onto retinal regions of low acuity, in the same way that we may see movement in our peripheral visual field and turn towards it to see, with our high-acuity central retinal region, what was moving. When a horse sees a movement in its peripheral visual field, it may react defensively. This may explain why a horse will suddenly raise its head and shy away from an object that has suddenly entered its field of view. In general, the farther an object is from the horse the less likely it is that the horse will perceive it as a threat and react adversely to it. Horses will react to stimuli appearing in their peripheral vision but, again, the greater the distance from the horse, the less the effect.

Control over aversive events

You will recall that in positive reinforcement the animal's behaviour is reinforced by a primary (e.g. food) and perhaps a secondary reinforcer (e.g. a clicking noise). It is easy to imagine the rewarding effects of providing an animal with something it likes. What, then, could be so reinforcing about aversive events? The answer lies in the animal being able to terminate, escape or avoid the aversive event. Where possible, running away provides the simplest solution for an animal faced with an aversive stimulus. This is known as *escape learning*, and in this case, it is not important where or how escape is achieved, escape itself is all that matters. Any aversive stimulus contingent upon some behaviour, and which effectively reduces that behaviour is, by definition, a punisher (McGreevy and Boakes, 2007). Control over aversive events is not necessarily bad. It is a fundamental characteristic of both natural and man-made contingencies that enables animals to operate optimally in their environments.

Through other associative learning processes, such as classical conditioning, neutral signals can evoke avoidance responses, provided their presentation is contiguous with the salient aversive stimulus (McLean and McGreevy, 2004). During training, horses are highly motivated to learn predictive cues about the aversive stimulus. For example, the characteristic actions of the rider's seat during deceleration herald aversive rein pressure. When the discriminative seat stimulus has

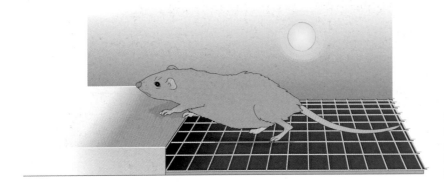

Figure 6.3 Rats show avoidance learning when they respond to a flashing light that heralds an electric shock from a grid beneath their feet.

been acquired and a sufficient response has been learned, the three elements of the operant contingency are easily identified: the discriminative stimulus (the seat), the operant response (the deceration), and the reinforcer (the cessation of the seat signal). In horse-training, as in all animal-training, the structural requirements of the operant contingency are the same whether they are motivated by attractive or aversive stimuli.

Avoidance learning

When a new signal becomes the trigger and so evokes an aversive response, it is described as a secondary punisher. Secondary punishers allow animals to learn to avoid punishing stimuli, which is known as *avoidance learning*. A trained rat will run off a grid that is about to be electrified because it has learned to associate a flashing light with an electric shock that follows (see Figure 6.3). So, in this example, a flashing light has taken on the properties of a secondary punisher. Avoidance learning is unique in that the learned response is persistent even in the absence of reinforcement. It is only possible when warning stimuli are available to signal pain-inducing events.

Active avoidance refers to movements learned in response to warning stimuli for the purpose of avoiding pain. *Inhibitory avoidance* refers to inaction, learned because action in the presence of the warning stimuli has previously led to pain. Our understanding of the neural tissues engaged in avoidance learning has come from studies of the effects of brain lesions (experimentally induced brain damage) and from brain-mapping stud-

ies such as positron emission tomography (PET) and magnetic resonance imaging (MRI) technology. Avoidance learning is studied primarily using rats, cats and rabbits that learn to jump over a hurdle or to enter an activity wheel to avoid a mild electric shock signalled by warning stimuli, such as a tone or light. If lesions are made in the medial dorsal and anterior nuclei of their limbic thalamus, the amygdala or in the cingulate cortical areas that receive input from these areas, the animals are incapable of active avoidance learning. Lesions in only one of the nuclei, or in the cingulate cortical projection field of a single nucleus, yield partial learning deficits (Gabriel, 1993). Inhibitory avoidance learning is prevented by hippocampal lesions. Successful performance in such tasks depends on the cognitive mapping functions of the hippocampus, including remembering whether particular environments are dangerous or safe (Nadel *et al.*, 1975).

The role of avoidance and escape learning in equitation is profound. It is not difficult to interpret the locomotory responses that occur as a result of the rein and leg signals in trained horses as examples of avoidance learning. Thus, avoidance learning and negative reinforcement can be seen to be allied processes.

Negative reinforcement

In negative reinforcement (NR), learning occurs because the stimulus is taken away, *subtracted* (Chance, 1993). Good examples are where a horse is motivated to remove itself from pain, discomfort or a predatory threat, but there are also more commonplace responses such as moving to the shade when the sun becomes too hot. The removal of the aversive stimulus reinforces the behaviour, thereby making it more likely in the future.

Negative reinforcement occurs in many subtle situations such as when you advance towards a horse and he retreats. As a result, there will be a learned response – the horse will retreat (i.e. remove you) earlier and earlier when he sees you approach. When the farrier goes to touch his hind-leg, the horse may swing away; if he does so, NR has occurred and the swing away will occur more rapidly the next time. Therefore, farriers, vets and all personnel need to learn that by such removal, habits of escape are rapidly acquired and elements of hyper-reactivity may also become attached to the response.

While many human–horse interactions begin with positive reinforcement, negative reinforcement forms the foundations of control. All responses in-hand and under-saddle begin with pressure but later come to be elicited by other signals. Thus, the reins, the rider's legs, whips, spurs, lead-reins and halters are all potential instruments of negative reinforcement (see Figure 6.4).

Releasing the pressure

It is the removal of pressure that initially trains the responses required in equitation, and this can take some time. Horses learn to stop in order to release rein tension, to turn to release turn-rein tension, to go forward to release pressure from both of the rider's legs, and to step sideways to release the rider's single-leg pressure. Similarly, in-hand, the horse learns to stop in order to remove the posterior lead-rein tension and to go forward to release the anterior lead-rein tension. With repetitions, horses learn to perform these manoeuvres from very light pressures because they perceive the initial increase of pressure of either rein or leg, and learn to respond to it in order to avoid the stronger pressure. Thus, in correct training practices, the application of all pressures must begin with very mild pressure. Soon, the horse perceives that stronger pressure can be avoided by reacting to the initial light pressure. Even though light pressure is the same modality as stronger pressure, this step arguably represents the conversion

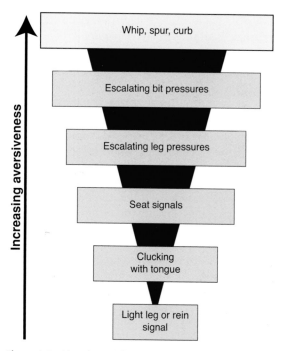

Figure 6.4 Negative reinforcement in training is unique because of its scalar properties where the potential exists to increase motivation through increasing pressure of reins, legs, spur or whip.

of response initiation from operant to classical conditioning (see Chapter 5, Learning II: Associative (attractive)).

Control and predictability

In any operant contingency, contiguity (the closeness of events in space or time) is essential (Lindsay, 2000). Horse-trainers refer to this as timing. In negative reinforcement, the behaviour learned by the horse is the one that predicts the release of pressure. This response is perceived by the horse as the one that solved the aversive problem, so it offers the same response more frequently in the future. From the horse's standpoint, offering responses that switch off aversive stimuli gives it *control* (McGreevy, 2004). As the animal increasingly responds to salient elements of the aversive pressure, such as the initial onset of pressure, it acquires a second element essential to its wellbeing and, as we discussed in the previous chapter, allows it efficient exploitation of its umwelt: *predictability* (Wiepkema, 1987).

Trialling responses

A key feature of operant conditioning is the tendency to trial a range of responses to solve the current challenge (hence, the alternate term of trial-and-error learning). When faced with an aversive stimulus (e.g. from the rider's leg when learning to go forward under-saddle), the horse may trial going backwards, kicking out or biting the rider's leg before it trials going forward, at which point the trainer must immediately release the pressure to reinforce the correct response. However, the trainer can set up the situation so that the horse is more likely to offer the correct response. For example, he or she may apply the first leg pressure only when the horse is standing with its hindquarters against a fence. This means that the horse's primary option is to offer a forward step.

Because of the tendency of animals to trial a raft of responses when presented with an aversive stimulus, it is interesting to investigate the range of responses an animal may offer to various pressures. McLean (2005b) conducted trials involving 50 young horses (Thoroughbreds and European Warmbloods) that were habituated to the presence of a rider astride but naïve to any locomotory responses. Horses offered an array of responses when the rider applied the go signal (closing/nudging both legs) on the horses' sides (Table 6.1).

Table 6.1   Distribution of trialled responses that arise from the closing pressure of the rider's legs

Response to leg pressure	Percentage of horses
No response within 5 seconds	32
Move neck and head up	18
Move head to side	14
Step back	6
Flight response (hunch back, buck, rear, spin)	8
Step laterally	10
Step forward	12

The large percentage of horses that do not step forward from the leg pressure of the rider suggests that stepping forward represents a learned association, trained by negative reinforcement when the trainer releases the pressure of the legs after the horse gives the correct response by going forward. In other words, the trainer maintains the pressure throughout the incorrect responses until a near-correct response is offered, whereupon the pressure is released. Interestingly and significantly, it is not difficult to understand how incorrect responses can be accidentally reinforced in early training, and that in such circumstances the young horse is at the mercy of the horse-breaker's knowledge or skills in the correct use of learning theory. Disturbingly, this highlights the ease with which a young horse can be transformed into an 'outlaw'.

How to use negative reinforcement

Stimulus control can be defined as the degree to which a response occurs in the presence of a specific stimulus and does not occur in the absence of this stimulus (McGreevy *et al.*, 2005). In horse-training, achieving stimulus control of the basic locomotory responses involves negative reinforcement, and the following steps have been proposed (McLean, 2005b):

1. The response to be trained is 'targeted' by the trainer. It is important that *only* the targeted behaviour results in the removal of pressure/discomfort.
2. The pressure (aversive stimulus) should be increased during the 'incorrect' behaviour until the targeted response emerges. During this phase, the pressure must not fluctuate or decrease because this constitutes a lowering of pressure and, thus, could be perceived as reinforcing.
3. If intermittent pressures are used (e.g. nudging by the rider's legs or tapping with a dressage whip), there should be no gaps greater than 1 second so that the horse does not perceive this transient relief as reinforcing.
4. At the *onset* of the targeted response, the aversive stimulus should immediately be removed. Removal of the aversive stimulus must be contingent upon the onset of the 'correct' behaviour.

A continuum of reinforcing possibilities

One of the interesting characteristics of negative reinforcement is the sliding scale of aversiveness (see Figure 6.5). If pressure B is greater than pressure A, then it follows that relief from pressure B is more reinforcing than relief from pressure A. For example, consider mouth pressures on a linear scale from 1 to 10, where 1 represents the mildest of aversive stimuli and 10 represents the most painful, fearful and unendurable level of aversiveness, intolerable even for the shortest duration. At some point along the scale lies a threshold where the tolerable escalates to the intolerable.

In practical horse-training, these mouth and body pressures are real; light cues occur in the lower scale, while the more motivating aversive pressures lie in the higher scale. Because equitation generally relies on a foundation of aversive stimuli, it is important to mention that, as most highly skilled trainers have noted, best practice is embodied in the use of the least aversive stimuli (the lightest cues). Furthermore, there are problems with using high levels of aversiveness be-cause of its associations with the amygdala (the brain's centre for processing emotional reactions). Fear and aversiveness are interconnected, and be-cause fear responses are resistant to erasure (Le Doux, 1994), trainers must be very cautious about invoking fear responses during training.

When horses have unfortunately habituated to the bit or to the rider's legs through incorrect neg-ative reinforcement, effective trainers can rehabil-itate such horses by increasing the motivation of the aversive pressure for a short duration and then releasing the pressure at the onset of the correct response. In other words, the operant contingency must be re-established. It is not sufficient to hope that horses might forget the aversiveness of stim-uli to which they have habituated. Re-training re-sponses that were incorrectly trained originally by negative reinforcement unfortunately requires deployment of greater motivational aversiveness than would otherwise be the case. This is why it is imperative that learning theory becomes part of every horse-trainer's education, so that it may be applied consistently both at the start and through-out every horse's training.

Negative reinforcement versus positive reinforcement

Many animal-trainers focus only on training via positive reinforcement (PR), because their subjects are required to perform at a distance and NR (typ-ically, by applying pressure) is irrelevant in these circumstances. Animals such as dolphins, seals, bears, zoo elephants and dogs to a large extent are trained via positive reinforcement. In positive re-inforcement, the trainer ignores errors made by the animal. If an animal takes fright during training for whatever reason, the trainer waits until the an-imal chooses to return to the training station. This presents no problem when the subject is at liberty, but when an animal flees with a rider astride, the situation is critically dangerous. Horse, camel and working elephant trainers almost universally use negative reinforcement because they can virtually 'force' the animal to turn, slow or go in adverse cir-cumstances. Herein lies a fundamental difference between positive and negative reinforcement: in NR, the trainer does not have to wait for the an-imal to offer the response – he can *contrive* it.

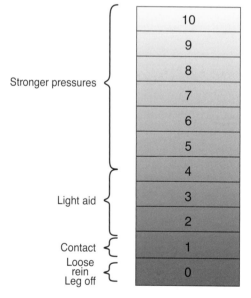

Figure 6.5   An arbitrary scale showing that the neutral stimulus, the discriminative stimulus (the light pressure signal) and the stronger motivating level of pressure can be imagined as a linear scale of pressure. (Illustration courtesy of Andrew and Manuela McLean.)

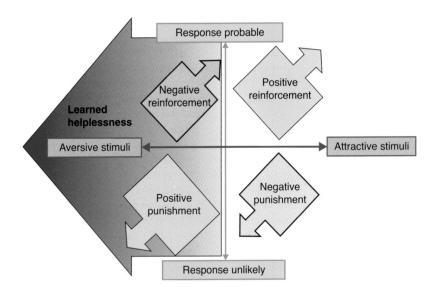

Figure 6.6 The likelihood of a horse in training offering a particular response is a result of the level of aversiveness or attractiveness of the stimulus. Within this structure lie all forms of reinforcement.

Does positive reinforcement equal positive training?

It is appropriate here to reiterate the use of positive and negative in terms of reinforcement and punishment (see Figure 6.6). Remember these terms were coined from their mathematical, as in *add* or *subtract*, rather than ethical associations. Yet, it is commonplace to hear, even from professional trainers and scientists, positive reinforcement referred to as 'positive training', implying that negative reinforcement is 'negative training'.

Prima facie, the distinction between positive and negative reinforcement is simple: one is concerned with attractive stimuli and the other relates to aversive stimuli. However, if we accept that both positive reinforcement and negative reinforcement are goal-directed behaviours concerned with drive reduction, we begin to see that there are elements of aversiveness embedded in positive reinforcement. For example, unless an animal is completely satiated, it is subject to varying degrees of hunger, which is an aversive state. Authors, such as Perone (2003), have rightly questioned whether the rat presses the lever because such behaviour produces food (the behaviour is positively reinforced) or because it reduces hunger (the behaviour is negatively reinforced). Such opposing, yet identical, propositions remind us that

compartmentalising processes assists our understanding of nature on the one hand but, on the other, also narrows our perception. The learning processes of animals are more seamless than our clumsy labels would suggest.

Is there an opposition reflex?

The horse typically moves *away* from an aversive stimulus. So, does it move away from hunger? Yes, in a sense, that is what keeps it moving across the pasture. In some sectors of popularised methodology of horsemanship, it is proposed that horses naturally move *towards* aversive stimuli (Wilson, 2004) and that horses need training to move away from aversive stimuli. The tendency to move towards aversive pressure is sometimes referred to as 'the opposition reflex'. It is totally implausible that horses or any other species would have evolved to move towards aversive stimuli. Under such circumstances, horses would be impaling themselves on all kinds of protruding objects in their environments. It is clearly adaptive to move away from pressure. However, it is feasible that under some conditions horses might be motivated to move towards pressure. For example, when they are moving through undergrowth, it might be adaptive to press on through.

Lindsay (2000) described this feature of dog behaviour, in which huskies naturally pull against the harness restraint around their necks. There may be a similar phenomenon in draught horses as a result of selective breeding. This example relates to pushing with only one part of the body, the chest. We know that there are other anatomical regions where horses are far less likely to push with (e.g. the groin or inguinal region, which is literally thin-skinned and typically sensitive or ticklish). Aside from limited examples, there is no adaptive significance in an opposition reflex. Certainly, it makes little sense for this to occur in the sensitive mouths of horses or on their sides where opposing naturally aversive objects could cause injury.

So, when the opposition reflex is believed to be occurring, what is actually happening? The most plausible explanation is trial-and-error learning (see Figure 6.7). A horse, when faced with a particular challenge will, through operant conditioning, trial various responses until it finds the solution that solves the problem. In the case of aversive pressures provided during training, the reaction that diminishes the aversiveness is not always as obvious to the horse as humans might imagine. For example, the horse's natural reaction to mouth pressure is most likely *not* to slow its legs but to run faster to flee from this source of pain.

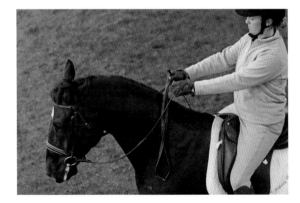

Figure 6.7 Horses learn to stop/slow from the release of pressure through trial and error. This highlights the need for trainers to release at the appropriate moment.

Round-pen as negative reinforcement

Round-pen work, such as has been popularised by the commercial methodology Join-up (Roberts, 2000), has been described as a method based on an element of the social ethogram of the horse in which a dominant member of a group will chase another to become its leader, force its compliance or win its respect. Unfortunately, this aspect of equine social behaviour has not been recorded outside anecdotal accounts and the methodology on which it is supposed to be based is rarely described in correct terms of learning processes. It is, rather, another example of negative reinforcement where the human in the centre of the round-pen pressures the horse to run around the pen but removes the pressure as soon as it slows. The horse's approaches towards the human in the centre of the round-pen are positively reinforced, and the approach behaviour is shaped through progressive improvements. However, if the horse stops approaching, the human punishes it by immediately chasing it away until it actively approaches the human again. Join-up can be established because it effectively utilises learning theory and, in particular, aversive conditioning.

Negative reinforcement in horse-training – In-hand

In-hand, the negative reinforcement process involves training the horse to lead forward, turn, stop and, sometimes, to step back. As far as leading forward is concerned, the aim is to train the horse to step forward from anterior lead pressure. However, horses are stronger than humans and when faced with the two choices of relenting or not to the forward lead pressure by stepping forward, many choose to tolerate and possibly habituate to the poll pressure. Most horsepeople, therefore, prefer to pressure the young horse slightly sideways (approximately 45 degrees) because this way, as the horse relents, it can be moved a fraction forward more easily (see Figure 6.8). When the horse steps forward, the lead-rein pressure is immediately released. This termination of pressure reinforces the embryonic step forward and the horse increasingly offers this response each time

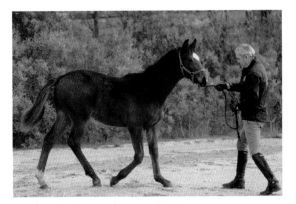

Figure 6.8 Training a naïve horse to lead involves reinforcing a single step slightly sideways of the forelegs. Sideways inhibits a backward resistance that may lead to rearing over backwards.

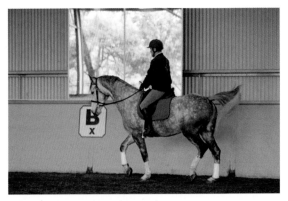

Figure 6.9 Shortening the strides can be trained by variations in the duration and magnitude of rein pressure that become associated with seat characteristics.

the lead forward pressure is presented in a similar context. Typically, the horse offers responses more consistently from anterior pressure and some time later will offer a number of steps and respond to increasingly light signals. As well as training the horse to lead in a straight line, the trainer using negative reinforcement in the form of pressure release may also reinforce faster or longer steps from subtle differences in the duration of anterior lead signals.

The stop and step-back responses are trained using negative reinforcement in the same way, except that pressure is delivered by the posterior facing lead-rein (rein towards the trachea). Here again, the pressure is released as soon as the animal gives the correct response and, again, the signal can be modified to elicit slowing and shortening of the stride responses. Similarly, during lungeing, the trainer negatively reinforces the horse's forward response using the lungeing whip for acceleration and the lunge rein for deceleration.

Negative reinforcement in horse-training – Under-saddle

Under-saddle, notwithstanding minor differences in equestrian pursuits, the following basic mobility alterations predominate: going forward, stopping, going backwards, changing direction with the forelegs or hindlegs and going sideways right or left. These variations in mobility are trained via negative reinforcement in that one or both reins or one or both of the rider's legs elicit the appropriate response through pressure and its release. Again, further developments can take place where the strides can be quickened, slowed, shortened or lengthened through the training of variations in pressures from rein or rider's leg (see Figure 6.9). These alterations typically involve variations in duration or magnitude of pressure. Horse-riders also use rein or leg pressure to effect alterations in head- and neck-carriage as well as body posture (longitudinal and lateral bend) and also to increase engagement.

Whips and spurs are used by many riders under the very same principles of negative reinforcement to effect control where the rider's legs fail to produce a sufficient response. When whips or spurs are used to trigger certain desirable behaviours, their intermittent pressure is maintained or increased until the desirable behaviour emerges (see Table 6.2). Intermittent pressures such as those from whips and spurs have two modes of interaction: their effect is a result of their magnitude and/or the frequency of use, both of which can be varied. The same is true for any intermittent pressure, such as the rider's legs (kick, squeeze, nudge) and the reins (pull, squeeze, vibrate). Similarly, curb bits with lever-action shanks (a first-class lever effect) produce a dramatic increase in pressure in the horse's mouth that depends largely on the length of the curb shank. Such technologies have been used for centuries because they

Table 6.2 Facilitating the learning of locomotory responses: the relationship between applying various aversive stimuli and the negative reinforcement of removing them

Required response	Aversive stimulus	Negative reinforcement
Acceleration and deceleration in-hand	Lead-rein signals	Removal of lead-rein pressures
Acceleration under-saddle	Leg signals	Removal of leg pressure
Acceleration under-saddle	Whip	Removal of whip
Acceleration under-saddle	Spur	Removal of spur
Deceleration under-saddle	Bit: via reins	Removal of mouth pressure

can inflict greater discomfort on the animal compared with standard, comparatively impotent rein and leg pressures. They are effective because they breach well into the pain threshold of practically all horses, regardless of sensitivity, overshadowing all other salient stimuli in the animal's immediate perception. They represent pressures that every horse will want to terminate.

Negative reinforcement in foundation training

The job of the foundation trainer or horse-breaker is to clearly install mobility responses by negative reinforcement so that the stimulus–response (S-R) associations develop to the point where they are elicited by diminutive versions of the relevant pressure signal. The training programs of all ridden animals, such as elephants, camelids and bovids, similarly centre on the use of negative reinforcement. With all these animals, humans have invented tools and techniques to increase the motivation of the animals, via aversive stimuli, to offer specific locomotory responses. For example, while nose rings and nose pegs are used to direct bulls and camels, a hook (called an *ankush*) of variable sharpness is typically used to train elephants in some parts of Asia.

A well-trained young horse may be described as having a perfect temperament, yet so much of the horse's future behaviour depends on the clarity of the early responses learned during foundation training. In fact, every domestic horse has a 'negative reinforcement profile' that is the sum total of all negative reinforcement interventions beginning with the first time a human touched it as a foal. If the foal ran away and, consequently, removed the human hand, this may feature as a fun-

damental lesson. A significant proportion of behavioural dysfunction is a result of incorrect negative reinforcement (McGreevy and McLean, 2005).

When negative reinforcement goes wrong

Negative reinforcement is also the responsible mechanism behind what are known as evasions. The word evasion is a euphemism for habituation and negative reinforcement gone wrong (see Chapter 13, Fight and flight responses and manifestations). Evasions represent the finest examples of horses training humans (see Table 6.3). Head-shy horses manage to stop having their heads touched by learning to throw their heads and remove a person's hand. Girth-shy horses, if they are successful, might manage to buck the saddle and girth off. Clipper-shy horses effectively remove clippers from their vicinity. Leg-shy horses remove human hands from their legs, and needle-shy horses remove vets with sharp needles. Whip-shy horses are effective at removing any hint of whip use and, sometimes, even the rider. Even if a rearing horse is not lucky enough to remove a rider, it generally does manage to render the rider helpless for a moment so that the reins go slack and the rider's legs slide back away from the sensitive site.

Fear associated with an experience results in associations being formed from single experiences and also results in recurring fearful reactions in subsequent similar situations. Horses are capable of one-trial learning (McGreevy, 2004) and discover in just a single attempt that bucking is effective, even if the rider is not removed. Bucking is additionally reinforced by the removal of the rider's control during the unhappy event.

Table 6.3 Learning various unwelcome behaviours: the relationship between various aversive stimuli and the negative reinforcement provided by their removal

Behaviour problem	Aversive stimulus	Negative reinforcement
Head-shy	Hands touching head	Removal of hands
Clipper-shy	Clippers	Removal of clippers
Needle-shy	Injections	Removal of injection
Leg-shy	Hands touching legs	Removal of hands
Bucking	Rider's control	Removal of rider
Shying	Rider's control	Removal of rider's control
Rearing	Rein and leg pressures	Removal of rider's control
Head tossing	Rein pressure	Removal of rein pressure
Refusing obstacle	Effort to clear obstacle	Removal of effort
Jogging	Rider's legs	Removal of rider's legs
Pulling back from tethering	Head restraint	Removal of head pressure

Similarly, during shying, the rider is dislodged and, thus, his or her control is temporarily removed. Because of the context-specific way in which the horse learns, it is likely that an identical reaction will occur at the same site in the near future. When horses swerve at jumping obstacles, the reaction is rapidly acquired because of the reinforcement provided by the escape.

Punishment

Punishment refers to the presentation of a stimulus that suppresses a behaviour (McGreevy *et al.*, 2005). It can be divided into two categories: positive punishment and negative punishment, depending on whether the punitive situation arises because of the addition or omission of an event. Smacking, slapping, whipping, punching and kicking are typical examples of positive punishment. However, the term also embraces even minor amounts of discomfort that suppress any behaviour. Withholding something attractive, such as food, is an example of punishment by omission. Negative punishment is usually not deliberately employed in horse-training, but it does occur inadvertently.

Animals being trained in some new behaviour will first attempt to offer an established response. The absence of reinforcement at that point makes repetition of this now-unwanted response less likely. Reinforcement has been omitted and, therefore, the animal has been negatively punished. However, defining punishment purely in terms of

its suppressive features is superficial. It is easy to imagine that at one time or another in training, regardless of the specific response that the trainer is intentionally rewarding or punishing, some behaviour is being thwarted at any given moment in favour of the one being performed. Labels such as punishment are therefore limiting. Punishment terminates the behaviour that it follows, but the behaviour that actually follows *after* the punisher is unimportant to the definition. However, in negative reinforcement, the contingent behaviour is identified and critical to the definition. Thus, the theoretical distinction between punishment and negative reinforcement becomes tenuous if the behaviour that always follows punishment is the same. For example, if the punishing stimulus results in the same behaviour each time, one could argue that negative reinforcement is taking place. Take the example of trailer loading. In some countries, horsepeople have been known to use a long whip or stock-whip on the animal's hindquarters when it refuses to go any farther. However, each time the whip is used, the horse runs backwards faster, the opposite effect to what was intended. What began as a futile exercise in punishment has now turned into a (more futile) process of negative reinforcement, where the use of the whip has trained the horse to run backwards. Unfortunately, the amount of violence characterised by punishment is often out of all proportion to the behaviour that it is intended to change.

Punishment is associated with certain emotional states, such as fear and frustration (Lindsay, 2000). Fear and anxiety can be adaptive in that they raise vigilance and promote attempts to regain control of aversive situations. Frustration enhances attempts at restoring instrumental control over available reinforcers. Kandel (2006) has pointed out something that Freud also reported: that while certain amounts of fear and frustration may actually enhance learning, high levels tend to depress it and may contribute to pathological emotional states, such as learned helplessness. Haag *et al.* (1980) found that punishment lowers a horse's tendency to trial novel responses to solve a problem. Mills (1998) summarised an array of problems associated with punishment, specifically, that punishment (see Figure 6.10):

1. is non-directive, suppressing but not enhancing alternative behaviours;

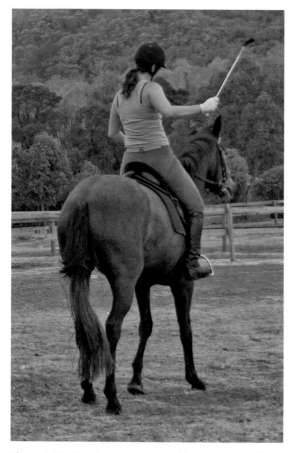

Figure 6.10 Punishment is replete with associated problems that range from a disinclination to trial new learned responses to the development of fearful associations with humans.

2. has the potential to desensitise an animal to the punishing stimulus if the punishment intensity is not optimal;
3. carries the risk of deleterious emotional changes that can interfere with attention and learning; and
4. may be associated by the animal with the person delivering it.

He concluded that punishment is best avoided as it presents a range of problems that amount to abuse. That said, it should be remembered that horse management frequently relies upon punishment. Consider an electric fence, for example. The electric fence is not only a positive punisher but also a highly aversive punisher; it may register as such a serious punitive event that an animal will scarcely venture to touch it a second time. As a punishing stimulus, an electric fence at least offers some controllability in the sense that the horse can actively choose to move away and release itself from the aversive stimulus. Compare this with an electric shock collar, where the controls are in human hands. Here, the animal has diminished control and is at the mercy of the skill and mood of the human. For this reason, many countries have outlawed the use of electric shock collars.

Punishment is commonly used when a horse bites or kicks a human, lunges towards a human or threatens to do so. McLean (2005b) has shown that biting and kicking correlate with specific dysfunctions of the go and stop signals in-hand and under-saddle; therefore, it follows that punishing the horse for biting and kicking may be inappropriate, compared with the therapy offered by re-training of the dysfunctional signals. Furthermore, punishment may not prevent future biting and kicking because it does not address the cause. This important caution must apply to all situations where punishment occurs. Punishment, therefore, may provide the wrong answer to a problem and may be too simplistic as a solution.

Non-contingent punishment

When horses behave dangerously, such as bucking, rearing, shying or bolting, trainers often feel justified in attempting punishment. Sometimes this may be effective, although it is difficult to conceive any practical way to punish bolting. There are two common issues in the use of punishment. Both relate to the belief, in some circles, that the horse's behaviour was deliberate and that he is aware of his misdemeanours. The first problem is the potential for excessive physical punishment (to 'teach him a lesson'), which has no place in a modern training program, and the second is the use of non-contingent punishment. For punishment to be effective it must be contingent – it must literally be connected to the offending behaviour. For example, when punishing a horse for kicking, the punishment must occur while the horse is kicking or at the precise moment the kick ends. The use of non-contingent punishment is confusing and frustrating for the animals concerned and, as it does with dogs (Lindsay, 2000), will most certainly have deleterious consequences. Because of such problems, punishment is best avoided.

When a jumping horse refuses an obstacle, it is not uncommon for trainers to use the whip as the horse stands motionless in front of the obstacle after its refusal. Punishment at that point is non-contingent and, therefore, devoid of any useful training effect. In some cases, the refusing horse is punished and then turned away for another presentation. When horses do attempt an obstacle after a random act of punishment, it is likely that increased anxiety levels make the horse run and, if the obstacle is in its path, it may well jump over it. At best, this is a haphazard training exercise, destined to have low, if any, efficiency. At worst, it simply trains the horse to default to a flight response in the presence of jumps.

Non-contingent punishment is ineffective. For example, a show-jumping horse that is pulling rails cannot be reformed by punishing it after it lands. In contrast, the importance of contingency has prompted some jumping trainers to resort to another technique: rapping. Rapping is an illegal practice (outlawed by the Fédération Equestre Internationale, FEI, Rules) that involves an assistant hitting a horse's forelegs as he clears a jumping obstacle. When this is done repeatedly, there is a temporary alteration in the horse's perception of the jumping effort required for a given height, so the horse makes a short-term increase in jumping effort. Because of the damaging effects of incorrect use, punishment should be used *only* when other avenues have been exhausted. In ad-

dition, it is best used in conjunction with an antecedent secondary punisher (such as the word 'No!') so that the primary punisher itself can be eliminated at some stage. The need for caution with regard to punishment underscores the importance of teaching horse-riding coaches the fundamentals of learning theory.

Experimental neurosis

Gaining control over aversive stimuli (e.g. escape or avoidance) is vitally important to animals. When escape is thwarted, control is lost, the animal's wellbeing is threatened and experimental neurosis may develop. Hence, extra care must be taken when using aversive stimuli to train animals because animals find it imperative to achieve control over such stimuli. Solomon (1964) showed that maladaptive behaviour arises when an aversive stimulus embodies these four conditions:

1. there are sustained raised levels of arousal;
2. the aversive stimulus is unpredictable;
3. the aversive stimulus is uncontrollable;
4. the aversive stimulus is inescapable.

Numerous studies attest to the problems that emerge when these conditions arise. Pavlov's (1941) experiments with dogs provided one of the earliest accounts of experimental neurosis, based on discrimination training (see Chapter 5, Learning II: Associative (attractive)). In one experiment, he rewarded dogs for associating a leg movement with a circular patch of light, but punished them with an electric shock when they responded to an elliptical one. When the dogs had learned these associations, he began some alterations to the experiment: the elliptical patch was made more circular. At some point, the dogs were unable to distinguish between a rewarded shape and a punished one. Some of the dogs became very aggressive while others tried to escape or gave up responding and fell asleep. Masserman (1950) performed a similar experiment on cats (see Figure 6.11). He trained cats to open a box for a food reward when signalled by a light. Later, when the cats opened the food box they sometimes received a blast of air. Again, some of the cats became excitable and hyper-reactive, while others became

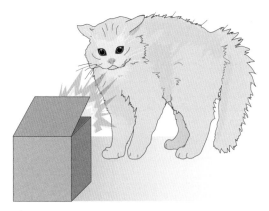

Figure 6.11 Masserman induced experimental neurosis in cats by punishing them with a blast of air after they had learned to open a box for a food reward.

dull and refused to move. These responses are examples of experimental neuroses.

Because of their reliance on stimuli based on aversiveness, horse-trainers should be very careful to ensure that the cues and pressures they use result in consistent, and preferably improved, learned responses. The prevalence of hyper-reactivity and dullness among trained horses suggests that at least some training methodologies pay scant regard to maintaining consistent operant contingencies throughout the horse's life. For example, in some dressage training systems, self-carriage (which implies the absence of aversive pressure) is seen as a phenomenon that may take years to develop. This suggests that the importance of the reinforcement component of negative reinforcement is either not understood or is ignored.

Learned helplessness

When animals are repeatedly exposed to pain as a result of sustained highly aversive stimuli, conditions such as experimental neurosis may escalate so that the animal loses all active control. When the highly aversive stimulus is totally inescapable, learned helplessness may set in. The important distinction here is that the animal no longer tries to cope – it simply gives up and becomes dull.

Learned helplessness was first identified by Seligman and Maier (1967; Maier *et al.*, 1969) as a result of their experiments with dogs (see Figure 6.12). After repeated exposure to inescapable aversive stimuli, these animals showed a deterioration of cognitive, emotional and motivational attributes. During the experiments, some dogs were trained to switch off an electric shock, administered to their feet, by moving their head sideways to contact a switch. Other dogs were similarly shocked but were unable to switch the electricity off. The next day, these two groups of dogs plus another unexposed group were subjected to electric shocks in a shuttle box apparatus, where the dogs could terminate the shocks by jumping a small hurdle. All dogs rapidly learned to jump the hurdle, except some of the group that were unable to avoid the shock during the experiment the previous day. Those dogs were helpless and instead of trialling a response to avoid the shocks, they showed intense hyper-reactivity and then became passive. More recently, Weinraub and Schulman (1980) proposed that it was the uncontrollability of the experience rather than the experience of shock itself that interfered with subsequent avoidance learning. It was noted that with sufficient exposures, diminished aggression and loss of appetite occurred and apathy persisted in these dogs long after the experiment.

Investigating the effects of previous exposure and controllable shock with rats, Seligman (1975) showed that past experience in dealing with escapable shock *immunised* subjects from the effects of learned helplessness when exposed to inescapable shock later on. On the other hand, naïve rats that had never been exposed to escapable shock became helpless after exposure to inescapable shock. Furthermore, Hannum *et al.* (1976) showed that rats that had previous experience in escaping shock early in their lives performed better in escape-learning tasks than did non-shocked controls. In dogs, it has been shown that individuals repeatedly exposed to excessive punishment, where they have learned to tolerate pain but not to benefit from it, gradually become unmoved by increasing pain (Lindsay, 2000). Previous exposure to correct pressure/release can partially immunise horses against subsequent bad riding, but bad foundation training can leave a lifetime legacy.

The symptoms of learned helplessness in rats and dogs that have been noted include anhedonia,

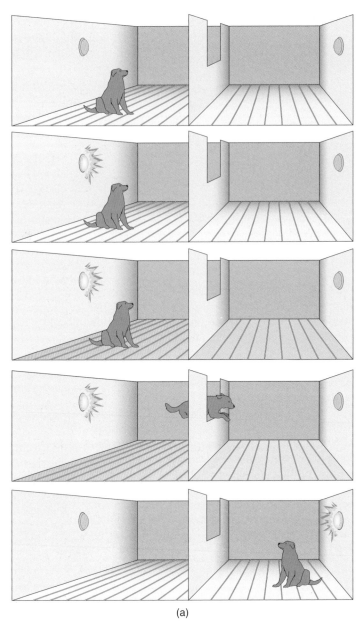

(a)

Figure 6.12   Seligman's dogs became apathetic when the warning light inconsistently predicted pain (See illustrations a and b) and avoidance became impossible.

depression and motivational, emotional and cognitive deficits (Seligman *et al.*, 1980; Pratt, 1980). Worse still, in the experiments carried out by Weiss *et al.* (1975) as well as Seligman and Maier (1967), several rats and dogs died as a direct result of the experimental treatments. These events confirm

the importance to animals of predictability and controllability, particularly when they are dealing with aversive stimuli. It is not surprising that learned helplessness has been used as an animal model of human depression and post-traumatic stress disorder (Hall *et al.*, 2007). The neural

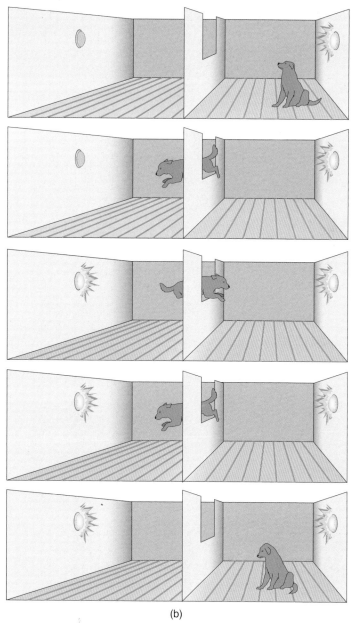

(b)

Figure 6.12   (Continued)

tissues responsible for generating experimental neurosis and learned helplessness are similar to human equivalents linked to depression (Cabib, 2006); their mechanisms seem to share a profound inhibition of dopamine release in the nucleus accumbens.

Learned helplessness in horses remains unresearched and subject to considerable speculation. However, many researchers have identified the possibility that learned helplessness in horses can be found (Ödberg, 1987; Lieberman, 1993; Ödberg and Bouissou, 1999). In a review of learned

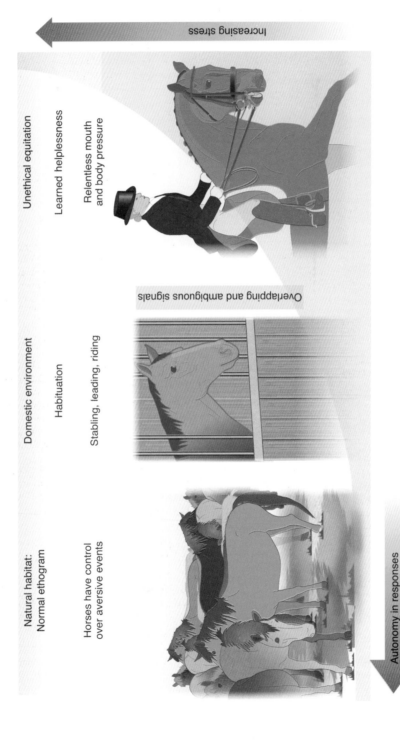

Figure 6.13 From the domestic horse's viewpoint, increasing amounts of losses of control followed by inescapable pain arising from poor equitation can lead to learned helplessness. This amounts to a major loss of predictability and controllability.

helplessness, Hall *et al.* (2007) indicated that some behavioural responses exhibited by the domestic horse are probably examples of learned helplessness. McLean and McGreevy (2004) pointed out that although many horsepeople assume that the loss of sensitivity in horses with 'hard mouths' and 'dead sides' is the result of accumulated scar tissue, it is more likely to reflect learned dullness. Just where this dullness emerges on the continuum that terminates in learned helplessness is not clear. However, the practice of using contradictory acceleration (leg/whip) and deceleration signals (bit via reins) simultaneously and indeed delivering these signals via amplifiers such as the (lever-action) curb-bit and rowelled spurs make the horse a likely candidate for learned helplessness (see Figure 6.13). Learned helplessness would show up only after the failure of active coping mechanisms, such as bucking and hyper-reactivity. Established learned helplessness may compromise horse welfare since an animal in this state has suffered a critical loss of control of its environment (Webster, 1994).

Conclusion

No matter how subtle it is, horse-training is largely based on the use of negative reinforcement. First principles in horse-training, therefore, are that pressure motivates the horse to respond, and its removal trains the response. Horses learn to stop, go and turn because these responses bring about the release of pressure associated with the rein or rider's leg, both in-hand and under-saddle. The anticipatory processes of classical conditioning result in the horse learning to respond to very light pressure or other cues.

Because the stimuli used in horse-training are based on aversiveness and because many disciplines of equitation may involve the use of severe bits and sometimes spurs, extra care should be taken to ensure that the cues and pressures are as light as possible. It is also a matter of importance for welfare that their use results in consistent learned responses and that these operant contingencies remain consistent over the animal's lifetime.

Take-home messages

- Avoidance learning and negative reinforcement are allied processes.
- Many human–horse interactions may begin with positive reinforcement, but negative reinforcement forms the foundations of control.
- First principles in horse-training are that the pressure motivates the horse to respond, and its removal trains the response. It is the removal of pressure that initially trains the responses required in equitation. The anticipatory processes of classical conditioning result in the horse learning to respond to very light versions of the motivating pressure or other cues.
- Fear and aversiveness are interconnected. It is imperative that fear responses be avoided at all costs because of their rapid acquisition and their resistance to erasure. It is also important to prevent fearful reactions recurring in subsequent similar contexts, so trainers must be very cautious about invoking fear responses during training.
- A significant proportion of behavioural dysfunction in the ridden horse is a result of incorrect negative reinforcement.
- The word evasion is a euphemism for habituation and negative reinforcement gone wrong.

Areas for future research

- Learned helplessness in horses.
- Longevity of pressure-based signals.

7 Applying Learning Theory

Introduction

Successful equitation relies upon non-associative and associative learning processes in the horse. What sets horse-riding apart from most other forms of animal-training is that the balance and position of the rider exert effects ranging from unobtrusive to a detraining outcome. For example, a well-balanced rider allows the horse to move unimpeded by the rider, whereas a poorly balanced rider may cause the horse to slow, quicken or drift sideways. For this reason, training in rider position has been the chief focus of equestrian coaching for centuries. Furthermore, because horsepeople were unaware of learning theory, they focussed heavily on the one objective and measurable facet of horsemanship: rider position. So, one might wonder how horses were trained without knowledge of learning processes, and the answer is most likely an heuristic explanation: that successful riders learned by trial and error themselves or by some kind of vicarious process from those skilled riders that were hailed as great horsemen or great masters. Thus, until now the application of learning theory to horse-training has been based on good fortune and shrouded in mystery, its only manifestation being in the effects of copying those that were more effective than others and cloaked in the dictums of rider-position teachings.

This chapter is dedicated to identifying how learning theory is correctly applied to training the ridden horse. It unapologetically describes the acquisition of trained responses in the horse aside from the effects of rider position. Other elements of equitation, including rider position and balance, are described in Chapter 8 (Training). Importantly, the process of correctly applying learning theory can be understood systematically by means of a set of principles that predict the success or failure of training, as well as its optimal efficiency. These are:

1. Train easy-to-discriminate signals.
2. Reduce negative reinforcement pressure (reins and legs) to very light versions of pressure (light signals).
3. Shape the components of responses progressively.
4. Train and subsequently elicit responses singularly.
5. Train only one response per signal.
6. Train all responses to be initiated and subsequently completed within a consistent composition and time-frame.
7. Train persistence of elicited responses.
8. Avoid and dissociate flight responses.

If trainers across all disciplines of equitation adopt the principles described in this chapter, some pressures, yet respond to others. For example, the horse has to habituate to low-pressure levels of rein, leg and seat contact, particularly in the sport of dressage. These low neutral pressures are known as *contact* (McGreevy *et al.*, 2005). When the variety of gaits is considered in relation to their effect on a rider, random variations in rider contact confound the horse's ability to discriminate between contact pressures and signal pressures.

Numerous signals from the rider are used to elicit the responses of go, stop, turn and sideways and their subsets of quickening or slowing the steps, lengthening and shortening the steps and changing the gait (walk, trot, canter and gallop). In the competition dressage horse, the number of responses is further increased when other movements and postures such as rein-back, lateral bend, lateral flexion are taken into account, altering the head and neck posture, collection, straightening the horse, lowering the hindquarters, as well as the movements of turn on the forehand (walk), pirouette (walk and canter), shoulder-in (trot), travers (trot), half-pass (trot and canter), piaffe and passage.

Despite the large number of responses, the limitations of the rider's interaction with the horse's body mean that there are insufficient sites on the horse's body in which to condition these responses. If a site is used to elicit several different responses, confusion can set in. For example, it is not uncommon for a rider's legs to stimulate

horses from sites on the horse's thorax not only to quicken, lengthen the strides, go sideways and canter but also to turn (instead of using the reins, for example). When it is considered that the normal scope of sites that the rider's leg stimulates is within the range of 10 cm to perhaps 20 cm, it makes the accurate discrimination of these four responses a difficult task, and the precise delivery of signals a great challenge for riders.

Similarly, across the range of equestrian disciplines, the bit in the horse's mouth is frequently used to elicit responses of slowing, shortening the strides, turning the forequarters or hindquarters, head raising, head lowering, neck shortening, straightening crooked necks and correcting tilting noses. The horse's back shows kinematics that are specific to each of the three gaits and these movements make the task of maintaining an even rein contact difficult in sports, such as dressage, that demand these criteria. Thus, the discrimination challenge for the horse is further complicated. Unsurprisingly, rider position and balance are typically the chief focus of equestrian coaching.

It should be mentioned, however, that some signals are less distinctive than others. Consider the seat, for example. The norm in most equestrian sports is to use saddles to disperse the weight of the rider and under-saddle padding (e.g. numnahs) to diffuse the saddle pressure so as to avoid back soreness in the horse (see Figure 7.13). The

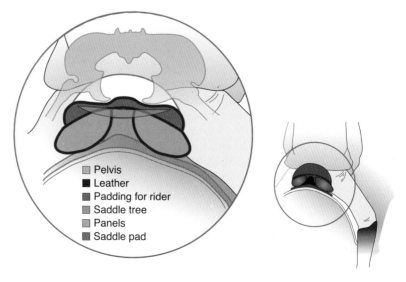
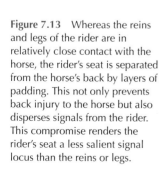

Figure 7.13   Whereas the reins and legs of the rider are in relatively close contact with the horse, the rider's seat is separated from the horse's back by layers of padding. This not only prevents back injury to the horse but also disperses signals from the rider. This compromise renders the rider's seat a less salient signal locus than the reins or legs.

☐ Pelvis
■ Leather
■ Padding for rider
☐ Saddle tree
☐ Panels
■ Saddle pad

saddle itself is padded or sometimes nowadays filled with air. The effect of this, however, is to dilute to some extent the signals of the seat. Another problem with the seat lies in its complex three-dimensional oscillations throughout the three gaits. Unpublished data (Clayton, personal communication, 2007) on using saddle pressure sensors suggest that seat signals for the same response (such as slowing) differ in all three gaits. So, even in best practice equitation, other signals, such as rein and leg signals, are likely to be more easily discriminated by the horse. Riders seeking to use subtle signals can shrink the rein and leg signals more easily than seat signals. This is probably the reason many riders believe that for downward transitions they do not use their reins at all but instead use their seat (yet, at the same time, they recognise that they are unable to relinquish rein contact). Perhaps the clearest use of the rider's seat insofar as the horse's discrimination is concerned is in its effect of maintaining the particular gait, speed and rhythm through its 'sweeping' and bouncing effect.

A solution to the disparity between responses and signal loci can be found in the various ways the signals can be combined from the following:

- the rider's legs can exert unilateral or bilateral pressure;
- the rider's legs can exert pressure from the upper leg (knee) calf and lower leg;
- the reins can exert pressure on the mouth unilaterally or bilaterally;
- the reins can be raised, lowered, opened away from the horse's neck or closed toward the neck;
- the reins can also exert lateral pressure on the horse's neck (neck-reining);
- the rider's legs can exert pressure that varies in duration (brief or more prolonged signals);
- the reins can exert pressure that varies in duration (brief or more prolonged signals);
- the rider's seat can express variations in site, lateral distribution, speed and range of motion;
- spurs used as a light signal can be precise in terms of site;
- verbal cues are sometimes used in equitation, although the use of the voice is forbidden in the sport of dressage (FEI, 2008).

These permutations emphasise the dual importance of rider position and training know-how in effectively achieving consistent responses in the horse.

Reducing negative reinforcement pressure (reins and legs) to very light versions of pressure (light signals)

Negative reinforcement (also known as pressure/release) is the most effective way to train reliable behaviours in the horse. When negative reinforcement is applied with a light antecedent discriminative stimulus (light pressure), the horse will increasingly offer the particular response from those light predictive signals. Therefore, the astute trainer will recognise the horse's anticipatory behaviour and the need for stronger motivating pressures will be obviated: signals will therefore reduce to light and subtle cues. Best practice training methodologies emphasise the importance of training the horse to respond to light signals.

When the horse responds from these lighter versions of pressure (after obedience level), positive reinforcement and secondary positive reinforcement should be incorporated to maintain responses and to help develop horse–human rapport. As mentioned earlier, positive reinforcement may be used concurrently with negative reinforcement, it makes sense to utilise positive reinforcement when negative reinforcement has reduced to light versions to avoid signal competition.

For efficient learning, the light antecedent signal should be contiguous with the reinforcement (release of pressure). If the light signal occurs too far away in time from the release, it may not be acquired as an eliciting signal. Therefore, optimally, the entire pressure/release scenario should be of no more than 3 seconds duration so that the horse is able to learn the light cue effectively.

Shape the components of responses progressively

The final desired responses required of horses in all disciplines are complex and each response, such as go, stop and turn, requires the trainer to recognise the earliest attempts by the horse to offer the correct response and then gradually shape them towards the goal response. Each stage should be consolidated to some extent before moving on the next piece to be shaped. Trainers should, therefore, not expect perfect responses to emerge from the onset of training but should gradually shape the horse's responses by careful successive approximations towards the training goal. Each stage of shaping should consist of a precise response that is *identifiable* for both horse and trainer in order to be repeated and reach consolidation (McLean and McLean, 2008). During the training of locomotion, developing steps, then strides, then the gait itself fulfils this requirement. A universal shaping scale is essential for acceptable modern horse-training in every discipline.

Train and subsequently elicit responses singularly

In training, the rider's legs and reins acquire learned associations with retraction, protraction, abduction and adduction of the horse's limbs in the stance or swing phase of the various gaits. These associations will be gradually extinguished if signals elicit responses that are impossible to fulfil because the horse's legs are in positions that make responding difficult (see Figure 7.14).

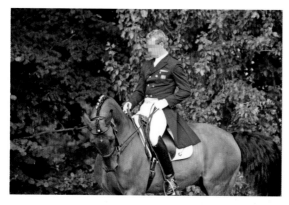

Figure 7.14   When both reins and leg signals are applied simultaneously, confusion sets in. Deterioration of one or both responses can also occur by overshadowing, which results in significant losses of responding to the reins or legs for stop or go. (Photo courtesy of EponaTV)

Even more impossible is when the reins and the rider's legs attempt to stimulate responses simultaneously, as seen in some contemporary training methodologies as a way of producing what is known as engagement. The horse cannot simultaneously retract and protract the same limbs and so is placed in a confused state. The horse's reactions depend on his genetic predispositions as well as the duration and intensity of the opposing signals. Such confusion may lead to:

- lowered responding to the individual signals;
- acute stress resulting in raised muscular tonus and fearful behaviours;
- conflict behaviours such as bucking, bolting, shying and rearing;
- chronic stress resulting in physiological and immunological deterioration;
- learned helplessness where the horse tolerates pain with severe welfare compromises;
- wastage where the horse is removed from the population (i.e. sent to the abattoir).

Pavlov (1927) described the situation that arises when two stimuli compete for salience. He defined the effects of this competition as resulting in 'overshadowing', where the more salient stimulus would outcompete the other. In the ridden horse, analogues of the overshadowing phenomenon manifest as habituation-like phenomena, where the horse may learn not to attend to the pressures of the bit (heaviness) and the rider's legs when simultaneously used during training (McLean, 2008). Anthropomorphically, the consequent dullness to the pressures may be interpreted as loss of 'willingness to please', laziness or, when conflict behaviours arise, sourness, resistance and evasion. For our purposes in this text, we use the term overshadowing to describe this parallel phenomenon, where one signal outcompetes another less salient stimulus.

It is now common for this important principle to be disregarded even at the highest levels of contemporary training practice; for example, the German National Equestrian Federation (1997) proposes that 'rein aids should only be given in conjunction with leg and weight aids'. Yet, Decarpentry (1949), one of the great masters of French equitation, maintained the importance of separating rein and leg cues with the famous French maxim *'hands without legs, legs without hands'*. This should be re-embraced as an important ideal that allows optimal learning and eliminates the potential for confusion for all equitation disciplines. Signals must be elicited singly and any set of signals should still be separated and elicited consecutively (Decarpentry, 1949).

The process of overshadowing results in one signal achieving salience while the other becomes habituated (McLean, 2008). This learning phenomenon is interesting because, while it appears that the horse is simply distracted momentarily from the weaker signal, the effects of overshadowing can be long lasting. So, while overshadowing one signal with another is detrimental to equitation, the process can be used to desensitise unwanted behaviours such as fearful behaviours to clippers, shoeing, worming, needles, girthing-up and head-shyness (McLean, 2008; see Figure 7.15). In these circumstances, overshadowing results from strengthening the effect of an in-hand locomotory signal in the face of the lowest threshold of the fearful behaviours. This protocol has direct analogues in the treatment of traumatic behaviours in humans in modalities known as power therapies (McLean, 2008).

Train only one consistent response per signal

A horse cannot be expected to know the intentions of its rider. It makes sense to recognise that confusion can also occur when a single signal has more than one response associated with it. For example, in equitation the stimulus of the single rein is the fundamental signal for the turn response. When riders attempt to bend the horse's neck laterally using the single rein, the horse can easily become confused between the dual response of either turning (changing direction) or lateral flexing of the neck: two responses from one signal. A similar confusion may result when both reins are used for altering the horse's head-carriage, because use of both reins together has an earlier fundamental association with slowing. McLean (2003) suggested that such confusions account for a significant number of conflict behaviours in the

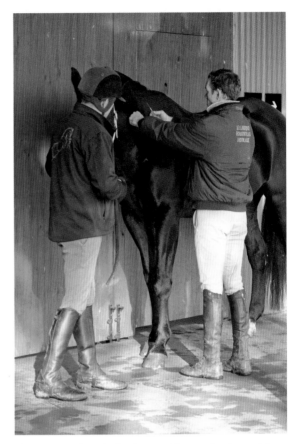

Figure 7.15   Overshadowing provides an effective tool for desensitising horses to needles, clippers and equestrian paraphernalia.

ridden horse and ipso facto add to behavioural wastage statistics.

Effective habit formation requires that a particular response must be elicited repeatedly. Discrete locomotory characteristics, such as the steps or strides of the horse, provide clear single units of responses that have an obvious beginning and end-point. Thus, it is useful for horse-trainers to be aware of the biomechanical characteristics of the horse's locomotion during acceleration, deceleration and turning. For example, when training basic (direct) turn responses, the most appropriate time to apply the signal for a right turn is when the right foreleg is beginning its swing phase (see Figure 7.16). If riders focus on this moment to elicit a response, the horse's acquisition rate is optimal. Many riders learn

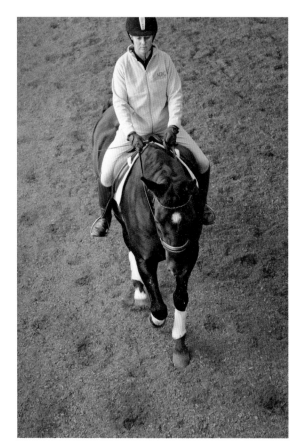

Figure 7.16 The rider should begin to signal the turn with the direct rein when the foreleg (on the side to which the horse is to turn) is leaving the ground.

At the same moment, the opposite forelimb in the stance phase propels the horse to that direction to a greater or lesser extent, depending on the signal strength. Trainers, therefore, need to be precise in eliciting and reinforcing the correct abduction response: signalling with the rein at the beginning of the swing phase of the limb. It follows that there are moments when such a turn is impossible: that is when the limb to be abducted is actually in the stance phase.

On the other hand, turns of the hindquarters (which lead to leg-yield and side-pass) should begin with an adduction, where one hindleg first crosses over the other (see Figure 7.17). For the same reasons as above, efficient training requires that the adduction response should be elicited at precisely the moment when the limb is about to begin the swing phase.

to feel these optimal moments with their seat, and this timing should be an important part of equestrian coaching. Similarly, the best time to decelerate is at the beginning of the swing phase of one of the forelimbs.

Turns of the forelimbs require even more astuteness on the part of the rider when it comes to eliciting an exact copy of a single response in early training. For example, a horse may turn its forelimbs by first either abducting the limbs or adducting the limbs. In dressage, the turn of the forelimbs requires abduction as the first reaction, but in any sport, training is expedited by reinforcing the same response each time. If the use of the rein is taken as the signal that elicits the turn of the forelimbs, then the rein should elicit an abduction of the same-side limb in the swing phase in which the limb moves to some extent laterally.

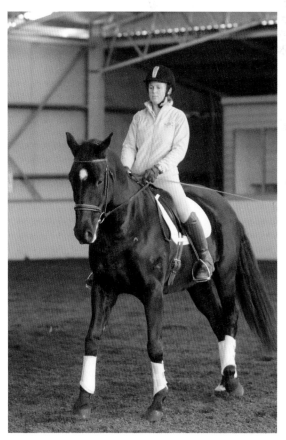

Figure 7.17 The rider should begin to signal the leg-yield with the leg signal when the hindleg (on the opposite side to which the horse is to yield) is leaving the ground.

Train all responses to be initiated and subsequently completed within a consistent composition and time-frame

It is recognised among horsepeople that the horse should initiate a response to the rider's signals immediately. This does not necessarily mean that the response should be completed immediately, but simply requires that the horse begins responding without delay. Because any learned response has definable features in terms of action and duration, it follows that transitions should be completed within consistent time-frames. In different horse sports, the structure of these transitions from one locomotory state to another may differ according to the requirements of the particular sport. In sports such as reining, because of its origins in cattle mustering, certain transitions must be so abrupt that the horse's legs immediately complete their response to the rider's cue (e.g. the horse may skid to a sliding stop). Turns must also be powerful and fast. These rapid transitions also characterise polo, polocrosse, racing, bull-fighting and, to some extent, show-jumping and cross-country jumping. In these sports, the transitions have a discrete structure with little room for confusion from that viewpoint.

On the other hand, in dressage and allied sports, transitions are not required to be completed abruptly, but instead should flow through a definable number of steps or time-frames. This is probably a result of its Middle Ages origin, where the weight of armour meant that any sudden accelerations, decelerations or turns could dislodge the rider. In addition, the combined weights of man and armour (on both horse and rider) placed extra weight on the horse's forehand, which already naturally carried around 15% more weight than the hindquarters, resulting in losses of power to the hindquarters. To counter this power loss, collection was developed where the hindquarters were trained to be carried lower, the hindfeet trained to be a little closer to the forefeet and transitions needed to flow in a rhythm to allow the hindquarters to continue to carry the weight as much as possible to facilitate maximum forward thrust.

Anecdotal observation of horses that are successful at the highest level of dressage suggests that transitions are completed within a stride or two and within about 2 to 3 seconds. Yet contemporary dressage texts do not define the time-frame or step/stride sequence surrounding transitions except to say that transitions should be within the rhythm of the strides (Decarpentry, 1949; Herbermann, 1980; German National Equestrian Federation, 1997). The absence of any clear prescription for transitions is an obstacle to the transmission of knowledge and inconsistency in reinforcing responses is likely to present as a source of confusion in the horse. This also hinders the process of habit formation, which is a relatively protracted process of neural maturation to the point of consolidation. Forming consistent habits imposes a strong obligation to train responses, including transitions, that are consistent in form and duration.

Given the characteristics of equine biomechanics and cognition, there are good grounds to suggest that the transitions can be consistently trained so that they become entities with definable aspects of locomotion and/or duration. For example, once the horse has learned a basically correct response to the rider's legs and reins, the alternating swing phases of both of the horse's forelegs (in the walk and the trot) can provide a definable framework to contain the three elements of the operant contingency: the discriminative stimulus (signal), the operant response and the reinforcer (release) (McGreevy and McLean, 2007; McLean and McLean, 2008). For example, during the development of acceleration, deceleration, abduction or adduction responses, the operant contingency can be exploited to align with the horse's forelegs. For the purposes of example, let us assume that the left foreleg is the first to swing:

1. the light signal is applied to coincide with the start of the swing phase of the left foreleg;
2. the period of increasing pressure to motivate the response coincides with the swing phase of the right foreleg; and
3. the immediate removal of the pressure coincides with the start of the swing phase of the left foreleg.

When the horse has learned to perform the transitions within three beats, the middle period of increasing pressure is no longer required and the

relaxation (Hölzel *et al.*, 1995). When the horse is trained to maintain its own tempo and rhythm, is straight (consistent footfalls) and its head and neck posture is consistent, it becomes calm and exhibits the quality known as 'looseness' (Hölzel *et al.*, 1995). Its locomotory behaviour is now under optimal stimulus control. Consistency of signals and responses confers the greatest level of predictability.

In-hand training

Habituation and familiarisation

Most domestic horses become familiar with humans early in their lives and may learn not to fear humans if they observe their mother being handled from time to time (Hausberger *et al.*, 2007b). With the foal at liberty, this process of gradual habituation is an important stage in early training and facilitates later foundation training. Furthermore, Ladewig *et al.* (2005) suggest that the more similar a horse's foalhood is to its adult life (including handling and management procedures), the easier the transition will be for it to its adult domestic situation. Young horses living in social groups rather than in isolation are likely to be easier to handle (Søndergaard and Ladewig, 2004). Foals often initiate contact early provided that they do not perceive humans as chasing them and,

more subtly, provided that humans do not negatively reinforce a flight response. Given that horses are adept at learning via negative reinforcement, the latter scenario is not uncommon. For example, handlers should be very mindful that when they lay hands on the naïve foal, if the foal should run or buck so that the human's hands are removed, the very first lessons in escape learning via negative reinforcement are embedded. The best scenario is, therefore, to touch the foal and remove the hands when the foal is immobile and relaxed and in this way the first lessons about human contact are *not* to remove it.

Approach

Making physical contact with horses of any age for the first time may be facilitated by knowledge of learning theory. Contemporary approaches such as the advance–retreat method (Wright, 1973) are based on the subtle use of negative reinforcement. Indeed, both successful and unsuccessful advance–retreat owe their results to negative reinforcement. For example, when used optimally, this method involves the handler advancing towards the wary horse but stopping as soon as the handler detects that the horse is about to escape, at which moment the handler takes a step back (see Figure 8.1). The handler then takes a couple of

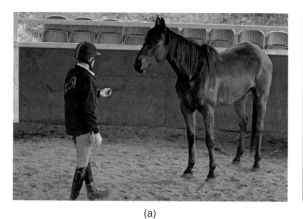
(a)

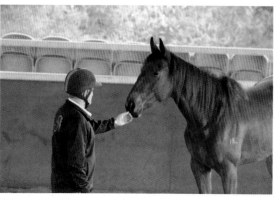
(b)

Figure 8.1   The advance–retreat method of catching horses is one of the most subtle examples of negative reinforcement. As the handler approaches the wary horse (a), the handler ensures that he or she retreats a step before the horse does. The handler can then take two or more steps towards the horse before having to retreat a step and, thus, he or she gradually closes in on the horse (b). The retreating (removal) of the handler negatively reinforces the horse's immobility.

steps towards the horse and again stops and steps back *before* the horse does. In this scenario, the handler gradually reduces the flight distance by negatively reinforcing the horse's immobility. If, however, the horse steps back and the handler also steps back, the horse's retreat is now negatively reinforced and the horse learns the wrong response – to step back on the approach of the human. This shows just how subtle negative reinforcement can be. For the horse's cognition, however, the process is abundantly clear.

Initial contact

Most horsepeople begin training foals at weaning time, and this is often the time that many foals make contact, habituate to a halter and train to lead for the first time (Hausberger *et al.*, 2007b). Typically, the mare with its foal at foot is led into an enclosure or stable. Successful first contact with the foal can occur through the gradual approach of the foal or using advance–retreat. Experienced trainers generally recognise that if the foal runs and the handler advances towards it or, worse still, rushes at it, damage is done to the foal–human relationship. In effect, the handler has negatively reinforced the foal's fear and it may take disproportionately longer to repair because fear responses are acquired so rapidly. Some trainers first touch a foal, young or naïve horse in a smaller enclosure, using a long pole, whip or broom, removing it as soon as the young horse is still. Then, the handler gradually moves closer, repeating the same touch–remove sequence until the handler is able to lay hands on the horse. Caressing the young horse at the base of the withers expedites relaxation and habituation to the handler.

Leading and control

To lead a horse, a lead-rope is generally attached to a head-collar, or reins attached to the bridle are used. Optimally, all equipment commonly used to lead the horse should be associated with thorough habituation. Training across all methodologies in-hand involves placing locomotory movements in all directions under stimulus control (see Chapter 7, Applying learning theory). Therefore, the horse is trained to go forward (including upward inter-gait and intra-gait transitions), to reverse, stop and slow (including downward inter-gait and intra-gait transitions) and to change directions with the forelegs or hindlegs.

Shaping

The optimal use of learning theory prescribes that these in-hand responses are progressively shaped. The beginning of training entails motivating the horse to go and stop and step back and rewarding any attempt in the correct direction. This is achieved through negatively reinforcing these transitions (increasing the pressure and then releasing) as soon as the horse responds. When the horse responds to light signals, the next step is to reinforce an increasing number of strides. A stride is defined as a complete cycle of the repetitive series of limb movements that characterise a particular gait (e.g. all four legs at walk; Back and Clayton, 2001). In all training, pressures should begin with the lightest versions, so that these act as discriminative stimuli and eventually elicit the transitions.

Further shaping involves maintaining the chosen directional line, whether it is a straight line (for acceleration and deceleration), or a curve (for turn). The final level of shaping in some methodologies involves reinforcing a consistent head, neck and body posture. The head, neck and body posture should be left as the last elements of the horse's biomechanics to reinforce because they are only associated with limb movements. Stimulus control of the head and neck posture is important because it is common for horses to associate random head and neck movements with locomotion, and such randomness and inconsistency may inhibit habit formation. Raising the head and contracting the back (hollowness) is generally associated with quickening, and lowering the head is associated with slowing (McLean, 2003). Stimulus control is achieved when these shaped elements are consistently incorporated into the learned responses for acceleration, deceleration, turn of the forequarters and (especially under-saddle) going sideways in various environments that the horse may encounter and at any time (see Table 8.1).

In all training, it is most efficient to begin shaping the smallest unit of a learned response and

Table 8.1 An example of shaping a response, in this case forward: go

Shaping component	Learned response	Effect
Step 1	Part of the correct stride from pressure	Horse steps forward
Step 2	A whole stride from signal	Horse steps a complete walk stride (4 steps in walk)
Step 3	Multiple strides from signal	Horse steps many strides
Step 4	Strides in the right direction from signal	Horse steps forward and maintains direction
Step 5	Strides with consistent posture from signal	Horse's posture is unchanged during forward locomotion
Step 6	Stimulus control	Horse goes everywhere and anywhere with above qualities

then target the smallest improvements so that in the end the animal is achieving the targeted learned response.

Inter-gait and intra-gait transitions

It is often necessary to train horses to shorten and lengthen steps in-hand, such as for the show-ring. Regardless of any competitive purpose, it is useful to train such responses because they elaborate training, giving the horse a greater set of cues and responses and helping create a predictable umwelt. To avoid problems in discrimination, characteristics of the lead-rein pressure may be altered to provide cues for longer versus faster steps (McLean and McLean, 2008). These pressure variations should be diminished during training to light versions of the pressure variations. Generally, the training of longer and shorter steps occurs later in training when the acceleration and deceleration responses are shaped and consolidated. As described above, the signals for faster or slower steps involve keeping them pressured, even if very lightly, for the duration of a stride, whereas for longer and shorter strides a *briefer* lead-rein signal is commonly used (brief pressure during a single step). Because the horse has already learned to maintain speed, the brief signal applied to one leg generally causes the same reaction in the contralateral foreleg. In the event that lengthening or shortening does not occur, the briefer rein signals are typically repeated.

Fortifying responses

Head-collars, snaffle-bits (on bridles) and halters can be rather blunt instruments. Sometimes the pressure exerted by head-collars, bridles or halters is not sufficient to motivate a horse to give the desired response. The motivation to remove the pressure on the poll can be outweighed by competing stimuli, such as the repelling effect of the float (trailer). In such cases, lead signals can be strengthened with the use of the long whip, tapping on the ribcage, but ceasing the instant the horse offers a single step forward. It is important that the horse is not afraid of the whip and does not react when the whip makes contact with its body. To habituate the horse to the whip, it is laid on the horse's body and is removed only when the horse ceases to react (see Figure 8.2). Alternatively, to overshadow an adverse reaction to the whip, it can be laid on the horse's body and the horse is then signalled to move back then forward repeatedly until its reaction to the whip subsides (McLean, 2008).

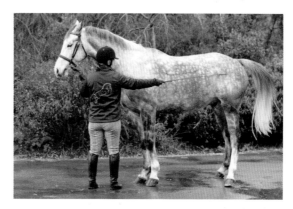

Figure 8.2 It is important to ensure that the sight of the whip or the approach of the whip is not a signal for movement. To do this, the whip is gently rubbed over the horse's body while simultaneously reinforcing immobility with the reins (overshadowing). This helps ensure calmness and responsiveness to the tapping of the whip as a useful signal.

During in-hand training, is it useful to use signals as similar as possible to those used under-saddle as this reduces the possibility of confusion. So, when the whip-tap is used to strengthen in-hand and under-saddle signals, the handler or rider should endeavour to tap the shoulder for turning, the sides for acceleration and the hindquarters for going sideways. Tapping the hindquarters for sideways rather than where the rider's legs press the horse's sides for sideways is common in dressage because of the difficulty in accurately tapping the ribcage on two distinct sites for forward and sideways (see Figure 6.8). In addition, discrimination can be further facilitated by shaping the training of the whip-tap for each of the three body sites in two ways: two taps for faster steps and one tap for longer steps.

The stop/slow signals of the lead-rein can be similarly strengthened with the correct use of the 'stallion bit' (rearing bit or chifney; see Chapter 10, Apparatus). As with the tapping whip, this is used in a continuous vibrating way until a single correct response occurs. With stallions, a stallion chain is sometimes used; this is attached to one side of the head-collar, brought underneath the stallion's mandible (lower jaw) and threaded through the head-collar to emerge on the opposite side or underneath. The stronger pressure exerted by this equipment can outweigh the strong social motivations of the stallion.

Alternative signals

Learning theory prescribes that there is a range of signals that can be used both in-hand and under-saddle; in other words, there are no necessarily correct or incorrect signals as long as the signals are specific, consistent and easily discriminated (McGreevy and McLean, 2007). Welfare considerations demand that every pressure signal should reduce to very light pressures that are released as soon as the animal responds.

Managing fear

Fearful, hyper-reactive responses should be very carefully managed. Dealing with fearful behaviours is examined in detail in Chapter 13

(Fight and flight responses and manifestations). Most fearful responses involve the horse quickening its legs and attempting to place distance between itself and the fearful stimulus. Both the quickening and the escape reinforce the association between the fearful stimulus and the escape response. Gradual habituation and overshadowing techniques (see Chapter 7, Applying learning theory) can be useful to alter the horse's reaction to the fearful stimulus (Christensen et al., 2006; McLean, 2008). On the other hand, flooding is sometimes used to prevent the expression of fear. For example, during foundation training, hobbles are sometimes used to prevent the horse's legs from moving in the face of aversive stimuli. Such practices can endanger the horse and are not recommended. In cases of milder expressions of fear, careful management involves using downward inter-gait and intra-gait transitions to inhibit fearful reactions.

Rewards

Positive reinforcement in the form of secondary positive reinforcement, such as clicker training (Chapter 5, Learning II: Associative (attractive)), can not only expedite training but may also serve to enhance the horse–human relationship. This form of reinforcement is, of course, more practical during in-hand than under-saddle training. Perhaps the optimal use of positive reinforcement, both in-hand and under-saddle, from the viewpoint of satiation and convenience is to caress the horse's withers (see Figure 2.7a, p. 13). This may also be used in the format of secondary reinforcement where a specific utterance such as 'good boy' serves as the secondary reinforcer, as described in the previous chapter. The optimal use of positive reinforcement is described in Figure 8.3.

Signals for acceleration (forward)

Training the horse to lead forward begins with operant conditioning (negative reinforcement) where increases in lead-rein pressure motivate the horse to move. The operant contingency begins with a cue of light lead-rein pressure *in the anterior direction* followed by a period of stronger

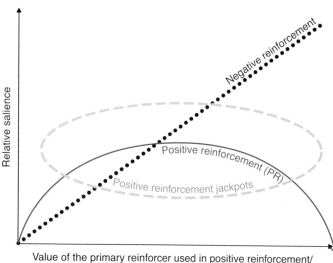

Figure 8.3 When positive and negative reinforcement are used concurrently, one may overshadow the other, depending on their relative salience. At low levels of negative reinforcement (rein/leg pressure) and high levels of positive reinforcement (jackpotting), positive reinforcement may be more salient, but as pressures increase, positive reinforcement may become less salient. This suggests that positive reinforcement is best used when negative reinforcement pressures have been converted to light signals.

pressure (see Figure 8.6a, p. 136), which is released when the horse offers the first sign of a correct or near-correct response (protraction of a forelimb in stance phase). When the horse has acquired the learned response of a visible but not perfect step in the forward direction, the trainer then targets reinforcing a single walk stride (a step of each of the four legs).

This anteriorly directed pressure acts on the poll (and dorsal parts of the mouth when a bridle is being used) and, in a broad sense, signals all upward inter-gait transitions in-hand as well as the intra-gait transitions of faster steps and longer steps. Many trainers make it easy for the naïve foal or horse to offer the desired response of walking forward when first cued by applying pressure slightly to one side instead of straight ahead (see Figure 6.8, p. 94). This lateral pressure causes a slight loss of balance so the horse steps to the side and the pressure is released. Through shaping, the horse learns to lead straight (see Table 8.2).

While the lead-rein itself, lightly pressured in the anterior direction, offers a clear classically conditioned cue for initiating forward steps, trainers sometimes unwittingly use a variety of cues. These range from voice commands to the handler's steps, which can initiate and maintain the horse's mobility. Provided the voice is used in a precise, standard and predictable way, it can be very effective and is only marred by the likelihood

that the horse is constantly subjected to words uttered by people and may previously have learned to ignore them. Effective users of the voice in animal training tend to use voice characteristics that are used only for training. Trainers who use their steps to elicit movement face more difficult hurdles. For the horse to discriminate when the steps of the human are meant to be a cue and when they are not is a major problem (see Figure 8.4). For example, when the handler moves around the horse during care and maintenance, the horse is generally expected to remain immobile, yet the handler's steps cue the horse to move. The horse may be punished for doing something it was cued to do. To solve this dilemma, some methods advocate that the handler adopts specific postures when cuing the horse to move. While this has some merit, it also becomes context-specific in that leading and non-leading postures of one person compared with another are not easily discriminated so that handing the horse over to another handler may result in confusion and apparent non-compliance. Another problem arises when humans are inconsistent and ineffective in adopting the specific posture. However, the handler's movement is not irrelevant for it may provide the most reliable cue for *maintaining* movement in the horse once elicited by other stimuli such as the lead-rein.

Lead-rein responses can be strengthened with a rhythmic whip-tap in the event that the lead-rein

Table 8.2 Stimulus–response characteristics of in-hand training

Targeted response	Targeted biomechanics	Operant discriminative stimulus	Motivation	Reinforcement	Other associated and maintaining cues	Possible verbal cue
Upward inter-gait transition and faster limbs	Accelerating protraction (swing) and retraction (stance)	Prolonged (2 steps) anterior lead-rein signal	Anterior lead-rein pressure/whip-taps on ribcage	Release pressure on improved step	Handler walking forward	'Walk on', 'trot on', 'canter', tongue click
Upward intra-gait transition: longer steps	Increased protraction (swing) and retraction (stance)	Brief (1 step) anterior lead-rein signal	Anterior lead-rein pressure/whip-taps on ribcage	Release pressure on improved step	Handler lengthening steps	Tongue click
Downward inter-gait transition and slower limbs	Decelerating protraction (stance) and retraction (swing)	Prolonged (2 steps) posterior lead-rein signal	Posterior lead-rein pressure	Release pressure on improved step	Handler slowing or stopping	'Whoa', 'stand', 'wa'alk', 'tro'ot'
Step backwards	Protraction (stance) and retraction (swing)	Posterior lead-rein signal	Posterior lead-rein pressure/whip-tap on chest or foreleg	Release pressure on improved step	Handler stepping backwards	'Back'
Downward intra-gait transition: shorter steps	Decreased protraction (stance) and retraction (swing)	Brief (1 step) posterior lead-rein signal	Posterior lead-rein pressure	Release pressure on improved step	Handler shortening steps	Brief 'whoa'
Turn forequarters	Abduction (swing), adduction (stance) then adductions	Lateral lead signal	Lateral lead pressure	Release pressure on improved step	Handler turning	Usually not used
Turn hindquarters and go sideways	Adduction (swing), adduction (stance) then abductions	Two whip-taps on hindquarters	Whip-tap pressure on sides of hindquarters	Release pressure on improved step	Handler stepping towards horse's hindquarters	'Over'

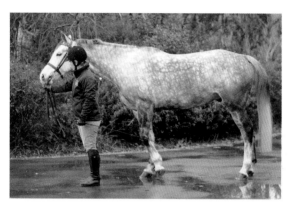

Figure 8.4   Horses are very adept at classical conditioning, so it is easy for a horse to learn to step forward when its handler takes a step. However, you do not want this to become the signal, as there are many occasions when the handler steps but requires the horse to remain in place. If signals are not consistent, confusion and conflict behaviours may set in. Therefore, it is important that the first signal for all in-hand locomotion is light lead-rein pressure in the appropriate direction.

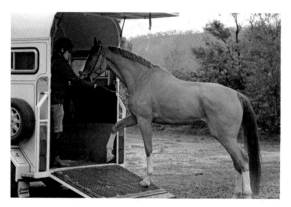

Figure 8.5   The whip-tap can fortify lead forward responses because it is more difficult to habituate to the whip-tap than to lead pressure.

signals fail to evoke a response. Whip-taps can be used to elicit various directional responses, so it is optimal to facilitate discrimination of the whip-tap signals. This is achieved by tapping on the ribcage in the same place where the horse will be tapped under-saddle. From the standpoints of welfare and optimal training, the whip should not be used to punish a horse for non-compliance to the handler's or rider's signals. The whip is as much a signal as any other stimulus and should be used simply to initiate responses (see Figure 8.5). Whip-taps are used in two ways in negative reinforcement: by varying their frequency and magnitude. To tap rhythmically and increase the frequency of taps rather than increasing the magnitude is the optimal method. Whip-taps should simply irritate the horse to react, not hurt him. The great usefulness of the whip is that it provides a larger range of aversive pressures than the lead-rein (or the rider's legs under-saddle), and within this range there is likely to be a specific pressure of whip-tap that will motivate most horses to react.

When stimulus control is achieved via the light signal or voice cue, the amount of negative reinforcement is dramatically diminished so the salience of the negative reinforcement is reduced

to the point where a positive reinforcer can now be salient. Because the timing and delivery of primary positive reinforcers, such as food or caressing at the withers, can sometimes be impractical, appropriate use of a secondary positive reinforcer can maintain the transition.

In-hand, most handlers aim for a number of specific qualities (mentioned in the previous chapter) in the final product of a forward response, and these can be achieved by shaping. When the horse has learned to lead forward a single step, it is then reinforced for leading a number of steps from a single light signal. The next quality to be reinforced is to maintain a particular direction. Trainers often negatively reinforce the direction by pressuring the lead-rein in the opposite direction of the drift. If the horse's head-carriage is too high or inconsistent, the horse may be motivated to lower its head from downward pressure, negatively reinforcing lowering of the head with release from the downward lead-rein pressure, and then shape this head-down response into its leading forward response so that the horse leads with a consistent head height. When all the qualities of the response desired by the trainer are incorporated into the horse's leading forward response, the horse's forward responses come under increasing stimulus control as the response becomes consolidated. As described earlier, the horse can be trained to offer longer strides from a brief lead-rein signal applied for one step of the walk. If the horse fails to respond, the pressure is briefly raised for further individual steps until the longer steps are elicited

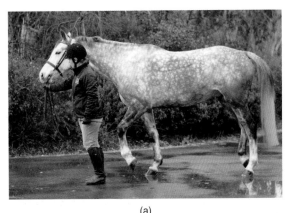
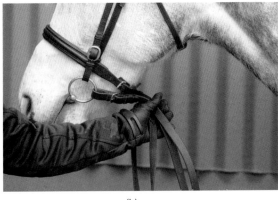

(a)   (b)

Figure 8.6   In-hand, the signal for going forward is lead-rein pressure in the anterior direction (a), while for stopping, slowing and stepping back, it is posterior lead-rein pressure (b). This difference is easily perceived by the horse.

from a brief light signal. From time to time, trainers may transiently increase the aversive pressure of the forward signals if the response wanes. However, in general, consistent responding can be optimally maintained by secondary positive reinforcement.

Signals for deceleration

Slowing (deceleration) or stopping the horse is signalled by a light pressure on the lead-rein, lead-rope or bridle reins, only this time *in the posterior direction* (see Figure 8.6b). The pressure from the lead-rein in the posterior direction is perceived by the horse principally on its nasal planum or, in the case of a bitted bridle, in its mouth (as in under-saddle). So, there is a fundamental difference in direction between acceleration and deceleration signals. This backward-facing signal is used to elicit all downward transitions, including slowing, shortening the steps, stopping and stepping backwards.

In early training and re-training, a basic attempt of slowing by the horse is initially reinforced. Then the trainer reinforces an entire stride of step-back (all four legs). The horse learns to associate the light signal with a subsequent period of stronger lead-rein pressure and so learns to respond from the light signal alone (McGreevy and McLean, 2007). Maintaining a slower speed and remaining immobile are also part of the shaping process of

the deceleration responses. As with the forward-leading responses, the slowing and shortening signals in-hand are usually further shaped so that they occur on a straight line and with a consistent head-carriage. To elicit shorter steps from brief lead-rein signals, pressure is applied for a portion of a step. The brief pressures are repeated from one step to another until the horse maintains shorter steps.

The slowing, shortening and stepping backwards responses can be thought of collectively because they all involve activation, in varying amounts, of protraction muscles in the stance phases and retraction in the swing phases of the steps of the particular transition. So, training the horse to step backwards simultaneously enhances the training of all the downward inter-gait and intra-gait transitions (see Figure 8.7). Deficits in the step-back transition have been reported to be associated with deficits in downward transitions (McLean, 2005b). Similar to the acceleration responses, the backwards response is triggered by escalating pressure, beginning with light pressure. The light pressure acts as a predictor of a period of stronger pressure and its subsequent release, so that the horse soon learns to respond to the light signals.

In the event of the lead-rein not triggering a sufficient step-back response, the horse can be motivated with whip-taps on the horse's forelegs or chest, or by squeezing the *brachiocephalic* muscle (McLean and McLean, 2008; see Figure 8.8a). (The

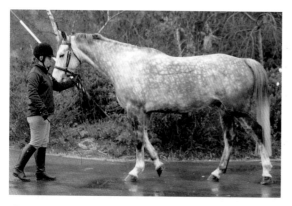

Figure 8.7 Training the horse to step-back in-hand enhances the stop and slow signals and provides a useful tool in re-training problems with the stop signals. This is because the neuromuscular coordination of stepping back is incorporated in all downward transitions to a greater or lesser extent.

horse should be habituated to the whip so that it is not fearful of it.) If the horse fails to respond, it makes sense to target a site that makes it most likely for the horse to offer the correct response so as to avoid prolonged tapping and confusion. The metacarpal (cannon) bone of the horse's foreleg provides an obvious site because one of the horse's legs must retract in the swing phase to begin the step-back.

Ideally, when cueing stepping back, the foreleg that is most anterior at any moment of immobility should be the one tapped, as that will be the first to move. The foreleg can be tapped at various fre-

quencies to ensure that the size and timing of the step is the required amount. As with forward, it is vital to cease tapping as soon as the horse offers the first correct or near-correct response (depending on its experience with the learned response). The train of events should begin with light lead pressure just before tapping the foreleg and should be contiguous with the whip-tap. Then, when the horse fails to step-back, the whip-tap can be used to evoke the response.

When the horse has learned to step-back from the light lead-rein signal, the response may come under the stimulus control of a discrete voice command such as 'back'. When this or any other response arises from cues or light pressures, it can be reinforced from time to time using secondary positive reinforcement. Reinforcing responses on a variable schedule of reinforcement helps build resistance to extinction.

Stepping backwards can also be shaped. As soon as the horse steps-back consistently from a cue or light lead-rein signal, a series of backward steps is reinforced. Further shaping of the step-back is sometimes considered necessary (Parelli, 1995; McLean and McLean, 2008) so as to deepen the deceleration responses across the board of training and to assist in the rehabilitation of horses with poor stop responses and so-called hard mouths. So, the series of backwards steps may be trained to occur in a straight line. As with the forward leading response in-hand, the backwards steps can be trained to include a consistent

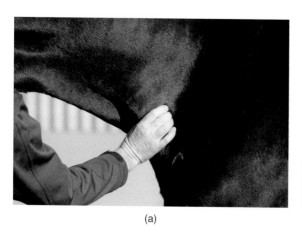

(a)

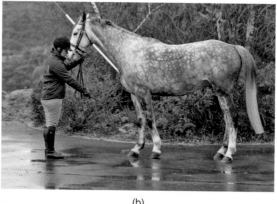

(b)

Figure 8.8 Training the step-back can be fortified by applying the light cue for step-back just before squeezing the *brachiocephalic* muscle (a) or just before tapping the *metacarpal* (cannon) bone of the foreleg that is likely to step first (b).

head height by lowering or raising the horse's head just before deceleration signals are applied.

In-hand, the deceleration signals from the reins are virtually identical to those under-saddle, so it is not surprising that the horse's deceleration responses can be 'pre-trained' in-hand ready for use under-saddle in the young horse. A horse with a problematic deceleration under-saddle can also be at least partially rehabilitated in-hand (McLean, 2005a).

Signals for turn of the forelegs

Training the horse to turn its forequarters is not only essential for the obvious reason of changing direction but also useful in correcting tendencies of the horse to drift to one side or the other. Horses typically swerve and shy using their forelegs rather than their hindlegs (McLean, 2005a). This directional predominance of the forelegs over the hindlegs indicates that placing the forelegs under stimulus control is a major component in training straightness (where the hindhooves step into the foretracks). It is likely that training turns in-hand pre-trains the same response under-saddle; indeed, ridden and handled horses tend to show the same errors in negative reinforcement of acceleration and deceleration responses in-hand as they do under-saddle (McLean, 2005b).

Fundamentally, the turn signal initially learned by the horse in-hand is the lateral lead-rein pressure exerted on the head-collar or bridle of the horse (see Figure 8.9). The effect of the rein pressure is to negatively reinforce lateral action of the forelegs conferred by alternating sequences of abduction and adduction (opening both forelegs then closing both forelegs; see Figure 11.6, p. 203) or vice versa. When the horse is standing upright and is bilaterally symmetrical, it tends to turn by abducting the forelegs before adduction. This is appropriate because, as established in the previous chapter, disciplines such as dressage require turns to be initiated by foreleg abductions followed by adduction. To maintain relaxation and consistency, trainers must be clear on the particular biomechanical response they seek and be diligent in reinforcing it.

Because most horses are usually led using a single lead-rein attached to the underside of the head-

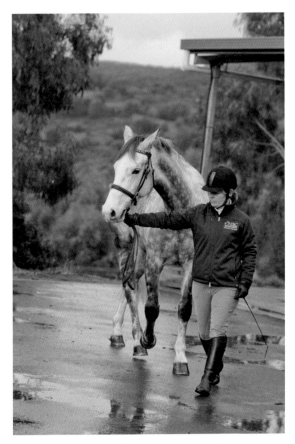

Figure 8.9 Training the horse to turn in-hand is useful in certain situations where the horse may veer to one side, such as loading the horse onto a float/trailer.

collar, there is generally no *discrete* lead-rein signal to turn the forelegs to either side because the turn signals tend to merge with the acceleration or deceleration signals. If the horse is walking at the speed of the handler or slower than the handler, the turn blends into the acceleration signal of the lead-rein. If the horse is walking faster than the handler, the turn signal merges into the deceleration signal. The negative reinforcement of the abduction/adduction sequence also *shapes* the turn response in terms of speed and directional line.

A training whip can be used to negatively reinforce turns, especially in situations where the lead-rein pressure is not sufficiently motivating. The horse is tapped rhythmically with the whip on its shoulder (the flat deltoid area over the humerus), which is the ideal site. The whip acts as an additional signal that can strengthen and sensitise other signals, such as the lead-rein signal for the turn response. The horse should be trained to respond from the whip-tap alone (with no lead-rein signal) so that it has a clear learned response to turn from the whip-tap on either shoulder as well as from the lead-rein. Turning from the whip-tap can be useful in training the horse to load into a trailer in the event it swerves.

Sometimes the horse may respond to the turn of the forelegs signal by turning only the hindlegs or turning the hindlegs too much (i.e. stepping out of the line of the foretracks). In such cases, careful use of lead-rein pressures or mild whip-taps on the appropriate shoulder corrects the forelegs. Achieving biomechanically consistent turns is important as it increases the efficiency of learning (long-term potentiation occurs more rapidly with identical responses) and, more important, lowers the potential for confusion and subsequent stress.

Signals for turn of the hindquarters

Turning the hindquarters is significant in some disciplines, such as dressage and reining, so training the horse in-hand to move its hindquarters laterally is useful as pre-training for under-saddle work. It is also useful to be able to move the hindquarters in situations where the hindquarters have veered to the side, such as during trailer loading or training a young racehorse to enter the starting gates. The hindquarter turn in-hand is, however, less important in terms of the totality of locomotory stimulus control than the more fundamental responses of acceleration, deceleration and turning the forelegs. When the horse is standing bilaterally symmetrical (upright), turns of the hindlegs tend to be effected by adduction before abduction (see Figure 11.8, p. 204). The sport of dressage follows this biomechanical predisposition and turns on the forehand and leg-yield are begun with an adduction step.

In some training methodologies, the cue for a turn of the hindlegs in-hand is often a touch or vibration of the fingers on the ribcage, while in others a voice command (such as 'over') is sometimes used. In order to elicit the response in early training, some trainers use whip-tapping on the hindquarters. In order to facilitate the horse's discrimination, the response is more easily achieved if the leg that is to be adducted is tapped around the hock area first. When the horse has learned to consistently adduct the tapped leg, the site of the whip-tap can be gradually moved up the hindleg to the lateral aspect of the rump (Figure 8.10). The subsequent shaping of the hindquarters response may include training the horse to respond to two light taps for faster steps and one light tap for a longer step, and transforming the signal to one or two vibrations of the fingers on the ribcage where

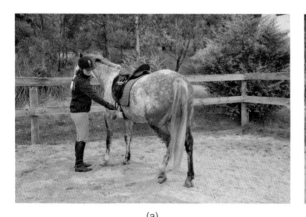
(a)

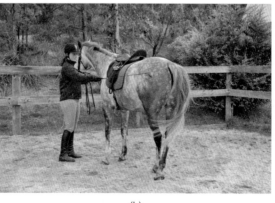
(b)

Figure 8.10   (a) Stepping sideways away from the whip-tap signal is facilitated by first tapping the horse's hock (where sideways is a more obvious reaction to the horse) and then (b) moving up the leg to the position of the rump. (Photos courtesy of Elke Hartmann.)

the rider's leg would elicit the same response. In this way, the sideways response under-saddle can be pre-trained in-hand.

Some trainers also shape the turn of the hindquarters response into a sideways response while going forward. This becomes an analogue of what is known as a 'leg-yield' and when this occurs, the trainer may shape various elements such as leg-yielding in a maintained speed, line and head-carriage.

Head lowering

Lowering the horse's head is a technique sometimes used by trainers to calm horses (Warren-Smith *et al.*, 2007b; see Figure 8.11). However, because a loss of calmness is frequently associated with poor use of negative reinforcement during acceleration and deceleration responses, lowering the head may give only temporary relief. When anxiety is caused by environmental events (such as leaves rustling in the wind), the effect of head-lowering in inducing calmness may be more lasting, possibly because of effects analogous to overshadowing.

Lowering the horse's head is useful as a shaping component when training locomotory responses. A high head-carriage is typically associated with hyper-reactive states and, furthermore, an inconsistent head-carriage impedes the development of consistent reactions to acceleration, deceleration and turn signals. So, training the horse to lower its head and shaping this into the go, stop and turn signals facilitates calmness and consistency, hastening the acquisition of long-term potentiation for these responses.

In dressage, the position of the horse's head has long been regarded as an essential feature of collection. This is because, as illustrated in Figure 8.12, simultaneously raising the head and shortening the neck is said to redistribute some of the horse's weight from the forequarters to the hindquarters (Karl, 2006).

Lungeing

Lungeing the horse often involves the use of a round-pen where the horse may move freely or

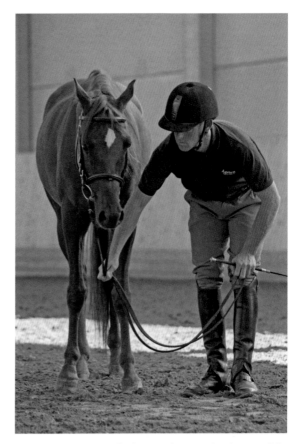

Figure 8.11 Training the horse to lower its head is a useful tool during in-hand interactions. It is important that this response is shaped gradually, beginning with initially reinforcing (release) for the smallest responses and gradually approximating the final targeted response where the horse will maintain his head lowered. (Photo courtesy of Elke Hartmann.)

be connected to the handler by a lungeing-rein attached to a lungeing-cavesson or bridle (Chapter 10, Apparatus). Training responses on the lunge and subsequently shaping them can be seen in the same format as other in-hand training (see Figure 8.13). It should be mentioned, however, that the slowing signal predominantly pressures only one side of the horse's head, and so bears little resemblance to the slowing signals used in-hand. For this reason, the slowing signals of lungeing must be trained via negative reinforcement. The lunge-line is used as a slowing signal by increasing vibrating/intermittent pressure and then releasing it when the horse offers slowing. The consistent

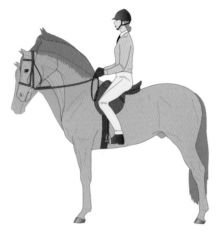

Figure 8.12 The redistribution of weight from front to back is thought to be facilitated by the elevation of the horse's head.

and correct release of pressure will enable lunge-line signals to be rapidly shrunk to light versions. The lungeing whip is used to trigger forward reactions, and these can be brought under the stimulus control of voice commands. Variations of both the type and amount of deceleration and acceleration signals can be used to motivate and train faster and longer inter-gait transitions.

During lungeing, when the handler in the centre of the lunge circle moves too far in front of the horse (so that the right angle represented by a line

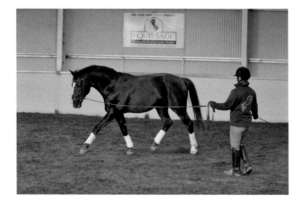

Figure 8.13 Lungeing is often used in training to assist in physical development, to help associate locomotory responses with signals and to exercise a horse. Trainers should bear in mind that continuously lungeing a flighty horse can create associations between humans and the flight response, which can be indelible.

drawn from the human to the longitudinal axis of the horse via the horse's shoulder is increased), the horse typically slows down. This is a typical ethological response to the horse perceiving that its escape forward is thwarted by a predator. On the other hand, if this critical angle (of handler to horse) diminishes to less than a right angle, the horse accelerates. Correct lungeing procedure requires effective use of these ethological phenomena.

Fundamentally, every flight response should be avoided because of its rapid acquisition and resistance to erasure (Seligman, 1971; Le Doux, 1994). When a horse shows a flight response on the lunge, it is important to slow the horse. Such slowing typically involves negative reinforcement where the rein pressure increasingly turns the horse until it slows; then, the pressure is immediately released. Soon, the horse slows from that turning signal. It is a matter of welfare that the horse is not put in a position of being 'chased' and expressing a flight response during lungeing. However, if the horse is quiet and consistently responding to the slowing signals (a good test!) or maintaining its speed, then lungeing is not detrimental. The same principles apply to round-pen work.

Under-saddle training

Foundation training

When the time for foundation training comes, the young horse is habituated to the appropriate equipment, such as bridle, saddle cloth, saddle and girth-strap pressure. This is often done on the lead-rein or lunge-line. Following successful habituation, the horse then also undergoes habituation to the presence of the rider either bareback or, after habituation, to the saddle and girth. Regardless of methodology, habituation is facilitated by progressing very slowly so that the process of sitting up on the horse may have a dozen or so intermediate steps, such as habituating the horse to a human jumping up and down beside it, then jumping a bit higher until lying on the horse and then habituating the horse to the arrival of the handler's leg over to the horse's off-side and then sitting up. For skilled horse people, it is

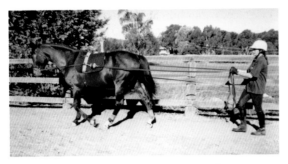

Figure 8.14   Long-reining the horse is a typical process in foundation training. Because the trainer's hands are at a considerable distance from the horse's mouth, skill is required to ensure smooth and consistent delivery of rein signals. It is also important to ensure that the driven horse does not perceive that he is being chased or else fearful, hyper-reactive associations can be incorporated into training. (Photo courtesy of Greg Jones.)

more efficient to habituate the horse to the rider bareback rather than saddled, in order to separate the mounting procedure from the girth pressure which many horses take time to habituate to.

Some trainers drive the young horse in long-reins once it has habituated to the saddle and bridle (see Figure 8.14). The disadvantages of this are that the young horse may perceive that it is being chased and develop a habituated mouth and hyper-reactive posture as it attempts to escape forward. It may also learn to associate some tension with horse–human interactions.

Signals used under-saddle

Under-saddle, there are three points of physical interaction between rider and horse: legs, seat and reins. Pressure from the rider's legs is universally used to signal acceleration responses by closing the legs against the horse's body. The legs, therefore, operate by negative reinforcement and in optimal training the pressures reduce to lighter versions. The rider's upper leg (femur) is often an acquired signal associated with turning the horse's forequarters. The rider's calves signal quickening of the horse's legs while the lower portion of the rider's lower leg typically signals longer strides. The rider's seat has less effect in terms of negative reinforcement since there is a limit to which the rider can increase the forces of the seat. On the

contrary, the seat is largely effective by classical conditioning: by association with the more powerful signals from the reins and rider's legs.

Equipment

The whip

The leg signals and seat signals for acceleration are typically fortified with the use of the long whip, the riding crop and the spurs. Whips should be used only as further signals and not as a punitive stimulus that, as believed in some circles, forces the horse to *pay attention* to a previous signal. Both are wrong for welfare reasons and the second is wrong also for unrealistic cognitive expectations (see Chapter 7, Applying learning theory).

Spurs

Spurs should be used only to make a signal more precise, not to inflict increasing pain on the horse's sides. Therefore, spurs should not be introduced until the horse's basic training is consolidated, in order to refine leg signals. Yet, it is not uncommon to see the use of spurs for young horses, for novice riders and for horses that are labelled 'lazy' (horses that are less motivated to go forward or that have been inadvertently reinforced for not going forward). The so-called laziness should not be thought of as a personality disorder but rather as a behaviour with a significant learned component.

Severe bits

The action of the bit can be fortified by the use of more severe bits. These tend to have an increased motivational effect through increasing pain; in other words, severe bits are effective as a result of their thinness, abrasiveness, corrugation, sharpness or via a lever effect. The lever effect is represented by the shank fixed on to the curb bit, which is a first-class lever (see Figure 10.6, p. 186).

It is crucial that riders recognise that the horse feels far more pressure inside its mouth from a curb bit than riders do in their hands, so 'feel' may be a rather inaccurate assessment tool. The importance of self-carriage (especially in horses in curb bits) and frequently testing for it by momentarily relinquishing the rein contact (for two strides) are of great importance for welfare reasons. This release for two strides is embodied in the German technique known as *Überstreichen*, and should be mandatory in all gaits and movements in dressage. Moreover, the enforced use of curb bits in Fédération Equestre Internationale (FEI) dressage tests and their use in reining competitions seems irrational and archaic and contributes to poor welfare. It appears that one of the reasons commonly given for using curb bits these days is that their use requires skill and is, thus, a further test of rider capability. However, since the expression of correct training is dependent on learned responses, it seems appropriate to use the simplest apparatus to demonstrate such skilled training rather than the harshest weaponry.

Posture and position of the rider

The presence of a rider affects the horse's kinematics (Sloet van Oldruitenborgh-Oosterbaan *et al.*, 1995) and the forces with which it impacts the ground (Clayton *et al.*, 1999). Research into impact forces at trot shows that the vertical oscillation of the vertebral column of the rider's body is subject to momentum and continues to descend until well after the reversal in the dorsoventral movement of the horse's back (Terada *et al.*, 2004) and these impacts have flow-on effects on the rider. Coordinated contractions of the rider's muscles not only stabilise the rider but they also synchronise with the horse's motion and, furthermore, can influence the horse's performance. So, the musculature of experienced riders coordinates with the rhythm of the horse's strides and each gait is characterised by a corresponding cyclic pattern of the rider's biomechanics. It has been shown that, at the sitting trot, novice riders tend to grip with their legs, using their *adductor magnus* muscles to maintain posture because they have not yet developed coordination between the *rectus abdominis* muscles (commonly known as the 'abs') and *erector spinae* muscles (the longitudinal back muscles), which is integral to the postural skills of experienced riders. Studies show that there is a brief but consistent burst of activity in the rider's *trapezius* muscles (shoulder blade) that possibly contributes to sta-

bilisation of the rider's head and neck during the impact phase of the horse's stride (Terada, 2000).

Increased intra-abdominal pressure in the rider's torso, due to *rectus abdominis* contraction during the mid-stance phase at trot, has also been documented, suggesting that the tightening of abdominal muscles assists in swinging the pelvis forward as the horse's dorsoventral oscillation reverses direction during mid-stance and begins to rise (Terada *et al.*, 2004). While these biomechanics are consistent among experienced riders, some variation is also shown in their musculature. For example, Terada (2000) showed that, among experienced riders, there is considerable variation in the range of motion in their hips and shoulders at trot. This may be explained by physical differences among riders or differences in coaching. Whichever way, it also suggests that while successful dressage equitation demands certain essential biomechanics, other aspects, such as the movements of the rider's hips and shoulders, allow for some deviation from the norm.

Novice riders tend to lean forward to compensate for the horse's motion, which sends the rider's trunk forward and back (see Figure 8.15). Terada (2000) reports that experienced riders adopt an almost vertical trunk orientation with a backward tilt of an average of 4 degrees. However, oscillations of the trunk occur in rhythm with the stride in the walk, rising trot and canter (Lovett *et al.*, 2004).

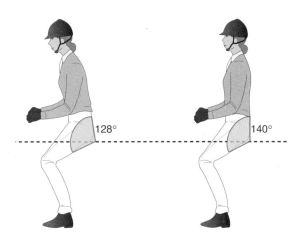

Figure 8.15 As riders become more experienced they tend to be able to sit more upright and their limb-torso angles open.

Equestrian coaches have long focussed on teaching their pupils to maintain their arms in a stable position beside their body. It is difficult to keep track of many body parts at one moment and human arms have shoulder joints, elbow joints and wrists that all provide different ranges of motion and, thus, can impede the acquisition of perfect balance if they are unstable or variable. Studies suggest that experienced riders maintain a consistent distance from wrist to the horse's mouth by adjusting the angles of their shoulder and elbow joints to compensate for the rocking motion of their bodies (Terada *et al.*, 2004).

Inter-gait and intra-gait transitions under-saddle

Under-saddle, longer and shorter strides are often required in addition to faster and slower ones. In a similar format to in-hand training, faster and slower strides are trained and consolidated to the point where they can be elicited by light signals before longer or shorter strides are trained. While faster and slower strides, including upward and downward transitions, are signalled for the duration of a stride (four steps for walk and two steps of the forelegs for trot, for example), lengthening and shortening involve brief signals. These brief signals or pressures are applied during a single step within a stride in walk and trot. Again, the contralateral foreleg step generally tends to shorten also, but if not, the brief pressure is repeated. In canter, the brief pressures are applied for a stride.

Signals for acceleration

Acceleration is the result of retraction of limbs in the stance phase and protraction in the swing phase (see Figure 11.2, p. 200). The fundamental signals for going forward under-saddle are provided by pressure from the rider's legs just behind the ventral thoracic (girth) region (i.e. where they hang vertically down the horse's sides; see Table 8.3). For optimal acquisition, the ideal moment to issue an acceleration signal is at the beginning of the stance phase of one hindleg footfall (which coincides with the beginning step of the contralateral

swing phase). In the early stages of negative reinforcement, the release occurs at the end of that step (Warren-Smith *et al.*, 2005b). As with all responses acquired by negative reinforcement, riders often resort to using the entire lower leg to motivate the naïve or poorly trained horse to go forward. Ideally, this pressure is preceded by the light pressure of the calves, and so these discriminative stimuli become the light signals in optimal training. This is typically accompanied by a 'sweeping' seat signal of similar duration. Increasing intra-gait speed can be differentiated from upward inter-gait transitions by pressure differences: by increasing the amount of leg pressure and differences in associated seat posture for upward inter-gait transitions. Further shaping of the acceleration responses entails eliciting an entire stride of the particular gait from a light signal of the calves. Multiple steps are then reinforced followed by the maintenance of directional line and body straightness and finally head and neck posture.

Longer steps are reinforced using brief pressure of the rider's legs for a portion of a single step and repeating until the horse learns to lengthen (see Figure 8.16). Should the horse quicken, the rider generally slows it with the reins and repeats the longer step signal. Under-saddle, the brief leg signals for longer strides often accompany an associated brief 'shoving' seat signal. Complete stimulus control occurs when the rider can go forward anywhere and everywhere within the normal domestic and training environment.

Longer steps are often established early in the horse's training because they assist in lowering and lengthening the horse's head and neck to promote relaxation. Lowering and lengthening of the cervical vertebrae are intricately associated with the lengthening of the stride. This biomechanical feature confers the first and most vital stage of training in many traditional dressage and reining methods: *longitudinal flexion* (see Figure 8.17), characterised by lowering of the poll, lowering and lengthening of the neck. In correct scientific terms, this posture should be termed longitudinal *extension*, since technically it involves more decontraction than flexion. Many training methodologies advocate this as the first major step of training because it promotes looseness of the musculature (Hölzel *et al.*, 1995; German National Equestrian Federation, 1997). However, many trainers ignore

trainers, use closing the knees to signal deceleration, which is learned by classical conditioning. Although the reins provide the only operant reinforcement for the deceleration responses undersaddle, it is worth considering the cognitive difficulty presented by this signal to the horse. The reins are physically distant from the part of the body that is intended to respond: the legs. This difficulty places considerable onus on the trainer to be aware of the actual leg movements that are to be reinforced. In shaping the deceleration response, the trainer initially reinforces a basic attempt, which may consist of any slowing, shortening or backward step. The next aspect to be shaped is an entire stride of the particular gait so that the release of rein pressure occurs as the horse offers the complete stride from a light version of the pressure signal. Multiple steps are also shaped as well as shortening the steps from a brief rein signal (pressured for a portion of a step). Finally, maintaining straightness and incorporating a consistent head and neck posture are trained. Shaping the rein responses is important and challenging: there are more conflict behaviours associated with rein responses than those with the rider's leg responses (McLean, 2005b).

At liberty, most of the horse's weight (around 60%) is carried on its forelegs, so deceleration places considerable force there. However, dressage practice revolves around the balance of the horse–human entity with the putative aim of transferring weight to the hindquarters of the horse. As described in Chapter 11 (Biomechanics), this involves a lowering of the horse's croup, which, in best practice, requires a heterogeneous closing of the joint angles of the hindlegs (Podhajsky, 1966). Biomechanically, this places more involvement of the hindhooves in deceleration. This occurs when the deceleration response involves a minimum of intermediate steps, which is characteristic of a highly trained horse (Argue and Clayton, 1993a, 1993b).

Where learning theory is incorrectly used in training, the horse's tongue often retracts to escape the pain (see Figure 8.20) and then is sometimes seen to droop flaccidly out of the mouth. This response may become habitual as soon as the bit is inserted into the horse's mouth. This is not uncommon in dressage and racing horses, where strong bit pressure may cause constant pain. Most likely the tongue drops out of the mouth as a result of tongue fatigue (the difficulty of sustaining the retraction) and there may well be a component of learned helplessness. In some horse-racing countries, it is legal to tie the tongue inside the mouth. It is imperative that lightness is the goal, unconditionally and throughout training. While moments of pressure may well be required to acquire certain responses, the horse should be free to travel in self-carriage.

Once again, we face the problem of the horse's ability to discriminate between the signals for alterations in stride speed and length: slowing and shortening. As with the acceleration signals, the problem is solved by using a consistent set of different rein pressures. For slowing the horse, including downward inter-gait transitions, the rein signal is more prolonged. For shortening the stride, the rein signal is relatively brief. The rein signal for downward inter-gait transitions is the same as for slowing, except that it is slightly but perceptibly stronger. In addition, there are associated seat signals for downward inter-gait transitions such as smoothly emphasising the bracing seat for a couple of beats of the rhythm. For the intra-gait transitions of shortening the steps, the bracing seat is stronger and brief.

Correct early training results in a horse maintaining its own rhythm, line and outline, culminating in a posture known as 'on the bit' (see Glossary and Figure 8.21). Sometimes a horse may constantly lean on the bit and the rider notices that the reins are heavy. While some consider that leaning on the bit is something the horse deliberately likes to do, a more enlightened interpretation suggests that such a horse has developed this habit as a result of poorly timed, insufficient or no negative reinforcement of the deceleration responses. In such cases, most horses accelerate when the reins are released. This places the horse in a confused state where the release of the reins that should reinforce slowing now elicits the opposite: acceleration.

Although it is common in dressage and eventing to insist on a rounded outline early on, this can lead to confusion and conflict behaviours when the horse is still requiring pressure from the rider's legs yet the rider is pressuring the reins to achieve a rounded outline. Because the muscles that provide acceleration are opposed to the ones that

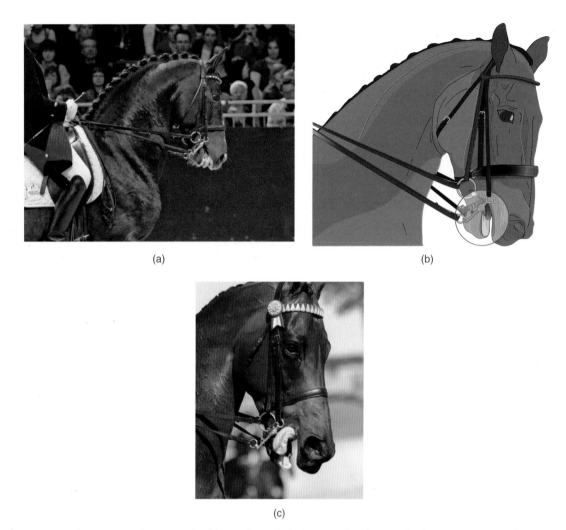

(a)

(b)

(c)

Figure 8.20   In best practice, the tongue should sit underneath the bit in a relaxed way. Relentless pressure across the tongue can restrict blood flow to the end of the tongue (a), a condition known as ischaemia that is characterized by a blue colour (Photo courtesy of Minna Tallberg.) (b) When the horse's tongue remains permanently retracted, it is a sign that the horse finds the bit aversive: mouth pressure is too strong and unrelenting. (c) When the tongue cannot escape highly aversive bit pressure by retraction, it may droop in a seemingly paralysed way. (Photo courtesy of Julie Wilson.)

provide deceleration, the signals must never clash and should be separated as outlined in the previous chapter. While it is common for riders to be taught to use leg pressures during all downward transitions, it must be recognised that this practice is inherently confusing for horses. If transitions are trained to be completed within the cycle of a single stride, the activity of the hindlegs remains and the rider's legs are obsolete at this moment.

Signals for turning the forelegs

Turning the forelegs typically facilitates changes of direction in equitation and results from consecutive abduction and adduction. In correct training, abductions and adductions are symmetrical: both forelegs open or close to the same degree, so that the horse's body is precisely upright and not leaning to one side. When turning, horses are trained

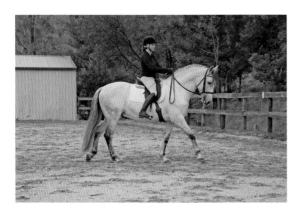

Figure 8.21   A horse under-saddle develops a rounded neck outline as a result of longitudinal, lateral and vertical flexion. From this position the horse gradually develops collection where the poll is at its highest point and there is increased arching of the neck.

so that the hindlegs also turn and follow the same path as the forelegs; however, when the forelegs are abducting, both hindlegs are adducting. Therefore, on curved lines this involves what is considered in dressage as *bend* along the vertebral column, although, as described in Chapter 11 (Biomechanics), the amount of vertebral bending is minimal in horses (Jeffcott and Dalin, 1980).

Turns may begin with either abduction or adduction. That said, sports such as dressage insist on abduction as the first response of a turn. Regardless, it is important that one or the other is *consistently* chosen to be elicited for the beginning of any turn in order to facilitate optimal long-term potentiation. When abduction comes first, the foreleg on the same side as the horse is turning abducts in the swing phase, while the contralateral foreleg abducts in the stance phase. When adduction comes first, the foreleg ipsilateral to the turn direction abducts in the swing phase, while the ipsilateral limb adducts in the stance phase.

Light pressure on the right rein is the fundamental signal for turning right, whereas pressure on the left rein is the main signal for the left turn. It is common to find that riders bring both hands slightly towards the right for a right turn or both slightly to the left for a left turn. When relatively greater pressure is applied to the rein that moves *away* from the horse's neck, it is known as a *direct turn* (see Figure 8.22a). Conversely, when relatively greater pressure is applied to the rein that

comes *closer* to the horse's neck, it is known as an *indirect turn* (see Figure 8.22b). The direct turn is generally the preferred turning method, but in cases when the horse's neck is laterally bending too much, or when the horse is drifting one way or the other, or the horse is vertically tilting one way or the other, the indirect turn is therapeutic. In best practice training, both direct rein and the indirect rein pressures are intended to negatively reinforce the stance phase abduction of the foreleg contralateral to the intended direction.

Following the initial training of the rein signals, the horse learns to discriminate the shift in the rider's position as he turns his shoulders towards the new direction. These postural signals are conditioned stimuli that have been acquired secondarily through the process of classical conditioning. Some trainers also use leg signals to turn, or use leg signals concurrently with rein signals. Both of these present difficulties for the horse. The first is difficult in terms of discrimination, as there are other responses elicited by the legs nearby (e.g. go, sideways and canter). The second is difficult because of signal salience – which signal should the horse pay attention to? One or both signals may therefore undergo habituation.

In foundation training, training the turn response begins with increased pressure on the single rein relative to the contralateral rein. The turn response is negatively reinforced until it is elicited from very light pressure. Usually, the trainer maintains somewhat less pressure on the opposite rein to prevent the horse learning the obvious yet incorrect response of bending its neck. When the horse has learned to turn from light rein signals, further shaping of the turn response involves training the horse to maintain its speed and step length, maintaining its line and straightness and maintaining a stable head and neck posture. Yet, more shaping occurs in dressage where the horse is trained to turn with lateral flexion (see Figure 8.23): the horse turns its head and looks in towards the direction of its turn and also tends to look down to some extent. For this reason, lateral flexion, along with longitudinal flexion, is a key component of training roundness and also being on the bit. Lateral flexion is facilitated by flexion of the cervical vertebrae at the atlanto-occipital junction, as well as C1, C2, and diminishing distally. When lateral flexion is consolidated as a shaped

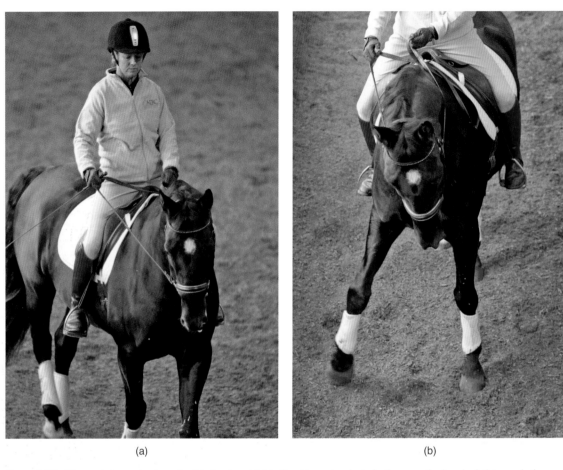

(a)   (b)

Figure 8.22 These photographs show the (a) direct and (b) indirect turn signals. In both cases, the hands shift towards the intended direction, but in the direct turn, the opening rein (moving away from the midline) is pressured, while in the indirect turn, the closing rein (rein moving towards the midline) is pressured.

component of the turn response, it is considered a precursor to what is known as lateral bend (described in Chapter 11, Biomechanics).

Typically, when horses shy, they suddenly change direction with their forelegs and this action is generally followed by a forward acceleration. Horses frequently learn to shy and these responses are then inadvertently negatively reinforced when the rider momentarily loses contact and position. Such reinforcement can be so powerful that features of the environment become salient and achieve stimulus control. So, placing the horse's direction under the stimulus control of the rider is of primary importance. While many trainers correct drifting by negatively reinforcing the

chosen direction using their legs, others prefer to use the reins. Because the forelegs are predominant in any alterations of direction (e.g. horses shy using their forelegs), it is preferable to interpret drifting primarily as a loss of stimulus control of the forelegs. At any rate, since losses of line are associated with losses of straightness (where the hindhooves no longer step into the foretracks), placing the forelegs under stimulus control is a vital component in shaping straightness of acceleration and deceleration responses.

Many movements have turn responses incorporated into them. For example, lateral movements such as leg-yield, half-pass, shoulder-in and pirouette in dressage, and side-pass in reining, all owe

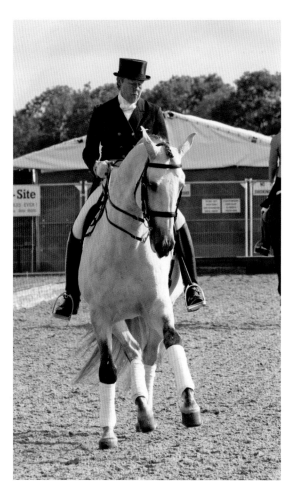

Figure 8.23   When the horse is moving on curved lines under-saddle in dressage, lateral flexion is required. This entails laterally flexing at the atlanto-occipital joint, as well as the joints surrounding C1, C2. A horizontal line across the nasal planum evenly bisects the curved line on which the horse is travelling. (Photo courtesy of Kyra Kyrklund.)

in order to establish consistent habits. For example, the horse may turn:

1. by abducting the forelegs first; or
2. by adducting the forelegs first; or
3. by turning the hindquarters and not turning the forelegs at all (This is by far the most confusing).

Another problem arises when horses make random turns in the form of drifting right or left during locomotion. On circles this is known as falling-in when the horse drifts out of the circle (see Figure 8.24). Other more subtle problems arise when horses abduct or adduct their forelegs asymmetrically. For example, during a turn right, the right foreleg abducts in swing phase and

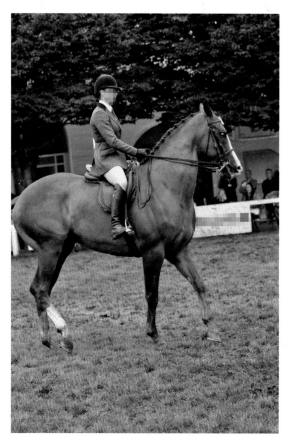

Figure 8.24   When the horse falls-in or falls-out, its head and neck are carried to one side, which becomes the concave side, while the horse drifts towards the convex side.

their quality in part at least to the correct training of turn responses. If the abduction in the swing and stance phases is not symmetrical, these movements can become poor and diminished or even appear lame. For example, if the swing phase leg is seen to lose its momentum or falter, the stance phase limb reciprocates and an unevenness of step occurs.

A number of problems arise as a result of incorrect training of turns. The horse may turn in three different ways, yet only one should be reinforced simultaneously the left foreleg abducts in stance phase. Any asymmetry results in losses of uprightness and balance where one foreleg deviates less than the other. Problems of this sort are most clearly evident in lateral movements, such as half-pass, where the horse may appear to travel sideways in small inexpressive steps or, worse, it may show alterations in rhythm that appear as lameness.

The (slightly) stronger the pressure on the turn rein, the smaller the circle becomes when the horse has learned proportional signal–response associations. Some trainers fortify the turn response using a single whip-tap on the outside shoulder at the beginning of its abduction in the stance phase just before the rein signals are issued. In this way, the rein response for turn can be classically conditioned in re-training.

Signals for turning the hindquarters and lateral movements

Under-saddle, turning the hindquarters without forward motion merges into going sideways when the horse is moving forward. Because the hindquarters largely drive the horse forward, they are not as involved in changes of direction as the forequarters; instead, they are involved in changing line. Therefore, training sideways movements begins with training the hindquarters to step to the right or left from a standstill (known as turn on the forehand). Then, when moving forward, this is transformed into what is known as leg-yield. In dressage, lateral movements that involve turns of the hindquarters include travers, renvers and half-pass (see Figure 8.25). Dressage requires that all lateral movements result in the horse going forward to some extent, but in other equestrian pursuits, such as reining, the horse may be trained to go completely sideways (full-pass) as well as sideways while going forward (side-pass). Clearly, in all sideways movements there is also an involvement to some extent of turning the forelegs.

Sideways movements are negatively reinforced by the rider's single leg. The discriminative stimulus is the light leg signal, which should coincide with the acquisition of an immediate response (McLean and McLean, 2008). Further shaping of sideways movements involves the horse persever-

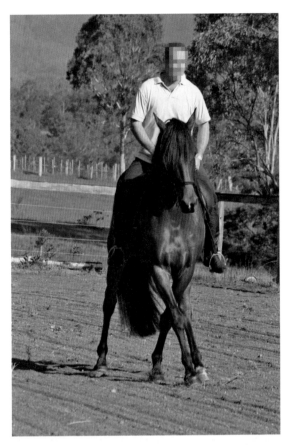

Figure 8.25 During lateral movements (including side-pass in reining), the sideways movement is conferred by consecutive abductions and adductions of the forelegs and hindlegs. To maintain balance, abduction of the forelegs can occur only during adduction of the hindlegs when the horse is going forward.

ing in going sideways and maintaining a consistent line. In dressage and reining, the postures of the horse's head and neck are also shaped.

Like turns of the forequarters, turning the hindquarters is conferred by consecutive adduction and abduction of the hindlegs. Adduction may occur first or second at liberty, but in dressage and reining, adduction is required before abduction, which is the opposite of the forelegs. Horses are not inclined to abduct the forelegs while abducting the hindlegs – this would present a significant balance problem. So, if abduction occurs in the forelegs, this is accompanied with adduction of the hindlegs and vice versa. When turning the hindquarters to the left, the right hindleg adducts in the swing phase while the left hindleg adducts in the stance phase. The amount of adduction required in equestrian sports is a function of the amount of sideways movement required. Half-passes and full-passes require that adduction occurs to the extent that the hindleg crosses the contralateral hindleg at the hock, whereas most lateral movements prescribe a lesser amount of crossover.

The typical signal for the sideways movement of leg-yield is light pressure of the rider's single leg. Generally, this single-leg pressure is applied farther behind the girth than the normal go signal (about 10–15 cm/4–6 in). However, some trainers simply train sideways from the application of a single leg signal at the same place as the go signals. The horse's resultant struggle to discriminate between these signals emphasises the importance of rider position and training. The correct moment to issue the leg-yield signal is at the onset of the swing phase of the leg contralateral to the direction to which the horse is moving.

Problems in sideways show up like problems in turns of the forelegs. The rider may have inadvertently reinforced abduction rather than adduction as the first steps of sideways, or the adductions may be asymmetrical, resulting in losses of uprightness of the hindquarters and shorter uneven steps.

Sideways movements can be fortified by the use of the whip-tap on the horse's hindquarters. Because the whip-tap is also a signal, it is important that the horse learns to respond to the whip-tap on the hindquarters alone so that it effectively fortifies the sideways reactions. When horses have habituated to the sideways signals and, thus, fail to respond sufficiently, the signals can be re-installed by classical conditioning where the leg signal is applied and contiguously followed by the whip-tap.

Other signals

The rider's seat as a signal

It is generally accepted that once signalled to respond, the trained horse should 'go on his own'. However, it is unrealistic to expect that the horse would go on ad infinitum without any signals. This is where the rider's seat has an important function: in *maintaining* the response. In the absence of stimuli to maintain responding in the horse, riders would have to rely on continuously eliciting the correct response. If they did this by 'nagging' with their legs, problems would begin to arise in the form of habituation and conflict behaviours. The same is true for any constant use of signals where associated responses are not forthcoming. For example, riders often click with their tongues incessantly, which dilutes the negative reinforcing effect of those signals, or they may overuse the term 'good boy' or other verbal praise which, if not connected to a primary reinforcer (e.g. food), diminishes the value of the praise as a secondary reinforcer.

The principle of training the horse to persist in its responding of speed, direction and posture is widely known and is embodied in the concept of 'self-carriage': the correctly trained horse should maintain his speed, line and head/neck outline without constant signalling from the reins or rider's legs. While the seat *follows* the movements of the horse's back in each gait, it is also associated with them. Through associative learning, the horse learns that when it does not align with the rider's seat, a leg or rein cue will follow. So, the horse learns to maintain the characteristics of its movement because of learned associations with the seat.

Because the horse's back moves in a distinct way in each gait, the rider is obliged to move his or her seat slightly differently in accordance with the defining characteristics of each gait. If the rider's seat is slower, faster, shorter or longer in its action than the movement of the horse's back, then the horse's locomotion is disturbed. For example, in the walk, the seat 'sweeps' forward and back as well as dipping a little forward at the most forward point as the horse's belly swings from one side to the other. When the walk is longer the seat movement is longer, and when the walk is short the seat's excursions are also shorter (Figure 8.26).

Similarly, during rising trot, if the rider increases or decreases the magnitude of the rising, then the horse's mobility is affected. Finally, if the rider's seat is not centrally balanced or if during the rising trot the rider lands in the saddle in different places, the horse's rhythm may be disrupted. On the other hand, if the horse randomly and disobediently

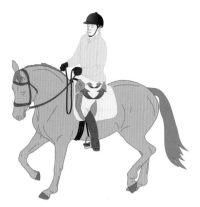

Figure 8.26   The rider's seat shows different characteristics with different gaits and stride lengths. For example, it has a long sweeping motion for longer strides (green arrow) and moves only a small amount for shorter strides (blue arrow).

alters its own rhythm or tempo, but the rider's seat remains in the original rhythm and tempo of a particular gait, then the horse is likely to resume the correct tempo. For this reason, the action of the rider's seat is a chief focus of equestrian coaching. The correctly moving seat of the rider in each gait provides a unique signal that can be operantly conditioned, to some degree, to maintain the locomotory activity.

During rising trot on a circle, equitation theory prescribes that the rider rises as the outside foreleg begins the swing phase and the seat intercepts the saddle at the start of the stance phase (see Figure 8.27a,b). This loads the diagonal pair of abducting outside foreleg and adducting inside hindleg with more weight and lightens the inside foreleg to facilitate turning.

At canter, the rider's seat 'sweeps' forward and back maintaining the tempo and stride length of the canter by lengthening/shortening or quickening/slowing the seat. There is also a lateral dipping of the seat towards the leading foreleg at its moment of maximum reach. This results in a slight asymmetry in the rider's seat movement that reflects the asymmetry in the gait itself. The seat is lighter in jumping because the rider's feet in the stirrups support more of the weight than in non-jumping equitation. In addition, the jumping rider may have a more forward-leaning upper body posture to counteract the shorter stirrups and greater accelerations.

The rider's seat is considered an important source of signals. If we were to rate the operant pressure-based signals according to their salience, we would note that signals issued to the horse's mouth have the highest degree of salience, because this is the most sensitive tissue, followed by signals issued to the horse's back and sides. Furthermore, the rider's legs are against the horse's sides, whereas the saddle and cloth separate the rider's seat from the horse. One would conclude that the horse's back receives more dispersed signals as a result of the presence of a saddle and a cloth,

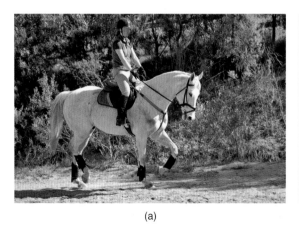

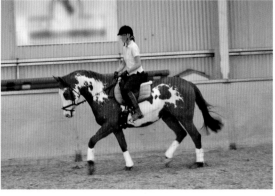

(a)   (b)

Figure 8.27   During the rising trot (i.e. when the rider rises within the beat of the trot), optimal balance is believed to occur when the rider rises (a) and falls (b) as the outside forelegs and inside hindleg undertake their swing and stance phases. Correct equitation involves refining this synchrony.

than the ribcage does from the rider's legs (see Figure 7.13, p. 119). This dispersion plus random and accidental alterations in weight and pressure from the rider in the various gaits (which vary according to skill level) make the seat a difficult cue to train and maintain in consistency. Thus, a considerable degree of habituation to the seat signals may occur for all but the most elite riders. The consequential effects on the horse's perception of seat cues means that a tiny rein signal would be as salient as a strong seat signal. Therefore, when a rider's feels that he or she is using his or her seat rather than the reins (especially with the lever effect of a curb bit), he or she is probably unaware of the differential perception of these signals by the horse. This is demonstrated when the reins are released and the horse is signalled to stop with the seat alone: in most cases, the horse will show no response or a diminished response to the seat. As signals for inter-gait and intra-gait responses, therefore, seat signals are most likely to be used in conjunction with subtle leg or rein signals. Nevertheless, in situations of optimal rider skill, it is plausible that small adjustments to the rider's seat can be perceived as signals.

Western horses show powerful downward transitions from the seat alone where the reins are entirely looped. These horses are ridden in curb bits with a high degree of lever action (see Chapter 10, Apparatus), so negative reinforcement is enhanced by a high degree of aversiveness. By classical conditioning, the seat becomes the discriminative stimulus and comes to elicit such responses by itself. The aversiveness of the curb rein also determines how long the seat remains a distinct discriminative stimulus without fortification from the reins. Clearly, when the operant conditioning is powerfully reinforced, a relatively benign discriminative stimulus achieves a high degree of salience.

Gait signals

Generally speaking, the signals for the upward and downward inter-gait transitions are the prolonged signals of the rider's calves and reins, respectively: they are similar to the signals for quickening and slowing but are of greater magnitude. These stronger signals are derived, logically, from the signals for faster or slower, since each upward

gait involves the legs going faster by around 20 beats per minute. Typically, the greater the speed change, the stronger the signals. So, a halt to trot signal is similar to but stronger than a halt to walk signal. The upward inter-gait transition to canter involves the same type of prolonged signal, but it also has a unique signal and preparation because it is an asymmetrical gait with leading and trailing forelegs and hindlegs. The leading leg is said to be on the inside because cantering and galloping quadrupeds universally tend to ensure that their leading forelegs are on the inside of their curved line. Therefore, the rider's signals are:

1. light signal of the inside rein;
2. inside leg in the normal position (girth region);
3. outside leg a few centimetres behind the girth (see Figure 8.28).

The inside rein is the preparation and the outside leg is the cue to canter (although some trainers cue it with the inside leg). Remember that the single rein is in fact the primary turning signal (see Signals for turning the forelegs, above) and should have stimulus control of the same-side foreleg. For canter, the inside rein signal stimulates lateral flexion (an integral component of turn). The turn rein signals the leading leg, as the leading leg is associated with the turn. In some methodologies, the presence of the rider's outside leg behind

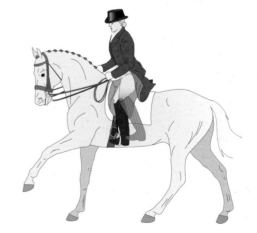

Figure 8.28   The canter is an asymmetrical gait characterised by leading foreleg and hindleg. The signals for canter require indicating to the horse the appropriate leg to lead with, and this is made possible by the altered outside leg position (further back).

the girth serves as a signal in conjunction with the seat in maintaining cantering.

Canter to canter (flying change)

One of the later gait change signals the horse learns is for the flying change. When changing lead from canter, the first leg to initiate the new canter configuration is the horse's *outside* hindleg; the change occurs following the period of suspension. For this reason, the fundamental signal for the flying change is the rider's outside leg. The difficulty for novice riders attempting their first flying changes involves the timing of exactly when to apply the signal in the ephemeral suspension phase. This is a good example of the utility of the school horse in enabling riders to learn more complex and precise aspects of equitation.

Horses are often reluctant to change from one leading leg to another under-saddle. This is partly because it is common to train counter-canter (where the leading leg is the outside foreleg) before flying changes (see Figure 8.29), and this unfortunately necessitates inhibiting flying changes to a greater or lesser extent. To train flying changes, some trainers use counter-canter on a small circle (perhaps only 15 m in diameter) to motivate a flying change as a result of the difficulty and effort of counter-canter on small circles. Others may use lateral movements, such as half-pass, towards a wall to motivate the change and still others use a pole on the ground where the horse canters over the pole and the change is signalled at the take-off stride before the pole. The whip-tap on the outside hindleg can more effectively replace the rider's outside leg in the event that it fails to elicit a change or the change is 'late behind' (the hindlegs change after, rather than at the same moment as the forelegs).

A canter is distinct from a gallop not only for differences in speed but when the uni-diagonal pair of legs separates to two individual leg beats while still retaining the moment of suspension. There is no specific signal for the gallop, partly because this moment of conversion from canter to gallop is not easily recognised. In some languages (such as French), there is no distinction between the words for canter and gallop. The prolonged pressure of the rider's legs in the canter configu-

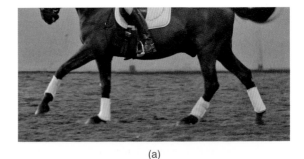

(a)

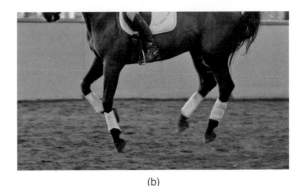

(b)

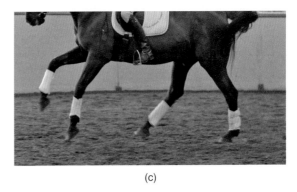

(c)

Figure 8.29   When the horse does a flying change (of leading leg), all four legs alter from leading/trailing to trailing/leading (a and c) during the moment of suspension (b). Skill is required to successfully elicit this at the optimal moment.

ration is the signal for the increased speed of the gallop.

Movements

When horsepeople fully grasp the profound significance of the four basic responses of go, slow, turn and sideways, they quickly appreciate that

Table 8.4   The basic responses that produce the movements in dressage

Movement	1st response component	2nd response component	3rd response component	Timing of signals
Shoulder-in	Direct rein turn forelegs	Indirect rein turn of forelegs (including bend)		One step apart
Travers	Indirect rein turn of forelegs	Turn hindlegs		One step apart
Renvers	Indirect rein turn of forelegs			One step apart
Half-pass	Shoulder-in components	Turn hindlegs		One step apart
Pirouette (walk and canter)	Shorten stride	Turn forelegs	Turn hindlegs a small step	One step apart
Piaffe	Shorten	Lengthen		Within the stride
Passage	Shorten	Lengthen		Within the stride

the so-called 'higher movements' consist of two or more of the four basic responses in a specific sequence (see Table 8.4). Therefore, once the basic responses are properly trained, the horse is generally able to perform at least a single step of a movement. Following this, the movements themselves require gradual shaping so they progress from a step to a stride and so forth. It follows that when movements fail, trainers should go back to repair faults that will be evident in the basic responses. The critical importance of separating the delivery of the signals when training or eliciting the higher movements cannot be overemphasised because of the possibility of confusion and negative welfare implications. Every composite movement in equitation is optimally elicited by closely spaced yet separated single signals. This separation coincides with the sequence of the various leg movements, diagonal pairs and different gaits surrounding the movements. For such reasons, the higher movements are the province of experienced and skilled riders. Also, only an experienced and correctly trained horse can respond to such closely spaced consecutive signals.

In an advanced horse, two signals can occur within a single step, provided they are separate enough to be salient. The closest that signals can be brought together is at the beginning and halfway through a single step. For example, in piaffe training, trainers may signal the horse with the go signal at the correct moment (when the hindleg begins its retraction in the stance phase) and then, halfway through that step, signal the horse to shorten so that the opposite diagonal couplet that are protracting in the swing phase are shortened.

That maximal proximity also applies to passage. For other movements, a cascade of signals is given at least a single step apart.

Some movements have precursors, for example, half-pass is a movement that involves a number of components. The horse has to go sideways, but with the added features of bending and laterally flexing into its turn direction, and leading with the foreleg. Thus, the half-pass is traditionally trained subsequent to the movement known as shoulder-in. Shoulder-in itself is a single step of direct turn followed by the indirect turn in which lateral flexion and bend are added as well as the laterally moving forelegs along the wall. So, the establishment of shoulder-in sets up the leading forequarters, bend and flexion. With these characteristics, the only additional signal that the rider is required to issue for the half-pass is the sideways signal of the outside leg.

In training all movements, trainers should recognise the importance of the principle of the exclusivity of signals (Chapter 7, Applying learning theory) and attempt to evaluate their training and deconstruct movements to their base components. They may then find that tension, hyper-reactive behaviours, dullness or conflict behaviours that appear in their work from time to time will disappear.

Higher steps – collection

It is generally recognised in dressage circles that the collected outline is not something that is trained per se, but is an emergent property of the process of engagement where the hindlegs step one hoofprint closer to the forelegs, which is first seen in transitions such as trot to halt. This causes lowering of the hindquarters during intra-gait transitions. German riding traditions describe this quality with the term *durchlässigkeit*, which translates as *thoroughness:* that quality in a horse that permits the signals (primarily the rein signals) to influence the hindlegs (USDF, 2002). Here, the desirable response is that hindlegs participate in slowing the horse by reaching forward to grip onto the ground more, which also lowers the hindquarters. In the development of collection, the steps of the horse are shortened, the poll raised and the steps become higher. Piaffe and passage also develop from shortening but raising the stride of the collected trot.

Piaffe, being on the spot, represents the ultimate collection of the trot, whereas in passage, the horse moves forward with shortened higher steps than the collected trot (see Figure 8.30). Piaffe also differs from passage and collected trot in that it has no period of suspension (German National Equestrian Federation, 1992). As the musculoskeletal system of the horse adapts to the stresses of the progressive biomechanical features of lowering the croup, the horse's physique alters as its topline musculature becomes more pronounced and its movement develops cadence: a rhythmic pause at the highest and lowest points of the step.

Take-home messages

The information summarised in Tables 8.2 and 8.3 serves as a virtual training 'tool box'. Horse-training is considered optimal and most likely to succeed when trainers:

- target a discrete biomechanical action such as retraction, protraction, abduction and adduction;
- use easily discriminated signals;
- use a separate signal for each response;
- use the operant contingency correctly;
- place the horse under the stimulus control of the handler/rider, not the environment;
- reinforce the first correct or near-correct response;
- gradually shape the response by adding one quality of a response at a time;
- reinforce transitions and movements using a variable schedule of positive reinforcement;
- disassociate from all training any expressions of flight response beyond that required for the gait.

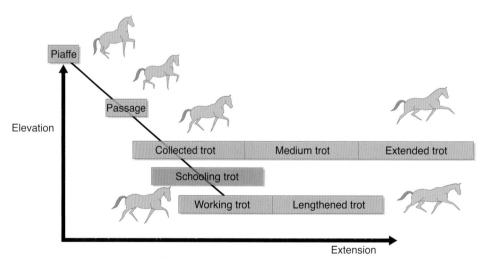

Figure 8.30   This graph shows the increased collection and simultaneous shortening of the stride as the horse becomes more educated towards piaffe.

Ethical considerations

- The whip and spurs should be used only to make signals more precise and not as punishment, or, in the erroneously held belief that they serve to make the horse attend to a preceding signal.
- The enforced use of curb bits in FEI dressage and reining competitions directly reduces horse welfare and should be reconsidered.
- Particular attention and care should be given to shaping the rein responses because there are more conflict behaviours associated with rein responses than with the rider's leg responses.

9 Horses in Sport and Work

Introduction

Every sporting discipline or field of work creates a different set of challenges for the horses involved; as well as the breeders, trainers, grooms and riders. This chapter not only explores the attributes of horses that excel in each of these contexts but also examines the way in which the application of learning theory can be customised to each discipline. Likely sources of conflict are also described for each discipline and the lessons to be learned from a particular pursuit are discussed (see Table 9.1).

A number of significant changes in the rules and structure of organised horse sports have emerged in response to concerns for horse welfare. For example, arduous elements of eventing prior to the cross-country phase have been removed chiefly because of concerns about horse exhaustion. It will be interesting to see how welfare concerns shape the future of some of these sports. Certainly, Equitation Science is poised to contribute substantially to the debates that surround any proposed changes.

Performance sports

Dressage forms the focus of many discussions throughout this book and so will be given only brief coverage here. The word 'dressage' comes from the French 'dresser' – to train (animals). With an emphasis on accurate execution of standard tests, dressage demands that all the horse's locomotory responses are under stimulus control. The subjective judgment of dressage leaves it open to criticism from both competitors and some scientists. Furthermore, since points can and should be deducted for a perceived lack of submission (although we encourage you to consider whether, to gain marks in this domain, the horse has to *submit* to signals or simply *respond* to them) and signs of resistance, it is not surprising that some elements of the welfare lobby are setting their sights on dressage. Practices during the warm-up, including hyper-flexion, have come under sustained surveillance and some criticism because they fail to align with what is considered acceptable in the competition arena itself (see Figure 9.1).

The problem here is that if the competition is all about training and producing inherent equine athleticism on demand, any training practices that fall outside the traditional appreciation of a powerful horse bearing a rider are questioned. It is possible that there may be some biomechanical benefit from hyper-flexing the neck, but if the horse cannot sustain this position without rein pressure, the practice is not likely to be wholly beneficial. From an ethological viewpoint, relentless pressure leads inexorably to all sorts of problems, not least

Table 9.1   Summary of the ethological and learning challenges offered by various sporting and working contexts

Work or sport	Ethological challenges	Learning and cognitive challenges
Dressage and equitation	Showing display behaviours out of context	Discriminating between physically similar pressure cues from riders
	Suppression of signals to conspecifics	Learning to respond to stop and go signals that are almost simultaneous
Show-jumping	Jumping obstacles that they would naturally go around	Learning to ignore novel colours and structures. Sizing-up on-approach unseen obstacles for both their height and width
		Learning to retain clean jumping style even when they have learned that fences fall when hit
Eventing	Combinations of the above two rows with speed and stamina	Combinations of the above two rows plus balancing the demand for boldness, fitness (for the jumping elements) with steadiness (for the dressage)
Racing on the flat (thoroughbreds, quarterhorses and Arabians)	Socially facilitated hyper-reactive responses	Maintaining learned response when fatigued or response is impossible
		Responding to jockey preceding and during flight response
Steeple-chasing and hurdling	As for all forms of racing (see above). Arriving at a fence simultaneously rather than with self-selected companions	Traversing obstacles and landing on unseen terrain. Learning to jump cleanly in gallop and when fatigued
	Socially facilitated launching at fences	
Harness racing (pacing and trotting)	As for all forms of racing	Learned inhibition of upward inter-gait transition (to canter).
		For pacers, if not inherently gaited, the need to modify 2-beat gait to lateral couplets within the constraints of the hobbles
Endurance	Entering unfamiliar areas	Combining attention to the rider and the novel challenges of the environment
	Sustaining speed despite fatigue	Also, remaining calm can represent a challenge to some horses, especially Arabians, most of which are predisposed to reactivity
		Negotiating entirely novel terrain
Gymkhana and mounted games, including tent-pegging, polo and polocrosse	Being among conspecifics that often travel at speed but in different directions	Learning the significance of various items of apparatus that cue 180 degree turns, changes of leg and abrupt halts
Stockwork, cutting and campdrafting	Approaching other herbivores at speed	Learning to take cues from both the cattle and the rider
		Anticipating the movements of the bovine protagonist
Reining	As for any horse working in isolation	Discrimination of classically conditioned positional cues from rider
Hunting	As with steeplechasing	Learning to remain under stimulus control despite socially facilitated cues that can prompt bolting

Table 9.1 (*Continued*)

Work or sport	Ethological challenges	Learning and cognitive challenges
Driving	Tolerating constant unseen auditory and physical presence to the rear. In teams (multiple configurations), there is a potential for socially facilitated bolting	Habituating to carriage and other pressures on the body while remaining responsive to rein and voice signals Reliance on rein tension as the chief means of communication by the human. Learning to maintain gait and rhythm without persistent cues
Breed and hack classes	Remaining calm in company, a challenge exacerbated by hyper-reactivity triggered by conspecific displays and high-energy diets	Responding to cues from riders, some of whom may be unfamiliar (e.g. judges who ride) and handlers in novel contexts
Side-saddle classes	As for all breed and hack classes (see above)	Learning to respond to unilateral leg pressures from rider when sitting to the side and then resuming responses in normal (astride) riding
Rodeo	Repeated anti-predator responses	Learning that the process is finite Unrelenting pressure from belly strap
Police work	Approaching humans who are behaving unpredictably	Sustained habituation to multiple, random cues as found in crowds. Learning to recognise those physical stimuli that come only from the rider
Horses in mining	Barren environment	Learning to respond to auditory cues from the handler and discriminate them from incidental conversations. The absence of a peripheral view (because of being in a tunnel) and of any depth to visual field (because of being in the dark)
Trail riding	Sometimes walking in single file in an enforced, rather than natural order	In hired horses that are exposed to many changes of rider, learned responses are likely to be fewer Navigating novel terrain

habituation, and the tendency for the horse to begin to travel with its neck too short. At elite levels, the rules of competitive dressage require that riders wear spurs and use a double bridle even though absolute lightness is valued in principle. These apparent contradictions are explored in Chapter 15 (The future of equitation science).

At the outset of training, **show-jumping** relies on the rider being able to make horses jump on cue. After that, most trainers expect a talented horse to use the obstacles themselves to gauge an appropriate take-off point. For responses to be predictable, they must be under stimulus control. Of all the critical qualities that must be under the rider's control, we propose that speed and line are paramount in show-jumping. The informed rider takes the opportunity to walk the course and map out the number of strides between obstacles, the take-off and landing spots for each fence and, as necessary, where time can be saved. All of these judgments contribute to success in show-jumping, in addition to a rider knowing his or her horse's idiosyncrasies (e.g. which jumps they are likely to be unfamiliar with or wary of).

Horses have evolved to skirt around ground-based obstacles and only jump if they have no other option. Jumping obstacles for sheer joie de vivre has not been recorded in free-ranging horses. In the domestic context, loose jumping (jumping without a rider) can give the illusion of the horse

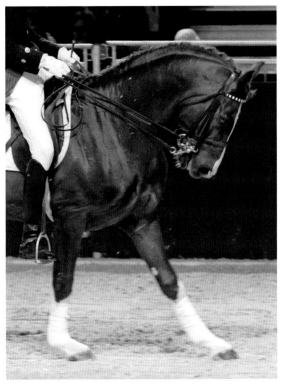

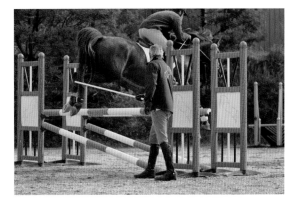

Figure 9.2   A horse about to be rapped.

Figure 9.1   A horse being hyperflexed. (Photo courtesy of Julie Taylor/EponaTV.)

exercising a choice to jump, but we should never overlook the effects of guiding rails, arena walls, jump-wings and the trainer's whip. That said, we *may* be breeding horses that are less fearful to the extent that some happily jump if there is a jump in front of them. Breed-specific data on this possibility would be extremely valuable.

When training horses over fences, trainers are giving horses opportunities to learn what they are capable of. This involves training them at slower speeds or gaits such as trot, as well as variables such as increasing the jump height and its appearance. According to the principles of shaping, it makes sense not to change more than one variable at a time when training. While gradual shaping is the goal, over-facing horses by failing to observe a gradual increase and instead presenting them with obstacles that are too high is a real possibility. Horses that run out have sometimes learned to do so because the rider turns the horse away after coming to a halt at a fence. Both the halt and the

turn away are reinforcing (see Chapter 8, Training). It is highly likely that the horse will repeat this response in future, even if it involves some pain in the mouth and sides as the rider attempts to suppress the response. Loss of line and subsequent steering failures also contribute to these evasions (see Chapter 13, Fight and flight responses and manifestations).

Jumping clean, rather than brushing the top rail with forelegs and hindlegs, is highly valued and is sometimes trained by a particular method of avoidance learning known as 'rapping' (see Figure 9.2). This involves an assistant striking the legs from a ventral angle as the horse crosses the top pole. The horse has committed to jump a certain height and then pays a price. It is struck whether or not it hits the pole. Rapping trains the horse to overcompensate at the zenith of its trajectory by jumping higher than it might have learned to do otherwise. This practice is banned by the Fédération Equestre Internationale (FEI) on welfare grounds, and is discussed further in Chapter 12 (Unorthodox techniques).

A popular way to train show-jumpers is to sensitise them to very light leg pressures and put them in a mildly controlled flight response. Keen show-jumpers often seem to have habituated to a holding rein and this may be why their riders seem inclined to change bits often or use more severe bits to give them the feeling of a more controlled power. Proponents say they want the horse to 'draw' to the fence, so if they release the reins the horse will go a little bit faster, even though this acceleration is minimal. They say that horses jump better this way than when in perfect self-carriage in terms of rhythm and tempo. In the light of this approach and the horse's adoption of a mild flight response, you can see why during training show-jumping riders prefer to use a running martingale more so than in other sports, such as dressage. This is because when the horse shows a mild flight response it tends to raise its head and become hollow in the back. The martingale tends to keep the head lower. One of the drawbacks is that the sensitivity to rein tensions required for slowing and turning can deteriorate if the reins are used for head-carriage but not slowing.

You have to wonder what might be going on with horses described as 'loving their jumping'. These horses do not maintain the rhythm and speed set by the rider's signals. Instead, they are under stimulus control of the fence itself, so they require few leg signals from their riders. By maintaining a tighter grip on the reins, riders usually end up detraining the stop response. The horse no longer responds to the more subtle signals of the reins because it has become habituated to a constant pressure. Horses may approach fences at increasing speed and give the impression of keenness when, in fact, they are simply rushing. Training horses to be under stimulus control of the rider's rein, leg and seat signals is an important feature of a well-trained jumping horse (McLean, 2005a). It is likely that these horses have experienced some pain from either the rider's hands or from hitting the top rail and then learned to run away. From this, they soon perceive the fence as stimulus for acceleration.

Horse trials or eventing, as it is sometimes known, combines the precision and obedience of dressage with the scope and athleticism of show-jumping and the stamina and so-called boldness of the cross-country phase. This combination emerged from military riding schools as a test of all-round obedience. The level of feeding and fitness required for successful performances in the cross-country phase can lead to horses that are highly reactive. This constitutes a serious challenge in the dressage phase.

Welfare concerns about horses injuring themselves on the solid fences of the cross-country course (see Figure 9.3) prompted a modification of fences in FEI competition. More technical fences (such as arrowheads and apexes) intended to test

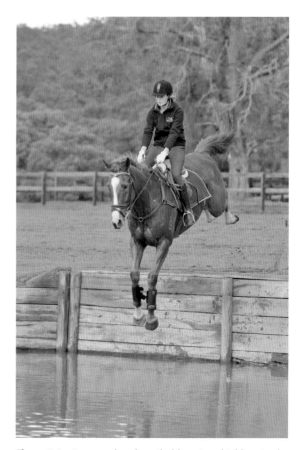

Figure 9.3 Eventers that show 'boldness' are highly prized.

accuracy also served to slow horses down. So, modern courses are characterised by these challenges rather than just big galloping-on fences. Frangible pins have been added so that jumps collapse on substantial vertical impact. All of this has led to a decline, in turn, in the popularity of rangy thoroughbred types in favour of Warmbloods.

The problem of solid fences is pivotal for the sport because the rider knows (better than the horse) that the fences are potentially lethal. This means that the rider's confidence and ability to ride according to his or her plan rather than the horse's immediate preference is largely what is being tested. Fence design will most likely continue to be moderated until fatalities of both riders and horses cannot be reduced any further without the discipline becoming a form of long-distance show-jumping. It is worth emphasising that despite extensive debate about rider deaths in eventing, the effects of course design and the demands of time limits, insufficient focus has been given to training the horse to maintain its speed and be under stimulus control by the rider. In contrast to horses that are under stimulus control, those that rush at solid fences and take off when in erratic speeds are at risk of flipping over the fences.

Racing

At first glance, traditional thoroughbred racing appears to be all about speed. But, most notably in non-sprint races, checking speed during the race is an integral skill if there is to be some energy left for the finish. Training the racehorse to accelerate at gallop and in the presence of other horses is a critical skill, but it must also be trained to decelerate from light signals in order to manoeuvre during the race. Some horses are said to be field-shy in that they are disinclined to enter a cluster of galloping horses or sometimes to gallop close to others. So, the acceleration and deceleration responses must be trained almost unconditionally to be under the stimulus control of the rider. Similarly, if the horse turns more poorly one way compared with the other (or if it turns poorly both ways), it will tend to drift. Drifting in racing is called lugging and, though very common, it has deleterious effects on speed. The resultant drifting as a result of poor steering tends to increase the distance to be covered, shorten the gallop stride and tire the horse. Lugging creates accusations of interference with other horses. This tendency is likely to be predisposed in horses with an innate motor or sensory bias to the left or the right (McGreevy and Rogers, 2005) and begs further study.

Around turns racehorses are biomechanically inclined to using their inside lead, for example, using the left lead stride pattern when running anticlockwise around a track (Adams, 1979). On straight sections of the track, where they can lead with either leg, they show a preference for one stride pattern over the other unless injured or fatigued. A study of thoroughbreds, Arabians and quarterhorses racing in the USA, where horses race around an oval racetrack in an anticlockwise direction, showed that 90% preferred their right lead stride pattern and 10% preferred the left (Williams and Norris, 2007).

Heterogeneous features in the surfaces used for racing can cause limb injuries (Fredricson et al., 1975). Most horses lead with the right leg when cantering and galloping to the right (i.e. in a clockwise direction; McGreevy, 1996), but fatal injuries on US racetracks are more likely to involve the left limb (Peloso et al., 1996). In any epidemiological assessment of this sort, it is critical that the direction in which horses are raced is factored in. Any lateralisation seen may not necessarily be an effect of training to work in one direction, since kinematic differences between the left and right limbs have been reported in 8-month-old standardbreds that have yet to be trained (Drevemo et al., 1987). Nevertheless, training and racing can influence asymmetries since it has been shown that, when moving around a turn, thoroughbreds strain the outside forelimb consistently more than the inside forelimb (Davies, 1996). This may reflect the extra abductive and retractive power required of the outside limb in canter and gallop on curved lines.

Most racehorses in training have little opportunity to canter (or gallop) in one direction spontaneously (i.e. without a rider) because they are stabled or kept in training pens that deny them the space to pick up sufficient speed to canter. However, prior to training and whenever they are turned out to pasture, they may demonstrate such a bias. Since the direction of racing for gallopers varies from track to track and state to state in many countries, including the UK, the USA and Australia (e.g. counterclockwise in New South Wales and clockwise in Victoria), and also from country to country (e.g. counterclockwise in Singapore and clockwise in Hong Kong), the relationship between motor biases and competitive success and wastage through injury may be important. The screening of individual horses for left and right motor bias may allow trainers to select horses more carefully for racing or other work. For example, horses with a left preference when grazing may be more efficient or faster in a race on a counterclockwise curve.

Preparing racehorses focuses chiefly on cardiovascular parameters, but physiological conditioning may be of no avail if behavioural conditioning is neglected. It is important to acknowledge that having horses' locomotory responses under clear stimulus control translates into effective acceleration. This demands that all riders must deliver acceleration signals (chiefly those from the legs and whip) effectively. They must not stop applying pressure until the correct response emerges, and stop when it does. Teaching personnel about learning theory would enhance racing success. While leaving the starting gates at speed is an important feature of a successful racehorse, simply increasing arousal in anticipation of the start is counterproductive. There is compelling evidence that horses that *lose* races tend to be more aroused and require greater control in the parade ring/mounting yard than winners (Hutson, 2002). Conversely, the calmer a horse is before the race, the more it will perform to its potential. For example, horses that are difficult to load into starting stalls are likely to perform far more poorly than their cardiovascular indicators at home have suggested (see Figure 9.4). It is recognised that nervousness in the parade ring may be a consequence of poor leading responses (McLean, 2003), so training to walk in-hand can have a significant impact on performance. Some of the more important dependent variables are summarised in Table 9.2.

The social dynamics within a group of racing horses have yet to be explored. Do they jostle for the lead? Or, do they jostle for safety? It is unlikely that horses have evolved to want to lead the herd, given that this is a vulnerable position that exposes them to potential threats. Understanding the cognitive aspects of horses during racing informs us about what is meant by the 'will to win' (see Figure 9.5). Perhaps thoroughbreds have been selected to be reinforced for running for its own proximate benefits over and above leading. Or perhaps it is a characteristic of horses in general to find running reinforcing. What does the finishing line represent to them? It is likely that with repetitions, horses learn to 'know' something about the finishing line, given that the rider changes his or her behaviour immediately after crossing it. That said, it seems unlikely that horses have evolved to have a concept of such a goal. How does this align with the evolutionary advantage of outrunning a predator or a conspecific during play?

It is important to recognise that current selection pressures in breeding only partially reflect those that created the original breeds. The modern show ring is the only environment in which conformation prevails in importance. Historically, breeding for different types of work would have placed more emphasis on behavioural tendencies than on

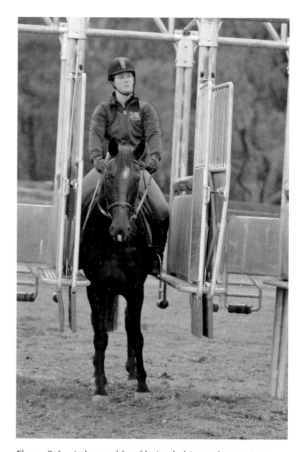

Figure 9.4 A thoroughbred being habituated to starting stalls.

conformation. There is some evidence of links between morphology and neural tissue (Evans and McGreevy, 2006), a finding that may predict behavioural tendencies. Selection for work shaped the horses considered typical of many breeds. We propose that, generally speaking, equine trainability and ease-of-habituation are characteristics that negatively correlate with each other. The horse that habituates rapidly becomes insensitive to pressure signals and therefore fails to discriminate between cues that differ only slightly in their location or intensity. These horses are not likely to excel in dressage or indeed most performance sports but may have a place as mounts for novices, assuming that they do not habituate to bit pressure and become unstoppable.

The hyper-reactivity of thoroughbreds is beyond dispute. They have been selected almost entirely for speed and the tendency to respond

Table 9.2   Some of the features of a racehorse's behaviour and presentation that can be used to predict poor performance (i.e. not winning)

Location	Variable	Extent to which this variable predicts poor performance
Stalls	Weaving and repetitive head movements	********
	Kicking	*****
	Pawing	**
Saddling enclosure/parade ring	Crossover (figure-of-eight or grackle) noseband	********
	Gaping mouth	****
	Twisting neck	***
	Nose roll (sheepskin noseband)	***
	Third metacarpal bandages	***
	Other bandages	**************
	Pacifiers (meshed eye protection)	**
Mounting yard	Slow gait	********
	Fast gait or circling	*****
	Bucking	*****
	Balking	****
	Courtship behaviours	***
	Ears pointing laterally or aborally	**
	Defecating	**
	Flicking ears	*
Track	Late	********
	Conflict behaviours	****

Source: Adapted from *Watching Racehorses*, with kind permission of Geoffrey Hutson.
Asterisks are used to depict the extent to which each variable predicts poor performance.

to the opening of the starting stalls and stimuli (hands, heels and whip) from the jockey. This is why thoroughbreds, in general, are not considered safe carriage horses. Imagine the weekly human death toll that would have been associated with using such a reactive breed in the shafts of horse-drawn vehicles.

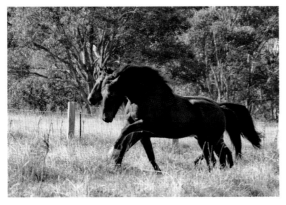

Figure 9.5   It is interesting to speculate whether horses have any concept of racing.

While some breeds are more reactive than others, some diets further increase reactivity (most notably in foals; Nicol *et al.*, 2005). These are the diets most often fed to the most reactive breed of horse, the thoroughbred. The mixture of breeding and feeding contributes to most of the dangers associated with racehorses. The other factor is social facilitation. One horse's flight response can trigger a flight response in conspecifics. From the authors' long-term experience in legal cases, the thoroughbred seems to have aggregated a larger human toll than any other breed.

Steeple-chasing and hurdling

When raced over fences, thoroughbreds are favoured for 'boldness' or 'bravery'. Outstanding steeple-chasers or hurdlers could alternatively be labelled 'oblivious to danger' or 'having a poor sense of self preservation'. Perhaps this reflects habituation or the horse learning that the threshold of aversiveness for environment is lower than the signals from their backs – so they go where they are pointed. As if jumping fences at speed is not dangerous enough, there is the additional challenge of jumping among a large gathering of other horses. This creates a further hazard: social facilitation on approach to a fence can trigger a premature leap, with horses landing on top of a fallen or falling horse or rider. In Australia, this dangerous tendency is called 'half-lengthing'.

Harness racing (pacing and trotting)

The relative calmness of standardbreds reflects selection not only for different gaits (trotting and pacing) but also for steadiness in a horse that is to be worked in **harness**, an aversive set of stimuli that may equate to being chased from behind. The calmness of standardbreds reflects the selection of horses that are sensitive enough to accelerate easily but do not run readily when being chased. This lowered flight response makes standardbreds great trail horses, especially suitable as beginner mounts. The pace is innate for some horses (e.g. Icelandic horses) but can be acquired by others. The progeny of pacers almost always pace, whereas only some 20% of the offspring of trotters are innate pacers (Cothran *et al.*, 1987).

The use of blinkers and sheepskin nosebands (see Figure 9.6) in racing and harness racing is interesting from a technical perspective since the wearer may be less distracted by lateral and ventral stimuli and the ground, and perhaps even its own forelegs. Reduced distractibility, at least in the first few outings, may not always equate with calmness, and it remains to be seen whether these devices are always calming. Given the high incidence of claustrophobia among horses, the reduced ability to maintain surveillance might be potentially threatening. Or perhaps, in this case, 'out of sight' *is* 'out of mind'.

Other forms of racing

Racing in other breeds, such as Arabians and quarterhorses (originally developed for stock work and now represented in both reactive racing and unflappable pastoral lines), follows the same training strategies to achieve swift acceleration and

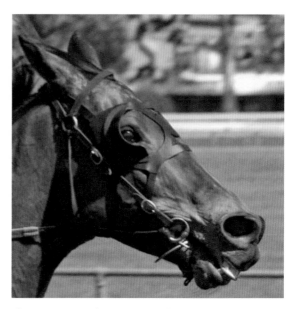

Figure 9.6   A racehorse wearing blinkers to modify its flight response and reduce distraction by other horses. (Photo courtesy of Sandra Jorgensen.)

straightness in response to pressure cues and shares a focus on producing young sprinters. This provides a platform for an interesting ethical discussion. The emphasis on youthful performers is fuelled chiefly by the industries that seek to encourage breeding by valuing the next great star, rather than longevity in individual horses. A high turnover of racing horses is in the interests of the breeding industry. However, if veteran races attracted significant prize money, there would be greater incentives to keep horses sound for longer, resulting in enhanced welfare for the racing population. Horses would not be rushed into racing as early as possible, which would allow more time to be spent in foundation training (breaking-in) young stock, an outcome that would probably make retired racehorses more useful and valued as riding horses.

In the case of **endurance racing**, the need for stringent welfare controls was accepted almost from the outset. Riding horses to exhaustion would never have been considered a sport and so veterinary checks (gates) are a fundamental element of the sport. Successful competitors select and produce horses that recover quickly from the physiological load that long-distance work

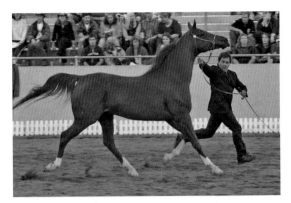

Figure 9.7   Arabian horse showing a big trot that is a characteristic of an endurance horse. (Photo courtesy of Julie Wilson.)

creates. Enforcement of the rules governing the sport does a great deal to prevent unsuitable and poorly prepared horses being entered for competition, but even at the highest level horses can succumb to exhaustion (EFA, 2003). And although riders in other equestrian sports may say that the gaits of the endurance horse are not ideal (a big trot is preferable to a slow canter for endurance horses; see Figure 9.7), the horses engaged in endurance riding seem to have a long working life.

Has this left us with ethical double standards when we compare traditional racing with endurance racing? If racing codes were emerging for the first time in the present day, what steps would be taken to ensure horse welfare? Would riders be allowed to whip horses that simply could not respond because of fatigue? These questions are explored further in Chapter 14 (Ethical equitation).

Mounted games

Polo and **polocrosse** have emerged from the ancient traditions of Chinese, Persian and Japanese mounted ball sports and the equally ancient pursuits of 'buskashi', involving the mounted dispute over decapitated goat carcasses (by Pashtuns) or the Tibetan tradition of hitting a recently bludgeoned muskrat. They rely on considerable horsemanship and balance because the rider must be able to lean out of the saddle, wrestle other rid-

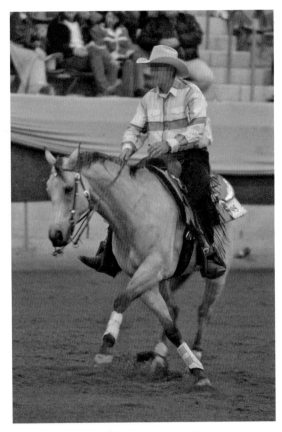

Figure 9.8   Neck-reining turn. (Photo courtesy of Julie Wilson.)

ers and execute hairpin turns at great speed all the while aiming to obtain or retain the team's possession of the 'ball'. From the horse's perspective, the challenges in this sport are considerable. Strong signals from the rider, and severe bits and bridles are commonplace. In addition, neck reining can lend itself to potential confusion (see Figure 9.8) on the part of the horse if the two rein signals (contralateral neck pressure and ipsilateral rein tension) are applied concurrently. The challenge for the discerning rider is to ensure that only one rein signal is given for the turn response. A single rein signal can be delivered with far greater clarity. Through a process of habituation this means that signals tend to get stronger. Against this backdrop, many polo stables exercise horses (as many as four per mounted rider) in-hand simultaneously. This may maintain cardiovascular fitness and may even have reinforcing properties for the horses if they

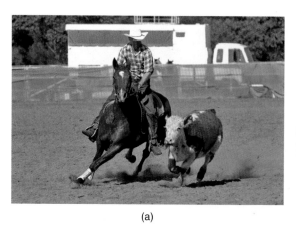 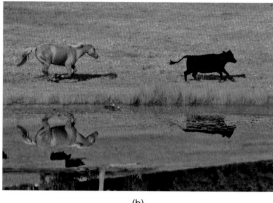

(a)   (b)

Figure 9.9   (a) Camp-drafting. (b) Cow sense is an innate trait found in some stock breeds, such as the quarterhorse. (Photos courtesy of (a) Julie Wilson and (b) Nic Ward.)

are a stable social group but does little to maintain shaped responses. The wastage in polo and, to a lesser extent, polocrosse is significant but it is more likely a product of trauma than behavioural issues.

Games such as **gymkhanas** and **mounted games** organised by pony clubs are designed to foster horsemanship and develop riding skills with far lower potential for confusion, habituation and trauma than the adult versions of mounted games: polo and polocrosse. Sometimes the ability to deliver signals with clarity is thwarted by the specific challenge of the activity but, as with the military and mounted police tradition of tent-pegging, the ability to maintain control of the horse while riding with one's centre of gravity to one side of it is highly valued.

Stock sports

The uniquely Australian sport of **camp-drafting** (see Figure 9.9a) similarly has a history based on utility in cattle farming. Camp-drafting involves separating (cutting out) a calf from a group and moving it into a small yard, called a *camp*, herding it through gates and around pegs in clockwise and anticlockwise directions.

The turns are facilitated by neck-reining but there is an added complication from other animals – the targeted calf and its herd-mates. The genetic trait of some horses to show 'cow-sense' (target,

chase and show agonistic behaviour towards an errant bovid) is a fascinating phenomenon (see Figure 9.9b). In Africa, however, it is not uncommon to see equids, such as zebras, chasing wildebeest, so this predisposition may possibly exist in the genome of the horse. It would be interesting to see what other behavioural traits are linked to this tendency and whether they can be harnessed for more traditional activities (see Figure 9.10). Could cow-sense, for instance, be associated with boldness in jumping or even in work as a police horse?

Reining competitions are now recognised by the FEI and can be seen as the western American version of dressage. With its voltes and sorties (which evolved from bull-fighting), reining is said to reflect the status of dressage at the end of the Middle Ages, the period in which Spanish conquistadors took equitation to the Americas. There is arguably more self-carriage in western riding than in modern dressage since the rein contacts are lighter. It carries with it the same theoretical requirements for training reliable responses to subtle signals in self-carriage. As the sport matures, it will be interesting to see how Equitation Science develops technologies that assist in the refinement of training and improvement of welfare.

Hunting

The use of horses in hunting has undergone some fundamental changes over the years because of the

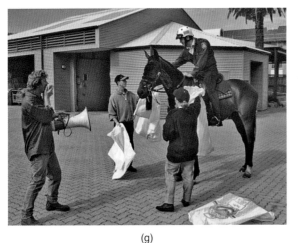

(g)

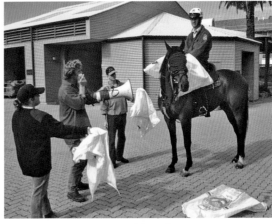

(h)

Figure 9.13   *(Continued)*

or a loud noise, is introduced to the horse when it is stationary, or by over-shadowing. Only once the horse appears to have acclimatised to the changed conditions, is it prompted to respond to simple, established signals (e.g. walk and halt) under the novel circumstances that are fabricated. The horse thus becomes habituated to responding despite the new stimuli. Further potential distracters are introduced in the same manner, until the horse is able to work in a wide range of situations.

The use of horses in **tourism** includes trailriding and carriage-driving in urban contexts. With **harness** horses, long working hours have a critical effect on the availability of water and food while at work. As with all horses working in urban contexts, those that have been hand-fed by passers-by are at risk of learning to nuzzle hands and pockets for food and, if not muzzled, may eventually become so-called muggers or even biters. Hard surfaces underfoot also predispose horses to concussive musculoskeletal disease such as ring-bone (Higgins and Wright, 1995). Providing shelter from sun and precipitation is important for horse welfare but overwork and the prevalence of poorly fitting harness are perhaps paramount.

Ponies used underground in **mining** activities were said to take some time to adjust to the light and to moving stimuli when brought back above ground. Blinkered, and often stabled underground, for months on end, they were not used to

seeing much other than miners, ponies and the occasional rat.

The exposure of trail-riding horses to incompetent riders is a concern for both welfare and behavioural reasons. Typically, their go, stop and turn responses are poor but they tend to have deeply ingrained following responses based on an ethological tendency to remain in the social group. Poor timing and failure to provide relief from pressure are likely to lead to habituation and the emergence of conflict behaviours. Clearly, hired horses are high risk for trialling undesirable responses and developing behaviour problems. The extent to which they can be remediated and indeed spared abusive handling depends largely on the frequency and quality of any supervision by the hirers and their staff. Operators who allow horses to be ridden without supervision place their horses at risk of inappropriate training that can amount to abuse.

Conclusion

The breadth of equestrian sporting activities and ways in which horses have been made to work for us serve to emphasise the species' tremendous behavioral flexibility. The qualities of breeds that specialise in various domains include their ability to meet the particular ethological, cognitive and learning challenges that these activities present.

Take-home messages

- Negative reinforcement is used in all examples of the horse at work and in sport.
- Despite the enormous variety in horse sports and equine work, only four basic responses are required of them all: stop, go, turn the forequarters and turn the hindquarters.
- Foundation training these basic responses allows horses to be trained with a customised plan that is specific to the discipline they are intended for, but also means that they can be re-trained for secondary work when their first career is over.
- Behavioural conditioning (improving the responsiveness) of racehorses is often overlooked in pursuit of cardiovascular fitness.

Ethical considerations

- Welfare is a reflection of usefulness, so should more emphasis be placed on ensuring that sport horses are under stimulus control?
- Should sentient beings be exposed to complete novices who are not simply learning to ride but are also learning to balance?
- Can competitions that use horses (and therefore aversive stimuli under a negative reinforcement framework) ever reward welfare above all else?

Areas for further research

- Evidence of communication among horses competing as a group has yet to be explored.
- Will an on-board device that measures fatigue and exhaustion ever be developed for riders to use and competition judges to check?

10 Apparatus

Introduction

The horse is as behaviourally flexible as any of the domestic species. This means that it tolerates sub-optimal conditions and so makes itself vulnerable to welfare insults. For an animal that has evolved to spend up to 16 hours a day grazing in the open and to expend considerable effort to avoid becoming trapped, the consequences of confinement and restraint for our convenience can be profound.

This chapter examines the various techniques and devices we use to contain and restrain horses. It asks how Equitation Science can be used to explain the effects of these traditions and innovations. It explains how Equitation Science can question items used solely because of tradition, and also highlights potential problems in training that emerge from the use of force rather than behavioural conditioning.

Stabling and feeding

We stable horses for our own convenience: it makes them easy to catch and keep warm and clean. But stabling obliges us to hand-feed. Dried foods are favoured because they are easy to store and transport, and concentrated cereals deliver nutrients in a form that more than meets the working horse's needs. Most horses bloom in coat and condition when fed at above their maintenance requirements and many show judges are quick to reward owners who present animals with unhealthy amounts of subcutaneous fat (see Figure 10.1). Unfortunately, many young horses are routinely overproduced to give the impression that they are well-grown for their age. The emergence of young horse championships in many disciplines also encourages levels of growth and training that may be too advanced and rushed.

Unfortunately, high-energy feeding can also trigger oral stereotypies, gastric ulceration and hyper-reactivity and, if feed is not reduced in anticipation of a smaller workload, some horses may be predisposed to develop exertional rhabdomyolysis (Valentine *et al.*, 1998). Explosive energy under-saddle often aligns poorly with training goals because calmness underpins clarity during response acquisition. Confinement in a stable is far removed from the horse's natural environment of cursorial grazing. Stabled horses can become so excitable when they emerge from confinement that they are prone to injure themselves in a frenzy of activity known as the post-inhibitory rebound (Figure 10.2). Although we struggle to measure it, many horses seem to find pleasure in exercise (Kiley-Worthington, 1987) and can find physically restricting environments stressful.

When mares confined for urine collection were released after six months in standing stalls, they

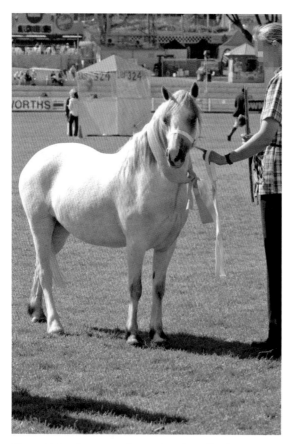

Figure 10.1   Show animals are often clinically obese yet, in the show ring, their owners are frequently rewarded for creating this condition. (Photo courtesy of Sandy Hannan.)

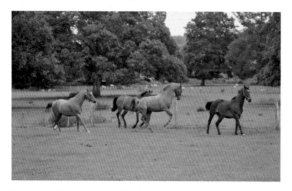

Figure 10.2   After periods of confinement and overfeeding, horses show a post-inhibitory rebound of locomotory responses.

showed a post-inhibitory rebound in locomotion (Houpt *et al.*, 2001), indicating that they were compensating for exercise deprivation in the same way that crib-biters show more of the behaviour after a period of deprivation (McGreevy and Nicol, 1998). So the heightened motivation for movement and indeed general activity (Mal *et al.*, 1991) can translate to unusually athletic manoeuvres and some injuries when confined horses are turned out. In addition, confined youngsters have less dense bone, and this may predispose them to pathological fractures and other harmful effects on the musculoskeletal system, which is generally in poor condition as a result of confinement (Bell *et al.*, 2001; Hiney *et al.*, 2004).

Confinement reduces spontaneous exercise, normal sensory stimulation and access to preferred conspecifics. It also imposes relative darkness. Horses in a dark stabled environment have demonstrated a preference for a lighted environment by learning to turn on lights by means of an operant device (trial-and-error conditioning; Houpt and Houpt, 1989). Being at pasture may be sufficiently enriching to account for data showing that training takes less time in pastured horses than in stabled horses (Rivera *et al.*, 2002). We know that horses make good associations with stables because that is where they are fed. Their inability to assess the long-term consequences of confinement is revealed by their willingness to enter stables for short-term gains. The same might be said of their decision to enter a float (trailer) that brings with it the added aversiveness of being on a moving platform. Indeed, anecdotal evidence suggests that even after they have endured traffic accidents in floats that have upturned, some horses still enter a new float seemingly willingly.

Apparatus used to distribute and apply pressure to horses

A range of saddlery items (tack) are discussed in this chapter, but this does not imply that the authors necessarily approve of their use or suggest that they are humane. Some might just as well appear in Chapter 12 (Unorthodox techniques). Our approach to the following discussion of equipment in horse-training assumes that the reader is conversant with learning theory (as described in Chapters 4–7).

Welfare is compromised by excessive pressure from apparatus. Pressure is a measure of the force exerted over a surface area and is usually expressed in Pascals (Pa) or pounds per square inch. For example, the pressure of the rider and saddle is the combined weight divided by the area of the horse's back they are in contact with. Therefore, with any piece of tack, the broader the area that touches the horse the less discomfort it causes and the less rewarding is its removal. In essence, all pressure-based training places the horse in a discriminatory dilemma. It has to respond to some pressures while habituating to others. When the pressures to which it must habituate are too great, the horse receiving them may be at risk of learned helplessness. Specific attributes of the interface between the human and the horse that can also compromise welfare include bits made of twisted or longitudinally ribbed (so-called bladed) metal or chain.

Saddles, treeless saddles, saddle pads, girths, cinches and surcingles

The premise of a saddle is twofold: to support the rider's position and to distribute the rider's weight across the musculature on either side of the horse's thoracic midline. The tree (rigid or semi-rigid framework) within a traditional saddle prevents the rider's weight from pinching the horse's back.

The still-evolving design of saddles remains purpose driven. The traditional 'selle a piquer' held the rider firmly and deeply in one place with his or her legs descending ventrally directly as they do in a modern dressage saddle. Earlier saddles from Spain and also American western riding saddles prompt riders to adopt a so-called chair seat in which the rider's legs are carried forward. They place the rider so that he or she sits on the horse's back, whereas in dressage the rider's weight goes directly down to the seat-bones and then to the feet. Jumping saddles have knee rolls that provide a forward buffer and are designed to be ridden with short stirrup leathers that tend to place the legs forward again. Racing saddles are tiny (weighing as little as 280 g) and the current trend,

regarded as dangerous by some observers, is for stirrups to become ever shorter.

Saddle-fitting is becoming more scientific as pressure-detection technology becomes more refined, which has allowed humans to meet the needs of the horse for comfort during its athletic work. However, the more padding a saddle includes, the greater the potential loss of what is known as 'feel'. The more widely the rider's weight is distributed across the horse's back, the less easily discriminated by the horse are precise signals from the seat.

Saddle pads are used to give unbalanced young riders rudimentary support, but they offer no protection to the horse's back. Treeless saddles are undergoing something of a renaissance because, without any rigidity, they are thought to be less likely to pinch. However, they may be less likely to support the rider's weight as successfully as a well-fitted traditional saddle and so may be seen as inadequate for performance sports that involve jumping and the high-speed descent of the rider into the saddle on landing. Ideally, treeless saddles will undergo rigorous empirical comparisons with traditional and cutting-edge designs (such as the so-called canti-levered saddle that flexes at the pommel) using pressure-detection technology to determine how the rider's weight is distributed at various gaits.

Saddles are now available with a wide variety of types of padding and even pneumatic cushions. In some instances, the angle of tree can be adjusted to suit horse backs of different widths, a potential boon to owners of horses that fluctuate in weight with the seasons. Straps prevent saddles from slipping: girths around the thorax, surcingles for both saddle and thorax, cinches or cinch-straps for the abdomen, breast-plates for the base of the neck and pectoral region and cruppers for the tail-head. If any of these are too tight or in contact with damaged or highly sensitised tissue, counter-predator responses may ensue (e.g. girth-shy horses are described in Chapter 13, Fight and flight responses and manifestations).

Bits, bridles, reins and nosebands

The horse's mouth never evolved to accommodate a bit and there is no convenient space in the buccal

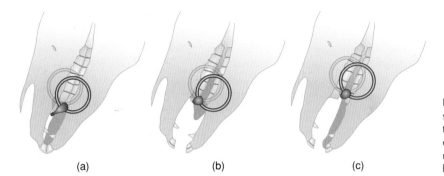

(a)   (b)   (c)

Figure 10.3 Fluoroscopic studies have revealed where the bit lies: (a) in the normal case; (b) when the tongue is retracted; and (c) when held between the molars.

cavity waiting to be filled by one. When the tongue is depressed by a bit, it does not fit in the narrow inter-mandibular space, so many bits press the tongue against the bars of the mouth (see Figure 10.3). Fluoroscopic studies show that the bit rests on the tongue, rather than the bars of the mouth, as was originally believed. The regular snaffle bit is designed to apply pressure broadly across the tongue and, some believe, also the upper palate. Jointed bits tend to form a peak as tension increases in the reins; these are said to have a nut-cracker action across the tongue and into the upper palate. In contrast, double-jointed snaffles are thought to reduce the tendency for the joint to travel dorsally when the reins are under tension (Clayton, 2005). Proponents claim the shape of the entire bit aligns better with the internal mouth shape. The tongue normally fills the oral cavity, so the bit sits on it but can easily press up on the bony, hard palate. When the horse relaxes the muscles of the tongue, the bit can simply indent the upper surface of the tongue. This relieves any bit pressure against the palate (Clayton, 2005). Certain types of bits may be associated with a reduction in swallowing frequency (Manfredi *et al.*, 2005) possibly by restricting the movements of the tongue necessary in deglutition.

The multiplicity of bits now on the market strongly suggests that bit designs are used to overcome training and performance issues, many of which probably reflect some deficits in training or riding.

Horses can be easily trained to pull against harnesses, breast-plates and collars in contact with well-muscled areas, such as the shoulders and pectoral regions, but are reluctant to fight pressure from bits in the mouth (especially if they touch only in small areas, as in the case of thin, bladed and twisted bits). When used only occasionally, chains in the curb groove or in the mouth are likely to have a strong effect, especially in the short-term. Bridles and bits of different basic design contact only small anatomical sites and the severity of their action is described in Table 10.1. It must be emphasised that the severity of action depends on various physical features of the equipment, such as tightness of the curb chain, the thickness of the bit and the length of shanks (see Figure 10.4).

Unrelenting pressure from a bit can prompt a horse to trial evasions (as described in Chapter 13, Fight and flight responses and manifestations). Unorthodox bits apply pressure with greater severity or to different parts of the mouth. Even though they can, and sometimes do, sever the tongue (Rollin, 2000), saw-chain bits (so-called mule bits and correction bits) are readily available to riders unable to produce a response in their horse with a milder bit.

In some equestrian cultures, hackamores and bosals are the preferred means of controlling the head; in others, they are used more often when traditional bits have proved ineffective. If changing or increasing mouth pressure is unsuccessful, riders and trainers may resort to an alternative or additional means of making the horse adopt the desired shape by applying pressure to other parts of the head. Typically, other 'training' devices employed include curb bits with chains, gags, draw reins, side reins, balancing reins and chambons

Table 10.1 The anatomical sites of negative reinforcement in which bridles and bits of different basic design can act. The severity of action (implied by the degree of shading) would depend on various factors, such as the tightness of curb chains, the thickness of the bits and the length of shanks

	Lips	Tongue	Bars of the mouth	Roof of the mouth	Ventral mandible	Nose	Cheeks	Poll
Head-collar/halter								
Bitless bridle								
Dually halter[a]								
Hackamore[b]								
Bosal[b]								
Unjointed snaffle								
Jointed snaffle								
Running gag[c]								
Dutch gag								
Curb bit without curb chain				*				
Curb bit with curb chain[d]				*				
Bit and bridoon								

[a] Increases the effectiveness of a standard halter by additional pressure on the maxillary and mandibular regions.
[b] Works outside the buccal cavity, by compressing the nose and/or mandible.
[c] The aversiveness of the bit is increased by pulling it towards the ears.
[d] Transforms bit into fulcrum, thus increasing its aversiveness.
*Depends on the presence of a joint.

(see Figure 10.5). Such devices generally use first-class levers that amplify the tension on the rein as a result of their lever action and so can create a misleading impression of mildness (see Figure 10.6). The length of the shank magnifies the leverage through the bit. Unfortunately, the tendency is to develop a reliance on these extra pulleys, rather than to use them solely for re-training.

Most naïve horses respond to humans as they would to a predator. They move away bodily or posturally to avoid physical or psychological pressure. While successful modification of these basic evasive responses can produce a highly responsive equine performer, inappropriate modification can make horses useless or dangerous. Horses that resist by fighting or ignoring pressure cues are often subjected to increased pressure via mechanical restraints and stimulants. However, as we have seen, horses rapidly habituate to aversive stimuli, so reaching for more severe bits is ill-advised and may lead to further desensitisation.

The perceived need in some equestrian sports to force horses into an 'outline' and make them work 'on the bit' can prompt trainers to use stronger

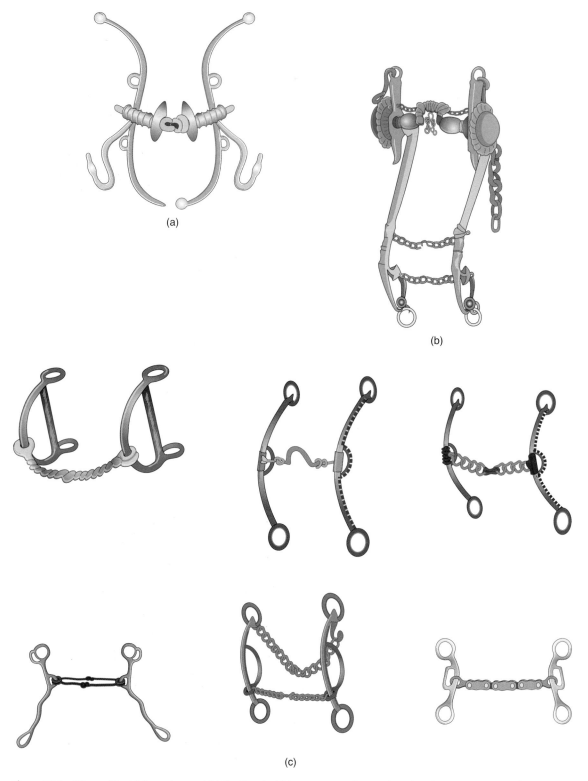

Figure 10.4   Bits used by (a) Xenophon and (b) the Classical Masters were at least as brutal as the most severe modern designs (c).

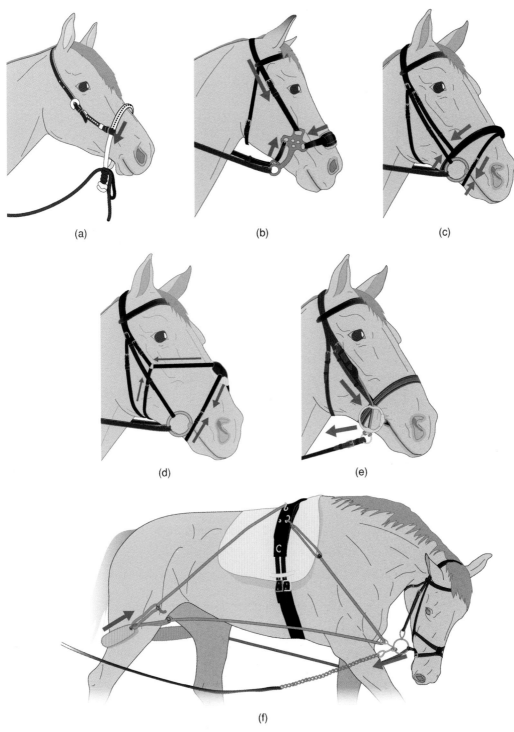

Figure 10.5   The action of various items of head gear (arrows show the direction of pressure). The illustrated items are: (a) Bosal; (b) Hackamore; (c) Flash noseband; (d) Figure-of-eight noseband; (e) Gag; (f) Pessoa.

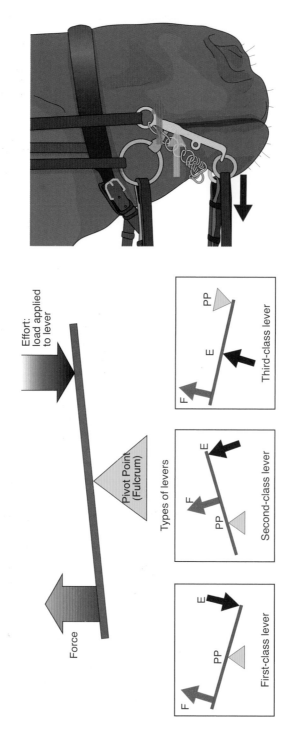

Figure 10.6 The classification of levers depends on the position of the pivot point or fulcrum and the direction of effort and force. The curb bit and chain act as a first-class lever that compresses the tongue and mandible, thus magnifying the horse's pain with little extra effort by the rider.

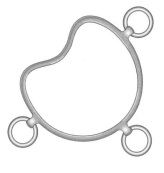 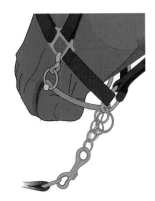

Figure 10.7   A rearing-bit with an inverted port bit presses the tongue onto the bars of the mouth.

bits as their first approach to achieving what is known as direct (or vertical) flexion. In contrast, enlightened trainers recognise that where aversive stimuli fail to elicit the desired response and begin to cause behavioural conflict, the application of more force should be avoided. Rather than applying a more severe bit, they aim to sensitise the horse to light pressures and to shape qualities such as a rounded outline as part of the training of stop and go responses.

When horses open their mouths to evade the bit, one short-term response by riders and trainers is to use a noseband that keeps the mouth tightly closed. Clearly, this does nothing to help the horse relax its jaw and is likely to act as an additional stressor. The same criticism can be levelled at tongue ties, since they restrict normal movement of the tongue such as during swallowing and also stop the horse finding comfort. As equestrian sports became more popular and competitive in the 1970s, dropped nosebands gave way to Hanoverian, crossover and grackle nosebands. Then in the 1980s, 'crank' nosebands emerged. These have an added feature: they can be tightened much further than regular nosebands due to a lever action. This highly aversive action seems to sensitise the horse's mouth, making the horse much more responsive to rein pressure and, to some, this gives the appearance of the horse becoming more 'submissive'.

Cheek pieces may prevent the bit from being pulled through the horse's mouth and equally may make turning pressures on the lateral aspect of the horse's lips clearer to the horse. Rearing-bits (also known as the chifney or stallion bit) also

have this feature but are generally thinner and have no joint; therefore, they have a more severe action than riding bits, such as a regular snaffle. The action of an rearing-bit presses the tongue against the bars and, not uncommonly, may cut the tongue itself (see Figure 10.7). Most rearing-bits have an inverted port in the middle and this is the most controversial feature of the bit as it drives the tongue into the cavity where it cannot fit and thus severely onto the bars of the mouth.

Rearing-bits without a tongue port work on the bars of the mouth rather than the tongue itself. Used correctly, these help to control particularly reactive animals such as naïve youngsters and fractious stallions that may readily toss their heads and stand up on their hindlegs. Again, the emphasis should be on using light pressure (so that the least amount of pressure creates the maximum effect) and, of course, the pressure must be released after every correct or near-correct response. These bits must never be used in attempts to punish a horse (e.g. by reefing on a lead rope).

Reins

The weight of the reins contributes to the neutral tension of contact. It has been suggested that reins long enough for long-reining may habituate horses to bit pressure simply because they are heavier than the reins used during riding (Warren-Smith *et al.*, 2007a). Equally, simply because of the distance the rider is from the horse, long-reins reduce the rider's ability to feel the horse's mouth.

The reins may act as a discriminative stimulus, too, so the feel of them against the neck can pre-empt turning. When turning, the outside rein can be drawn medially against and across the horse's neck to help train the neck to remain straight during turning. When it comes to turning, different disciplines apply pressure differently to the bit. In some sports, horses are trained to turn through such a neck-reining technique where the outside rein presses against and over the neck.

The reins used in reining competition are necessarily heavy so that they hang away from the horse's neck when not applying pressure to it. Long riding reins hang redundantly from the withers and are sometimes used to trigger forward motion by striking them across the horse's shoulder. Using the reins in this way (where one side is struck more than the other, often as a function of the handedness of the rider) can train a horse to travel in other than a straight line.

The breadth of the bit that has contact with the mouth (or other part of the head) and the action of any levers will also affect the way rein tension is translated to the horse. But bitless bridles are not necessarily a panacea for horses, since they rely on negative reinforcement (and therefore the horse's motivation to remove the pressure) as much as any bitted bridle and may sometimes lack the ability to deliver the clear lateral pressure needed for turns, tending instead to tighten on the horse's head before effecting a turn. They do however, avoid oral conflicts. It is, therefore, important that when equitation scientists report studies of rein tension, they must specify the dimension and design of the gear used.

Side-reins, martingales and tie-downs

Side-reins (see Figure 10.8), martingales and tie-downs that apply pressure to the nasal planum via the noseband (in the case of the standing martingale and tie-downs) or the mouth via the reins (in the case of the running martingale or draw reins) prevent evasive raising of the head (see Table 10.2). The rider can use the lever action of the running martingale to pull the head lower. Critics rightly point out that these gadgets force the horse into an outline rather than train self-carriage through lightness. Rather, when the head is forced down-

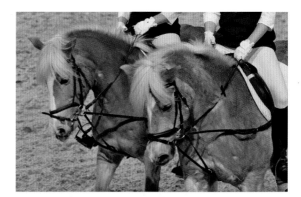

Figure 10.8   Side reins and draw reins are used to coerce the horse to adopt a rounder outline, compromising the stop/slow response. (Photo courtesy of Minna Tallberg.)

wards, the muscles of the neck and topline are not 'suspending' the head and neck but, instead, the horse is attempting to raise its head against aversive pressure. We know this because as soon as one releases the reins on a horse with a device such as a martingale on, it raises its head immediately. Gadgets that fix the head position deny the horse's need to move its head forwards and backwards in the walk and the canter, which consequently become stilted.

The position of the horse's head and neck is pivotal in balance and so the effect of the martingale on locomotion should not be underestimated. Standing martingales should never be used for jumping but running martingales may be justified in the case of racehorses that toss their heads vigorously when literally fighting for their heads and may, in the process, hit their jockeys in the face.

The straps between the rings and girth on a running martingale and the noseband and girth on a standing martingale can be tightened to the extent that the horse is forced to carry its head in a low position, receiving negative reinforcement by lowering its head. These devices defeat any attempt to achieve self-carriage and, because the horse rapidly adopts a new posture that riders become accustomed to, they are rarely dispensed with. If this device is to be used at all, the length of the straps of a running martingale should be adjusted so that they engage only when the poll is extended vertically.

Standing (fixed) or running martingales should not be confused with Irish martingales that simply

Table 10.2 The sites in which various devices are attached. The severity of action (implied by the degree of shading) would depend on various factors such as the tightness of nosebands, the length of straps and the inclusion of elastic

	Ventral girth	Lateral surcingle	Bit	Noseband (upper)	Noseband (lower)	Reins	Browband/ crown piece	Gaskin
Side reins[a]		▨	▨					
Draw reins[a]	▨		▨					
Standing martingale	▨			▨				
Running martingale	▨					▨		
Chambon[b]	▨					▨	▨	
Market Harborough[c]	▨					▨		
Pessoa[d]		▨						▨
Dropped noseband					▨			
Hanoverian noseband (including grackle, figure-of-eight, crossover)				▨	▨			
Crank noseband				▨	*			

[a]Used by trainers who prioritise outline before lightness and rhythm. At best, these devices use negative reinforcement to arch and shorten the neck and give the impression of correct training, but they force the wrong muscles to carry the neck, which usually results in a contracted neck.

[b]Uses negative reinforcement to train the horse to lower its head, thus reducing hollowness or hyper-reactivity and facilitating rounder topline. Possibly replicates postural calmness (see discussion in Warren-Smith et al., 2007b).

[c]Uses force to obtain head-carriage for trainers who struggle to obtain lightness and roundness with dorsal muscle groups.

[d]Causes intermittent pressure on the horse's mouth, from its hindleg action, to force it into a rounder outline.

*May include secondary lower strap.

join the reins under the horse's neck to reduce the chance of the reins falling over the neck and being trodden on.

Dentition and mouth pain

The horse's comfort, especially when ridden, can be profoundly affected by its dentition. Put simply, horses have not evolved to accommodate a bit (of whatever volume) in the mouth, so the intra-oral presence of the bit requires the tongue to move into a more-or-less abnormal position. This, and the need in some disciplines to maintain a contact, can reduce the horse's own ability to keep its cheek and tongue away from a sharp element of its dental arcade. The result is resistance (see Chapter 13, Fight and flight responses and manifestations) and a narrowing of the margin that represents neutral contact. In essence, the horse becomes more difficult to maintain in speed, line and posture.

Mouth pain may also be associated with heavy-handed riding or inappropriate gear. For example, some jointed bits can cause pinching between the second premolar and the labial commissures. Wolf teeth, especially those with loose roots and

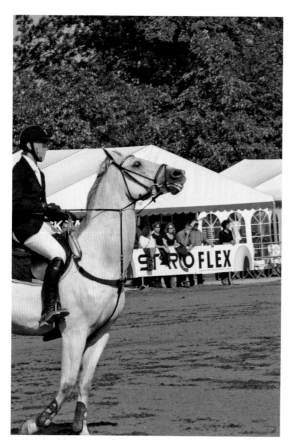

Figure 10.9   Horses often toss their heads upwards in an attempt to resolve inescapable mouth pain. (Photo courtesy of Julie Taylor.)

cusps that are directed towards the seat of the bit, may make the horse reluctant to accept the bit and may trigger it to reef the reins out of the rider's hands. This can rapidly escalate into head-tossing (see Chapter 14, Ethical equitation and Chapter 13, Fight and flight responses and manifestations; see Figure 10.9). The reinforcing nature of this activity seems obvious and is likely to be most profound if the rider usually yields. In the event of a horse fighting the bit, some veterinarians and equine dentists are prepared to remove an appreciable portion of the second premolar to create a 'bit seat' or 'cheek seat', which is supposed to improve comfort in this part of the mouth (Wilewski and Rubin, 1999). While one study reported improved athletic performance in most horses after the creation of bit seats (Wilewski and Rubin, 1999), an abiding question is whether a simple change of riding tech-

nique or bits (e.g. to an unjointed design) would have been equally effective.

Whips and spurs

If a horse fails to show sufficient forward movement or impulsion, trainers direct their attention to the sides where they can increase the pressure by using whips and spurs and more effectively send the horse forward (or, simply, away from the rider's leg). Although, for some, these stimulants are distasteful, they are not necessarily contraindicated. They can be introduced so that they can be used minimally and with accuracy to ensure consistency and be employed transiently to fortify the rider's leg signals. That said, whips fortify only if the horse has a clear learned response to the whip, so it is very useful to train the whip/go response without leg first.

Apparatus used in restraint

The practice and principles of physical restraint

Among veterinary professionals, physical restraint of horses (e.g. with twitches or hobbles) during painful procedures is often possible but rarely preferable to chemical restraint. This is legitimate, if the alternative is a brutal struggle or an opportunity for the horse to learn dangerous evasions. Fundamentally, force can escalate the aversiveness of the procedure and is ultimately likely to compromise the horse–human interaction and make the horse less compliant for future procedures. Numerous handling problems are the legacy of previous mistakes in timing and consistency. Others can have proximate causes in physical pathologies, so handlers should always consider seeking veterinary advice before embarking on any course of behaviour modification. For example, a horse that is reluctant to step backwards must be checked for back pain (referred or otherwise) or for specific problems such as wobbler syndrome (Moore *et al.*, 1994).

Once a flight response starts, most naïve horses when restrained by the head will continue to struggle until the pressure around it is released. This explains why horses should be tied up with a secure halter (or head-collar) and rope and never by the reins or a lead attached to the bit. The rope can be tied to a length of baling twine, which is attached to a solid object. Baling twine and quick-release knots will be safer if a struggle ensues because it will break or release more readily than regular lead-ropes and reins. However, there is a paradox here, because a quick escape is reinforcing for the horse so future struggles become more likely. A preferred approach is to first teach the horse to come forward from lead pressure, then tie its lead-rope to a car inner tube firmly attached to a secure point where the ground surface is safe. In those rare cases that the horse does resist, the inner tube acts like a strong hand.

Even if they are secured by so-called quick-release knots, releasing panic-stricken horses can be very dangerous, especially when more than one horse is tied up and motivated by socially facilitated hysteria. It is worth noting also that quick-release knots do not untie readily once they are under pressure and, in such cases, bowline knots are preferable. Tying horses at nose height maximises normal head movement within the limits set by the length of rope, which should be short enough to prevent the horse putting its leg over the rope and long enough to allow the horse to turn its head to examine objects that would otherwise be in its blind spot. Horses will work to remove themselves from the threat of discomfort. The danger of horses fighting against physical restraint by blindly paddling their limbs in pursuit of freedom means that hobbles and ropes as means of restraint should be avoided wherever possible. Rope-burns and even fractures can result from roping, strapping and hobbling techniques, even under conditions of best practice.

Roping techniques used to pacify horses during aversive interventions are described exhaustively elsewhere (e.g. Waring, 1983; Fraser, 1992; Rose and Hodgson, 1993). Generally, these have been superseded by chemical agents since there is no justification for allowing horses to fight against physical restraint when there is no evidence that they can predict that the episode will end. If, during a handling procedure, a horse is not likely to learn good associations with personnel, then we should avoid it learning anything. The use of overshadowing techniques to reduce fearful responses to interventions such as farriery, clipping and in-

jections is yet to be empirically explored but holds tremendous promise in the hands of skilled practitioners (McLean, 2008).

Horses show an early-morning peak in their plasma beta-endorphin concentrations (Hamra *et al.*, 1993) and so are likely to be least sensitive to noxious stimuli at this time of day. As a result, it has been suggested that this may be the preferred time to undertake elective aversive procedures. The natural inclination of horses to flee from threats makes them difficult to deal with in the open and even attempts to corner them in a field or yard for interventions are ill-judged if a stable with a non-slip surface is available. Before any invasive handling or veterinary procedure, anything that may get in the way during a struggle or a forced retreat by the handler, most notably water buckets, should be removed from the stable.

Stables with low ceilings are sometime helpful when handling horses that are inclined to rear or have learned to throw their heads up to avoid a twitch. The presence of the ceiling prevents the horse from gaining momentum as it swings its head up. Though the horse might throw its head up once, it probably feels the ceiling with its ears, and rarely does so a second time. Only ceilings with no projections (such as jutting beams) that might damage a horse's head or neck are suitable for this purpose. That said, good handling should place the horse under stimulus control and remove the need for the horse to learn the 'hard' way.

When handling fractious and naïve horses, it may be helpful to use calm horses as 'tutors' (because of the social facilitation effect). In cattle, the reverse has been demonstrated, and it has been shown that alarm substances in the urine of stressed conspecifics increase reactivity to aversive events (Boissy, 1998). It would be interesting to learn whether any equivalent messaging occurs among horses. Such substances may linger in transport areas such as holding pens and trailers, or even in areas used for aversive procedures such as veterinary interventions.

Physical restraint should not be used in ways that directly compromise horse welfare. Tying horses up for aversive procedures is inadvisable since their tendency to fight against such restraint precipitates attempts to flee and so increases fear and the likelihood of damage to equipment or, worse still, injury to themselves or personnel. Restraining horses effectively with a halter has more to do with timing than force and appropriate behaviour must be negatively reinforced with the release of pressure and then positively by stroking the animal in anatomical areas previously or intrinsically associated with stress reduction, including the forehead, neck and withers. Fear reactions generally manifest as locomotory responses, so gaining control over the horse's legs is very useful. Overshadowing techniques that centre on gaining stimulus control of the horse's legs are important here (see Chapter 6, Learning III: Associative (aversive)).

Cupping a hand over a horse's eye on the side on which it is being treated is often helpful for needle-shy horses. The same principle seems to apply when blinkers, shades (pacifiers) or sheepskin nosebands are used on racehorses. The idea is to reduce the number of fear-eliciting stimuli the horse has to cope with. This can have the effect of moderating arousal levels and maintaining the horse's flight response under the control of the rider rather than the environment. In a similar way, covering a horse's eyes in a fire allows you to lead it out of a burning stable – 'out of sight' seems to mean 'out of mind'. Originally, pacifiers were made of fly-mesh and were primarily used to stop dust and sand getting in a horse's eyes during track-work. However, trainers soon noticed a serendipitous feature: when horses wore these screens, they were much quieter and less reactive to environmental stimuli. It may be that, to an animal that is unable to extrapolate, the fly-mesh cross-hatching radically turned down the volume on visual signals that had reliably triggered hyper-reactivity in the past.

When increased restraint is required, it sometimes takes the form of hobbles, a tail rope or service hobbles, but these dubious techniques should be seen as emergency measures rather than routine approaches. Distracting the animal with the use of a twitch or rope gag may occasionally prove useful when dealing with the hindquarters of a fearful horse, but again, overshadowing via the bit is preferable (McLean, 2008). At least in the short-term, the distraction caused by the twitch or rope gag is chiefly pain, even though it may be rapidly modified by endorphins (Lagerweij et al., 1984).

Head restraints

Halters are designed to be placed on the horse from the near side. They should be tight enough to prevent the horse from removing them, low enough to assist in control of the head's direction and high enough to avoid fracturing the nasal bone or cartilage. The noseband should be loose enough to allow the horse to open its mouth and chew. Halters designed to tighten around the head if the horse resists work well when used with the correct technique of negative reinforcement within the pressure/release framework, but the horse should not be tethered by one. The Dually™ halter and stallion chains use a similar principle, tightening and applying pressure around the nose if the horse struggles. Stallion chains can be confusing to the horse because the eccentric chain pressure tends to result in neck shortening rather than slowing the legs.

Although horses generally lead better from the near side, this is simply a convention and fails to recognise that there are left- and right-preferent horses (McGreevy and Rogers, 2005). Horses with a motor preference that manifests as left- or right-hoofedness are likely to be under the influence of one brain hemisphere more than the other. Although yet to be studied empirically, this may translate to sensory dominance of one side over the other. So when leading horses from their off-side, as is the convention, the influence of the right visual field may be compromised more than the left. Leading horses from both left and right sides will determine which side suits the horse better.

The latest generation of head-collars (such as the Parelli halter and the Dually™ halter) are strong; they tend to exert more pressure than regular head-collars because they are made with thinner webbing and tighten under pressure.

Horses are best controlled if the handler is standing midway between the horse's head and shoulder. With this approach, accelerating and decelerating signals can easily be issued via the lead-rein. In addition, a flighty horse can be controlled in an open space as its momentum can be deviated by a sharp tug on the lead-rope. However, when doing so, the horse's hindquarters will tend to swing out away from the handler, so there is a possibility of a collision with objects to the side.

Tryptophan

Serotonin (5-HT) – or its precursor, 5-hydroxytryptophan (5-HTP) – may induce sleep and, importantly, appears to reduce anxiety. It is produced chiefly by neurons in the rostral pons and midbrain. It is synthesised from the amino acid tryptophan, so oral supplementation with tryptophan may increase serotonin concentrations in the brain (Hahn, 2004). Dietary tryptophan has been used to mildly 'sedate' horses, but this is a topic of some debate since it has also been shown to stimulate horses (Bagshaw *et al.*, 1994). The 5-HT system is the mediator of learned and sustained fear responses, and decreased 5-HT concentrations have been associated with violent psychopathological behaviour in humans (Lee and Coccaro, 2001).

Reserpine

Reserpine is a product of the root of *Rauwolfia serpentine*, an Indian climbing shrub. It depletes amine concentrations in the brain, including serotonin, noradrenaline and dopamine. Noradrenaline is an excitatory neurohormone in the brain, so its depletion explains the calming or tranquillising effect of reserpine in the horse (Tobin, 1978). Its calming properties have been exploited for management and training purposes. The lasting nature of the drug (up to 10 days) accounts for its appeal to those seeking to modulate equine flight responses, especially during traditional 'breaking'. There is considerable variability in the pharmacokinetics of reserpine in horses, with reports of adverse reactions (especially among stallions), including erratic behaviour. It has lost favour among veterinarians because of its role in anaesthesia deaths because of hypotension.

Take-home messages

- Pressure is a function of force applied to a given surface area and is ubiquitous in horse training. Force applied to a small area can result in very high pressure.
- Tack is designed to either disperse pressure (e.g. in the case of the saddle) or direct pressure (e.g. in the case of head restraint).
- In tack designed to direct pressure, the narrower the interface with the horse, the more severe the apparatus and the greater is the need for excellent timing in pressure-release.
- Safety considerations are paramount when restraining horses.
- Good technique is more sustainable than instruments or equipment that allows handlers to apply more force.

Ethical considerations

- Devices that generate endorphins and ultimately restrain horses may do so through the intermediacy of pain and, therefore, may be less ethical than pharmacological restraint or behaviour therapy.
- Technological advances may facilitate restraint without due regard for welfare.

Areas for further research

- Animal welfare science must address the possibility of learned helplessness resulting from radical restraining techniques.
- The emergence of polymers and so-called smart materials may yet enhance the effectiveness of traditional items of saddlery.
- The development of materials to be placed in the mouths of horses merits particularly close scrutiny.

11 Biomechanics

Introduction

This chapter is not intended as a definitive work on equine biomechanics – this subject is more thoroughly treated in appropriate texts (e.g. Back and Clayton, 2001). Rather, this text will describe the limb movements in sufficient detail to explain the nature of the locomotory requirements that the handler and rider's signals are intended to control during equitation. As discussed in Chapter 8 (Training), the rider's cues should target a discrete biomechanical action such as retraction, protraction, adduction or abduction, and therefore a working knowledge of equine biomechanics is advantageous for optimal training.

Locomotion

While kinematic features of equine locomotion have been extensively studied (especially forward locomotion), very few data are available on the neural basis of movement in horses, so much of what we know about locomotion stems from laboratory studies of rats and cats. However, there are good grounds on which to extrapolate these data to horses (Gramsbergen, 2001).

Neuromuscular coordination of locomotion is complex yet predictable. Just as an orchestra's strength is the result of individual contributions by the musicians, the horse's mobility can be traced to individual components. The locomotory responses that allow horses to go forward, backwards, faster, slower, sideways, and to turn result from individual muscles. They comprise the basic responses that riders endeavour to place under the control of their signals (a process known as *stimulus control*, see Chapter 7, Applying learning theory). These locomotory responses can be broken down into four basic ways of moving that can be thought of as building blocks for all movements in-hand and under-saddle in all equestrian disciplines (see Figure 11.1):

- Acceleration,
- Deceleration (including reverse),
- Turning with the forelimbs,
- Turning with the hindlimbs.

When we consider the possible directions the horse's limbs can take to allow the four basic responses listed above, it follows that different muscles or muscle groups account for each one. Biomechanics identifies the four main ways in which limbs can move that result in locomotion (Back, 2001; see Figure 11.2):

- Protraction (moving the leg forward),
- Retraction (moving the leg backwards),

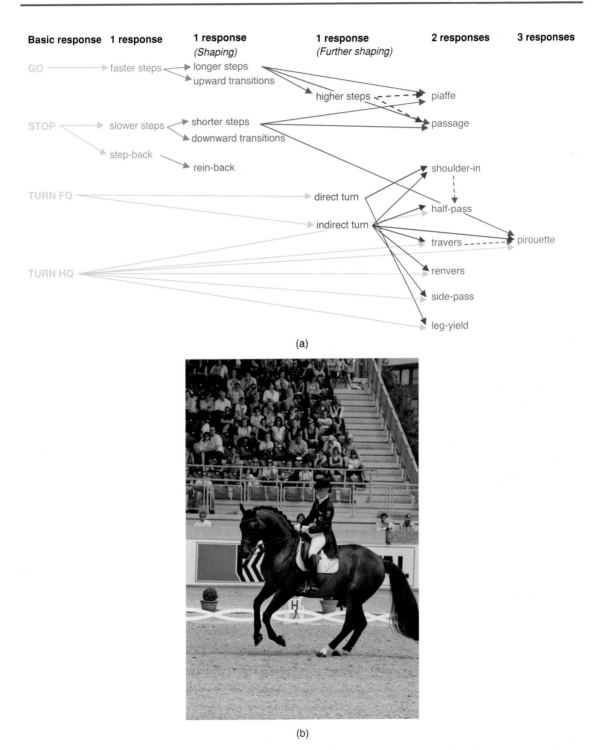

Figure 11.1 (a) All movements required of trained horses are derived from the basic responses of acceleration, deceleration, turning the forequarters (FQ) and turning the hindquarters (HQ). Dotted arrows refer to shaped preparatory movements that usually precede elicitation of the targeted movements (b). In dressage, the canter pirouette represents a movement that consists of a cascade of the largest number of single responses: shortened canter, turn of the forelegs and turn of the hindlegs. (Photo courtesy of *The Horse Magazine*.)

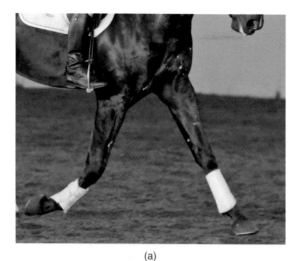

(a)

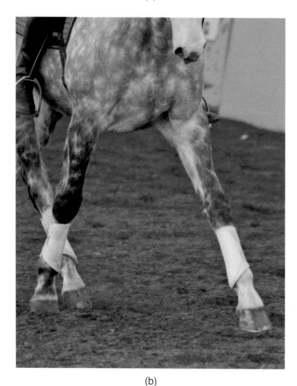

(b)

Figure 11.2 (a) Training the horse to go forward or backwards is a matter of reinforcing the biomechanical responses of protraction and retraction of the limbs. (b) Training the horse to turn the forelimbs, hindlimbs or both requires reinforcement of abduction and adduction of the limbs.

- Abduction (moving the limb away from the medial plane),
- Adduction (moving the limb towards the medial plane).

Protraction and retraction account for acceleration and deceleration, while abduction and adduction produce changes of direction and lateral movements (McLean and McLean, 2008). The relative amounts of these four limb movements at any moment provide the precise direction of travel. All movements therefore can be described as having specific amounts of retraction, protraction, abduction and adduction, depending on the direction of the limb in the stance phase, as compared with the swing phase (see Figure 11.3).

The stance phase and the swing phase

When the limb is in contact with the ground, it is said to be in the *stance phase*. This phase begins at impact and ends at lift-off (Clayton, 1989) and refers to any moment of ground contact that occurs during locomotion (see Figure 11.3). The stance phase supplies the power for locomotion. Locomotion results from the horse exerting forces against the ground produced by the action of the muscles. Generally, the angle of the limb to the ground in the stance phase is an indicator of the direction in which the hoof is pushing against the ground. Friction between the hoof and the ground allows locomotion to happen. Gaits are characterised by repetitive cycles of limb movements known as strides (Clayton, 1989). In biomechanics, the event demarcating the start and end of successive strides is the moment of impact of a hindlimb on the ground.

The *swing phase* defines the period when the leg is not in contact with the ground (see Figure 11.3). While the swing phase supplies no power to the horse's locomotion, it nonetheless has an important effect on locomotion in that its velocity and magnitude can vary so that the power of the subsequent stance phase is altered. Additionally, in the symmetrical gaits of walk and trot, the swing phase is concurrent with the stance phase of the contralateral limb. Thus, the velocity and magnitude of the swing phase reflect changes in impact velocity and power of the contralateral

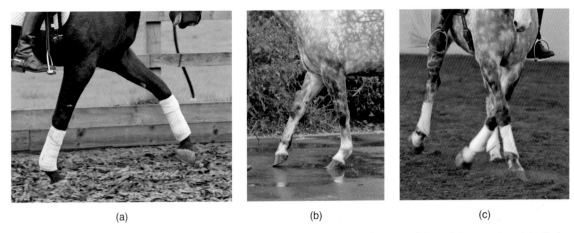

(a)   (b)   (c)

Figure 11.3   (a) When the horse goes forward, protraction of the limbs occurs in the swing phase, while retraction of the limbs occurs in the stance phase. (b) When the horse steps backwards, the opposite occurs. (c) On the other hand, going sideways is conferred by consecutive abductions and adductions of the fore- and hind-limbs in swing and stance phases.

limb in the stance phase (unless the horse is lame). In the asymmetrical gaits such as canter, the swing phase may have a more independent character. The larger swing phase of the leading forelimb at canter, for example, reflects the greater power of the non-leading forelimb in effecting turns towards the direction of the leading leg.

Stabilising muscles

Some muscles that contract for specific movements are *mostly* responsible for that movement, with a number of other muscles playing a lesser role. If you think of protraction as the opposite to retraction and abduction as the opposite to adduc-

tion, it is easy to understand that during stance-phase retraction, the protractive muscles are not flaccid but are active to some extent in that they stabilise the limbs (see Figure 11.4). During stance-phase protraction, the retraction muscles stabilise the limb. The same stabilising effect occurs during abduction and adduction. Without the antagonist muscles, the limbs would be unstable and uncontrollable.

The mechanics of locomotion

Going forward, backwards, changing direction and going sideways are a result of what the limbs are actually doing when they make contact with

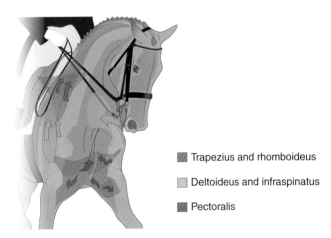

■ Trapezius and rhomboideus

☐ Deltoideus and infraspinatus

■ Pectoralis

Figure 11.4   Locomotion requires particular muscles to move the limbs and other associated muscles to stabilise them.

the ground. Furthermore, when horses increase speed, they eventually change gait, which gives maximum energetic efficiency for a particular speed. It is now time to look more closely at the mechanisms that provide changes of speed, direction and line.

Forward and reverse

Going forward implies retraction in the stance phase and protraction in the swing phase. When going forward, retraction has already begun before the limb makes ground contact (Back and Clayton, 2001; Pilliner *et al.*, 2002). This allows some limb velocity to be generated before ground contact so as to minimise losses of power when contact is first made with the ground. On the other hand, reversing means that the protracting limb is in the stance phase while the retracting limb is in the swing phase.

It is likely that, while slowing down, horses may decelerate relatively passively in that their momentum simply peters out with each stride. Alternatively, the horse may slow using the energy of *active protraction in the stance phase* (see Figure 11.5). Such active transitions may occur with

abrupt deceleration (e.g. a sliding stop). These are necessary in sports such as polo, campdrafting, cutting, reining, and mounted games. The biomechanics of reversing and actively slowing are little studied. In dressage, transitions are typically required in a smooth rhythm within three beats of the relevant gait (McGreevy and McLean, 2007). Argue and Clayton (1993a, 1993b) describe transitions in dressage as either Type 1, where there are no intermediate steps in between, say, walk and trot, or Type 2, where there may be some intermediate steps, such as a shorter broken trot step. They found that in walk and trot transitions, Type 1 transitions characterise the more highly trained dressage horse, whereas Type 2 transitions between trot and canter showed no association with level of training. More research needs to be undertaken here, where the transitions are signalled by the rider at precisely the same moment. For example, if the rider were to initiate the transitions when the outside foreleg began the stance or swing phase, it is likely that the number of footfalls could be measured from the beginning to the completion of the transitions. This would allow a standardised measurement of the transition from initiation to completion for research purposes.

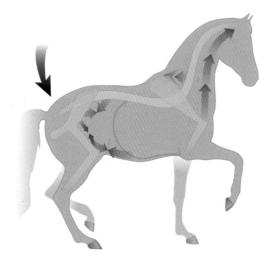

Figure 11.5 The lowering of the croup that is the hallmark of collection is first seen in the stop response when the hindlegs increase their role in deceleration. The muscle groups used are the sub-spinal, sub-lumbar, abdominals and others, such as the *iliacus* and the *psoas*. In addition, the raised head in collection raises the foreleg through the connection of the *brachiocephalic* muscle to the humerus of the foreleg.

Changing direction: turns of the forelegs

Turning with the forelegs allows changing direction and moving on curved lines, including circles. Alterations in direction generally result from recurring sequences of abduction/adduction or adduction/abduction of the forelegs. At any moment during a turn of the forelegs, one of the pair that is abducting or adducting will be in the swing phase while the other is in the stance phase.

However, there may be associated differential alterations in acceleration and deceleration that may also facilitate turning. Horses may lean in when turning and this may be especially apparent in the faster gaits, such as canter and gallop. When horses turn by leaning in, the actions of the legs involve acceleration rather than significant amounts of abduction and adduction. In sports that require turns at high speeds, such as reining, campdrafting, polo, all racing codes and games, leaning in may be the predominant form of turns instead of or including large degrees of abduction and adduction of the forelimbs (and hindlimbs).

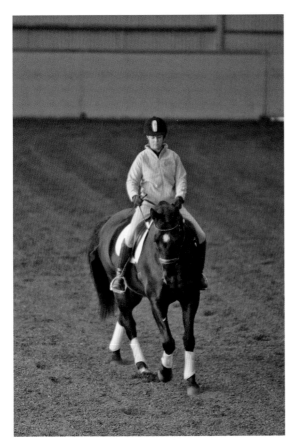

Figure 11.6 Turning the forelegs involves consecutive abductions and adductions. Smooth turns are a result of a consistent tempo and stride length during these biomechanical actions.

crete biomechanics of the turn of the forelegs require the use of the reins for optimal achievement of stimulus control.

In the forequarters of the horse, powerful abduction muscles facilitate fast turns at speed; the horse drives itself in a turn from the large muscles of the outside shoulder (the *trapezius, rhomboideus, deltoid* and *infra-spinatus* muscles) by abducting the limb opposite to the direction of the turn. Reining, campdrafting and polo horses owe their abilities to turn suddenly to the powerful abduction muscles; this explains the heavily built shoulders that characterise the best of these equine athletes. This greater power of abduction in the horse's forelimbs contrasts with primates (including humans), who required greater adductive power for arboreal locomotion. Unlike humans, horses do not have clavicles (collarbones) for attachment of the adductors. The horse does not require a collarbone as its limbs move predominantly fore and aft. In equids, the clavicle is represented by a tendon within the *brachiocephalic* muscle.

On a curved line or a circle greater than six metres in diameter, what is known to dressage trainers as 'bend' occurs when the hindlegs fall into the line of the foretracks (see Figure 11.7). On circles smaller than six metres it is difficult for the hindlegs to step into the foretracks owing to the poor ability of the horse to bend its thoracic and lumbar vertebrae. Of course, commensurate with the tightness of the turn, there is generally a

Training a horse for the sport of dressage requires an upright horse (on the vertical plane) at all times and leaning in is avoided: each hoof should make contact with the ground squarely. The cavalry history of this sport meant that armoured soldiers required horses to stay vertical and carry as much weight as possible on the hindquarters. So dressage training requires that turns begin with abduction before adduction so that the execution of movements such as half-pass and pirouette begin appropriately. For example, during a correct turn to the right, the first step is an abduction of the right forelimb in the swing phase with a simultaneous abduction in the stance phase of the left forelimb (this limb drives the turn). The next step involves the right forelimb adducting in the stance phase while the left forelimb adducts in the swing phase (Figure 11.6). In dressage, the dis-

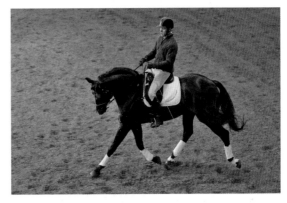

Figure 11.7 In the sport of dressage, horses are required to step into their foretrack line with their hindhooves on all curved lines greater than 6 m in diameter. This means that the vertebral column of the horse should show some flexion, which is known in dressage nomenclature as 'bend'.

symphony of protraction/retraction blended with abduction/adduction.

Changing direction: turns of the hindlegs

The horse is also able to change direction by turning its hindlegs. When hindlegs and forelegs turn simultaneously, turns are more rapid because the degree of direction change is increased. These dual turning abilities are adaptive for a prey animal during escape procedures. Such turns characterise sports that require rapid alterations of direction, such as reining, campdrafting and polo. However, in dressage, simultaneously opposing turns of the forelimbs and hindlimbs are not prescribed because of the requirement to maintain a significant proportion of weight directly on the hindquarters, a central precept of the sport.

For correct hindquarter turns in dressage training, adduction of hindlimbs must come before abduction. The first step of a hindlimb turn begins with a simultaneous adduction of both hindlimbs, one during the swing phase and the other during the stance phase. Adduction of the hindlimbs is then followed by abduction, and so on (see Figure 11.8). In other words, the hindlegs cross and then open. Note that turns of the hindlimbs differ from those of the forelimbs in that forelimb turns involve abduction first, whereas hindlimb turns involve adduction first. Again, the direction is a result of whether the adductions and abductions are in the swing phase or in the stance phase. For example, stepping sideways with the hindlimbs

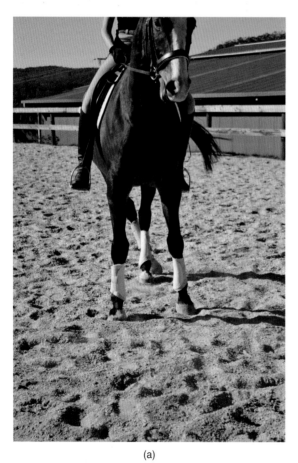
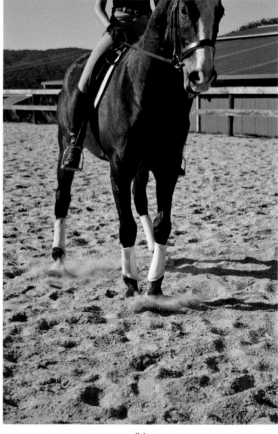

(a)   (b)

Figure 11.8 Turning with the hindlegs or going sideways involves consecutive adductions (a) and abductions (b) (Photos courtesy of Amelia Martin.)

to the left involves a simultaneous adduction in the swing phase of the left hindlimb with an adduction in the stance phase of the right hindlimb, followed by abduction.

Changing line: sideways

When forelimbs and hindlimbs turn in the same direction and to the same extent, the horse goes sideways (i.e. it changes line but does not change direction). Because going sideways results from turns of both fore and hindlegs, it has the combined biomechanical characteristics of those turns. Therefore, the individual turns of the forelimbs and hindlimbs are generally trained first.

In reining, pleasure and trail classes, going sideways is called a side-pass, while in dressage training it is known as leg-yield. Sideways movements, such as leg-yield, that involve some forward movement as well as going sideways require a blend of abduction, adduction, retraction and protraction; the relative amounts of each depend on the steepness of the sideways movement. Early dressage training of leg-yield requires that the tracks from each hoofprint follow a 22-degree diagonal line (see Figure 11.9). (A 22-degree line is represented by the KXM, HXF diagonal lines of the standard 60 m × 20 m dressage arena.) In more

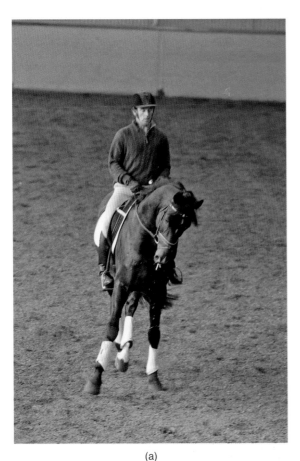

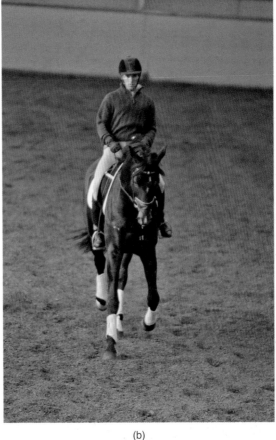

(a)   (b)

Figure 11.9 As with all training, it is much more efficient to shape and consolidate the required behaviour gradually. Therefore, when the horse is learning to leg-yield, simply going sideways is rewarded at first, regardless of whether the horse is straight in its vertebral column or not (a). Straightening is dealt with at a later time (b). (Photos courtesy of Amelia Martin.)

advanced training, the angle of lateral movements becomes steeper.

Consider a leg-yield to the left at walk. Because the walk begins with a foreleg, the first step of a left leg-yield will be by the abduction of the left foreleg in the swing phase and the simultaneous abduction of the right forelimb in the stance phase. Immediately following the abduction of the left forelimb, adduction during the swing phase of the right hindlimb occurs as well as the simultaneous adduction in the stance phase of the left hindlimb.

Transitions

The horse can make significant speed alterations by changing from one gait to another through walk, trot, canter and gallop. These alterations are termed *inter-gait transitions* (McGreevy and McLean, 2007). The horse is also able to effect speed changes within the gait either by altering the speed of the legs or, alternatively, by lengthening or shortening the stride. These are termed *intra-gait transitions* (McGreevy and McLean, 2007). Riders and trainers generally and collectively group these transitions as either *upward* or *downward* transitions.

The gaits

The purpose of the gaits is to provide speed within the parameters of energy efficiency. A gait can be defined as 'a complex and strictly coordinated, rhythmic and automatic movement of the limbs and the entire body length of the animal, which results in the production of progressive movements' (Barrey, 2001). Gaits can be classified according to symmetry. Walking and trotting are symmetrical gaits, where left and right footfalls are evenly spaced in time. In contrast, canter and gallop are asymmetrical gaits, where the right and left limbs move in a dissimilar way. Gaits can also be defined by the presence or absence of a suspension phase (Barrey, 2001). Suspension is the period when all four limbs are in the swing phase (Clayton, 1989). Walking gaits have no suspension phase.

Gaits are described as 2-beat (trot), 3-beat (canter) or 4-beat (walk and gallop), which cor-

responds with the number of footfalls or beats that can be heard within each stride. Most riding horses have four natural gaits (see Figure 11.10):

Walk (a four-beat gait),
Trot (a two-beat gait),
Canter (a three-beat gait),
Gallop (a four-beat gait).

Some breeds, known as gaited breeds, have been selectively bred and trained to exhibit other gaits, such as pacing (an alternating bilateral two-beat gait), tolting (in Icelandic horses, a rapid alternating unidiagonal four-beat gait similar to the walk), and racking (similar to tolting and found in some breeds in the Americas). Horses change from one gait to the next, because of the increasing metabolic cost of speed and as a result of ground forces on the limbs reaching a threshold force. In the absence of human interference, when carrying increased weight, inter-gait transitions occur at progressively lower speeds (Farley and Taylor, 1991).

Walk

The walk is an alternating transverse four-beat gait. When the horse is standing relatively squarely, the first leg to leave the ground is a foreleg. Beginning with the left foreleg, the sequence of steps is LF, RH, RF and LH (see Figure 11.11). In the walk, each limb typically strikes the ground at a rate ranging from 50 to 60 beats per minute. In synchrony with the walk, the horse's neck extends and contracts. For this reason, the rider's hands follow this movement and should also move forward and back, otherwise, the walk becomes stilted. In a stilted walk, the flexions of the limb joints are differentially altered. With a longer walk, such as in a free or extended walk, the rider's hands should show the largest magnitude of movement.

Trot

The trot is a symmetrical, diagonal two-beat gait in which the limbs form diagonal pairs. There is a period of suspension between each diagonal pair

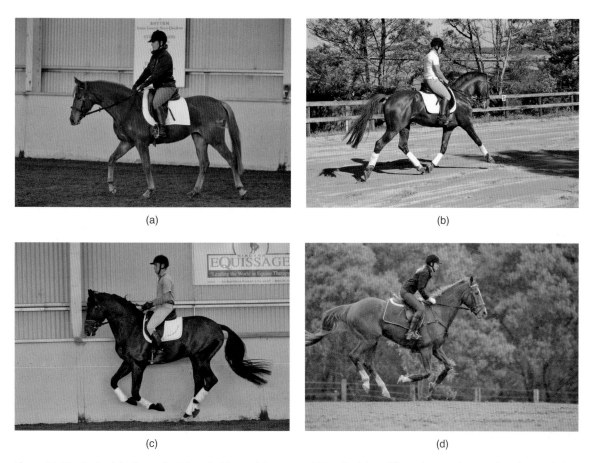

(a)

(b)

(c)

(d)

Figure 11.10 Each of the four gaits ((a) walk; (b) trot; (c) canter and (d) gallop) has different beat and suspension characteristics. (Photos courtesy of Amelia Martin.)

of limbs. The sequence of footfalls is RH+LF and LH+RF. In some specific postures and circumstances, the diagonal pairings are slightly asynchronous; this is known as diagonal advanced placement (DAP) and is discussed later. At trot, each pair of limbs typically strikes the ground at a rate ranging from 70 to 80 beats per minute. In the trot, the neck does not extend or contract during locomotion as it does in the walk and canter.

Canter

The canter is an alternating uni-/bi-diagonal three-beat gait with a period of suspension after the third beat. The footfalls of the canter, with the right foreleg leading, are RF, LH and RH+LF. As

in the trot, there may also be some diagonal advanced placement of the single diagonal pair of limbs under certain conditions. In canter speeds required for dressage, the limbs or the pair of limbs strikes the ground at rates ranging from 70 to 110 beats per minute. The canter is thus the most variable gait in speed.

The canter is an asymmetrical gait, because the three beats comprise a leading hindleg, then a diagonal pair (foreleg + hindleg), followed by the leading foreleg and terminating with a moment of suspension. When horses at liberty turn in the canter (or gallop), they generally prefer to lead with the inside foreleg. The non-leading foreleg has a shorter swing phase than the leading foreleg and this asymmetry probably confers different stance phase characteristics on the forelegs.

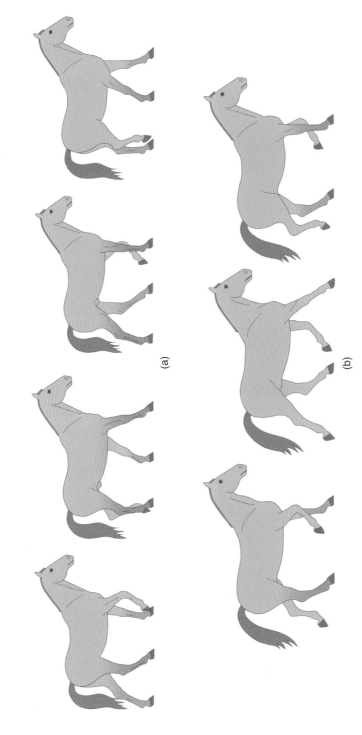

(a)

(b)

Figure 11.11 The cycle of limb movements at walk (a), trot (b), canter (c) and transverse gallop (d). Colour coding shows right and left weight-bearing limbs.

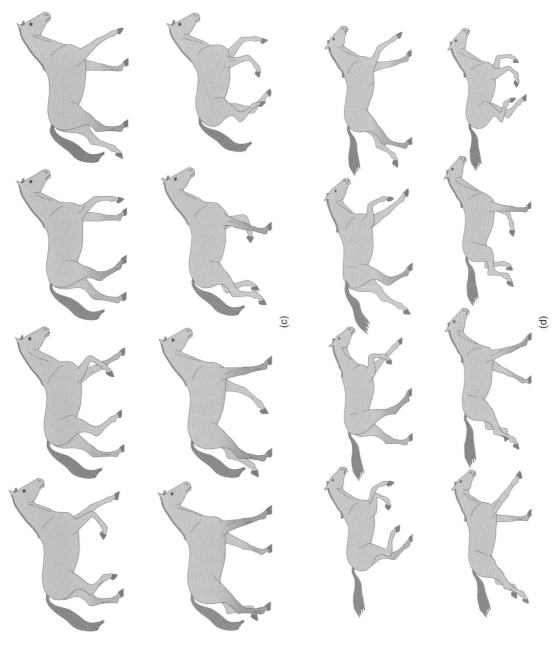

(c)

(d)

Figure 11.11 (continued)

It is likely that this arrangement facilitates efficient turning, since counter-canter (cantering on a circle with a leading *outside* leg) is difficult for most horses. Counter-canter is more difficult to achieve under-saddle than 'true canter', because during counter-canter the leading foreleg now takes the role of abduction in the stance phase.

In the changes of various gaits into the canter, the initial limb to begin the canter differs. Decarpentry (1949), with the benefit of moving film, was the first to describe this. For example, he found that when the horse makes the transition from trot to canter, the first limb to begin the canter is the leading forelimb. However, when the horse makes the change from one leading leg to the other in the canter (a flying change), the first limb to begin the new canter is the outside hind. This has implications for the signals used in training and re-training. For example, to execute a flying change, any signal should target the new outside hindleg immediately following the suspension phase.

Gallop

The gallop is a four-beat gait derived from the preceding gait, the canter. It is similar to the canter except that the speed is greater and the diagonal pair of legs is separated. Speed is the product of the dual components of stride frequency (SF) and stride length (SL) and can be estimated as follows: Speed = SF × SL (Barrey, 2001). Stride length increases linearly with the speed of the gait, while stride frequency increases non-linearly (Leach and Cymbaluk, 1986).

The sequence of the limbs in the gallop is generally transverse (Figure 11.12); however, in fatigued horses or where the forelimbs change before the hindlegs, rotary gallops may be seen (Barrey, 2001). In both rotary and transverse gallops, the hindlegs follow each other sequentially; in a transverse gallop, the third limb placement following the preceding hindleg is the opposite foreleg, followed by the final foreleg. Thus, the first foreleg is contralateral to the preceding hindleg. A typical transverse gallop sequence with the right foreleg leading is LH, RH, LF and RF. A transverse gallop on the left lead is RH, LH, RF and LF. A rotary gallop, on the other hand, follows a rotary sequence of footfalls and can be clockwise or counterclockwise depending on the

leading leg. A rotary gallop with a leading right foreleg has a clockwise sequence of RH, LH, LF and RF, while a rotary gallop with a leading left foreleg is counterclockwise, LH, RH, RF and LF.

Jumping

Jumping obstacles occurs mostly at the canter and gallop although riding at the trot is important to establish self-carriage and good technique. Clayton (1989) describes three functional phases of the jumping effort: the approach phase; the jump phase (including take-off, jump suspension and landing subsets); and the move-off phase (Figure 11.13). She proposed that the approach strides themselves can be labelled so that approach stride 2 precedes approach stride 1, and so on. Similarly, the move-off strides can be labelled as move-off stride 1, 2, and so forth. This approach allows for a systematic analysis of jumping kinematics. For example, labelling each stride allows description of the characteristics of a precise stride.

Barrey (2001) described the footfalls of the jumping effort as the trailing hindleg and leading hindleg at take-off, the airborne phase, followed by the trailing foreleg, then leading foreleg in the landing phase. At the take-off, the canter or gallop mechanics are altered so that the hindlegs are more synchronised than before to allow more power in the take-off (Barrey, 2001). The airborne phase is a long dissociation of the diagonal during which a lead change can take place. Many jump trainers, as well as dressage trainers, use this phase in training flying changes. Indeed, some trainers use a pole on the ground to increase the period of suspension to increase the likelihood that a flying change will occur when the trailing hindleg is stimulated by the rider's new outside leg or whip-tap to initiate a new canter stride. The trailing hindleg is the first leg to begin the new canter stride (Back and Clayton, 2001).

The correct posture of the horse during the jumping effort should be parabolic (see Figure 11.14) so that the topline is involved in the jumping arc. A good jumper raises both knees evenly, and evenly flexes both knee joints of the front legs. A lowered foreleg is thought to be associated with errors such as unevenness in rein contact. The hindlegs should tuck up high and, at the peak of jumping elevation, the horse may kick out

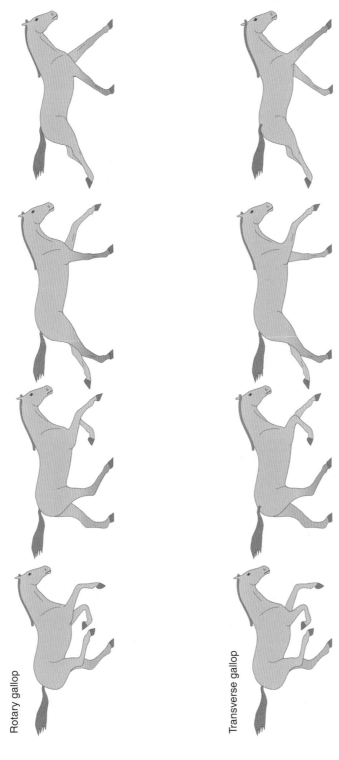

Rotary gallop

Transverse gallop

Figure 11.12 Horses may make a transition from a transverse to a rotary gallop during fatigue or when lead changes are initiated by the forelimbs. The footfall sequences of a rotary gallop are similar to those of a disunited canter.

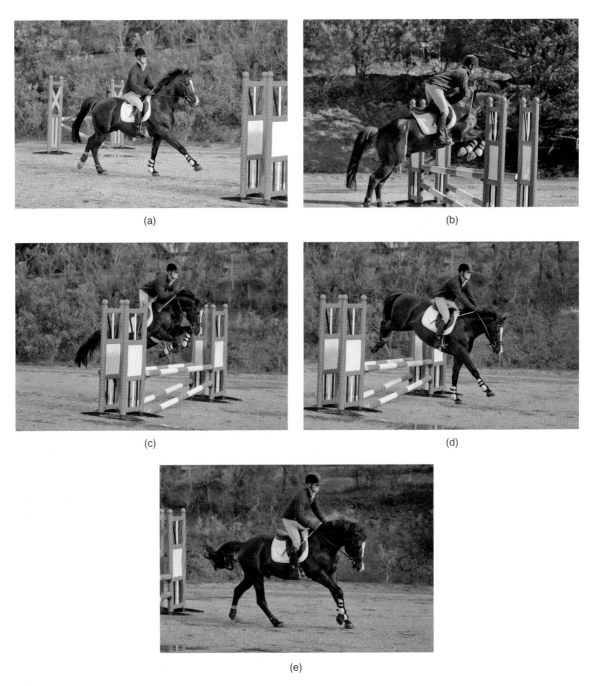

Figure 11.13   The three phases of jumping: (a) the approach phase, the jump phase (including (b) take-off, (c) jump suspension and (d) landing subsets) and (e) the move-off phase.

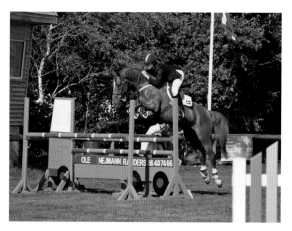

Figure 11.14 Show-jumping trainers aim to train horses to take off close to the obstacle and thus to make the shape of the jumping effort parabolic rather than longer and flatter. This shape (also known as a bascule) requires the horse to arch his neck and flex his back and allows him to jump as athletically as possible. (Photo courtesy of Susan Kjaergard.)

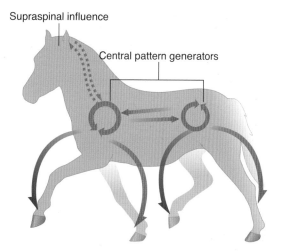

Figure 11.15 The central pattern generators are directly responsible for the precise synchronisation of the limbs in each gait. For example, in the trot they coordinate the alternating sequence of diagonal couplets.

with both hindlegs. Mistakes with the hindlegs are thought to be associated with the rider's seat and posture such as sitting up too early.

The central pattern generator

When a foal is born, the gaits are already present. The diagonal pairs are also in place in the trot and canter. The diagonal connections of the horse's legs apply further, so that in all gaits, there is more or less some diagonal duplication. For example, in the four-beat walk, a longer stride of the right hindleg is associated with a longer stride in the left foreleg, and so on. Similarly, during turns, when the right foreleg abducts, the contralateral hindleg also tends to adduct. Thus, a sharp left turn of the forelegs results in a sharp right turn of the hindlegs. Though undesirable in dressage for reasons mentioned earlier, this diagonal synchrony is clearly adaptive for wild equids under predatory pressure in that it confers faster changes of direction. Trainers, coaches and riders are often aware of this diagonal mirroring effect: in a trained horse, a certain threshold of tension on a rein will turn the forelegs one way and hindlegs the other.

The diagonal connectedness and maintenance of gait rely on a type of neural circuitry, called a neural oscillator, which coordinates limb movements. These neural oscillators are also known as central pattern generators (CPGs; Gramsbergen,

2001; see Figure 11.15). CPGs are independent to some extent from the brain. It has long been known that when the spinal cord is severed, alternating trunk and limb movements can still occur. Gramsbergen (2001) reports that while locomotion is initiated in the mesencephalic brain stem, fibres project to the CPGs located in the spinal cord itself. He surmises that CPGs are among the first neural circuits to develop in neuro-ontogeny and largely tend to remain unaltered throughout life.

The existence of CPGs implies that movements in the forelimbs are more or less reflected in the hindlimbs. Furthermore, the forelimbs may have greater significance in locomotion than is currently believed by modern horse-trainers in that the CPG of the forelimbs directs the hindlimbs. For example, studies in altricial neonates, such as rats, suggest that forelimb locomotion precedes hindlimb locomotion (Gramsbergen, 2001), which is known as the cephalocaudal gradient. This may have implications in quadrupedal ungulates such as horses in the neural connections and sequences of the various gaits. For example, many dressage trainers attempt to maintain the hindquarters behind the forelegs to achieve straightness (hind-hooves into foretracks), instead of the approach of more enlightened trainers who recognise that gaining precise stimulus control of the forelegs in deceleration and turns automatically results in straightness (Kyrklund, 1998; McGreevy and McLean, 2007; McLean and McLean, 2008).

The vertebral column

The amount of mobility of the horse's vertebral column is a significant issue for equitation. The cervical vertebrae of the horse's neck are very mobile laterally and dorsoventrally. It is well known in the discipline of dressage that problems of balance arise when the horse's neck is carried to one side. Because the head and neck make up around 10% of the horse's total body weight, a neck bent and carried to one side adds extra weight to that foreleg adding to its adductive power in the stance phase and causing falling-in or out. For this reason, neck straightness is a high goal in dressage and many trainers adhere to the maxim that the neck should not express more bend than the rest of the horse's vertebral column.

The thoracic and lumbar spine of the horse is much less flexible than generally believed (Jeffcott and Dalin, 1980). While objective studies on the degree to which a horse is capable of bending are lacking, Faber *et al.* (1999, 2000, 2001a, 2001b) studied the dorsoventral bending, lateral bending and axial rotation characteristics of the equine spine at walk, trot and canter (see Figure 11.16). They reported that lateral bending of the thoracolumbar vertebral column occurred only to a small degree and that the amount varied with the gait.

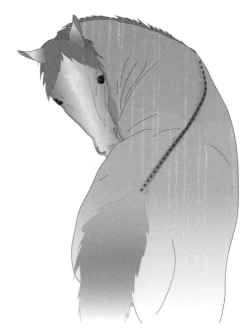

Figure 11.17   Horses have difficulty in scratching their rumps with their teeth owing to the limitations of lateral bending of the thoracic and lumbar vertebrae compared with the cervical vertebrae.

Dorsoventral movement was greatest in the canter while lateral bending was greatest in the walk. The greatest amount of axial rotation was found to occur at walk. In studies of canter conducted on a treadmill they reported that bending occurs chiefly in two places: T10 and L1 (with less consequential movement at S3). While dressage prescribes that horses should laterally bend the vertebral column when ridden on curved lines, we should be mindful of the variable bending capabilities of different sections of the vertebral column (see Figure 11.17).

Roundness

Roundness refers to the arched head, neck and apparent dorsoventrally rounded body posture acquired by the horse in correct dressage training. It is characterised by self-carriage where the horse has learned to persist in his speed, directional line and head, neck and body posture without support from the rider. However, roundness is frequently a forced response where the rider increases tension on the reins until the horse shortens its neck or

Maximal ranges of motion

Spinal Movement	Walk	Trot	Canter
Dorsoventral + 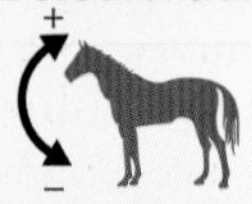 −	7°	5°	16°
Lateral + 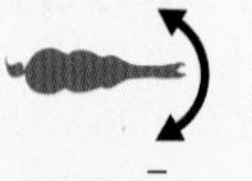 −	5.5°	3.5°	5°
Axial + 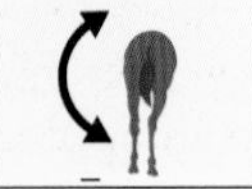 −	13°	3°	8°

Figure 11.16   Dorsoventral flexion/extension, lateral bending and axial rotation are characteristics of the equine thoracolumbar column in walk, trot and canter.

uses concurrent rein and leg pressures to 'drive the horse onto the bit' (see Chapter 12, Unorthodox techniques). Although this is contrary to the tenets of classical dressage, it provides the illusion of roundness and collection and is known as false collection. Dressage experts, however, can readily perceive the incorrect outline, where the neck is shortened and the loins are hollow. The result is that the rider's tight control on the reins to maintain this posture and the incorrect neck and back muscles involved prevent correct development of the topline. There are significant welfare issues surrounding such training, which manifest in a raft of problems ranging from tension and conflict behaviours to wastage. In correct training, the horse's head should be suspended from his withers in self-carriage and the weight in the rider's hands should be the weight of the reins and a light connection to the lips and tongue of the horse. Such lightness is the putative goal of Baroque training styles and modern classical training. It is imperative that, from the horse's viewpoint, pain is escapable and controllable, so lightness of course is important for the horse at every stage of training, and those methodologies that embrace correct roundness training and constant self-carriage are more correctly aligned with the correct application of learning theory than coercive methods.

Collection

The horse at liberty carries most of its weight on the forelegs, so untrained horses carry themselves on the forehand in an apparent downhill way of going. Collection implies an uphill way of going (Clayton, 2004). It is characterised by a highly arched neck where the poll is the highest point and the topline physique of the horse is highly developed. The collected horse has learned to lower its hindquarters using a combination of muscles, including the abdominal and sub-lumbar muscles, which increases the engagement of the hindquarters (Clayton, 2004). The development of collection redresses the previously mentioned downhill situation, where the hindquarters now step in advance of a line dropped from the stifle (Pilliner *et al.*, 2002) and lower. This is said to

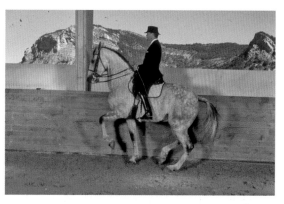

Figure 11.18   Collection involves a shift of weight from the horse's forehand to its hindquarters. This shift is a function of altered stride kinematics and joint flexion of the hindlegs, flexion of the horse's lumbar vertebrae and raising the head and neck. This posture is a prerequisite for all higher dressage movements. (Photo courtesy of Cadmos Verlag and Philippe Karl.)

put the horse in a stronger position to engage its hindlegs while carrying a rider (see Figure 11.18).

While it has generally been supposed that collection is mainly a product of the hindquarters being lowered, Clayton (2004) points out the greater significance of the sling muscles (*serratus ventralis*, *pectorals* and *subclavius*) of the horse's forequarters and the muscles in the upper part of the forelimbs. Tension in these muscles raises the forequarters, increasing the uphill posture of collection.

The relevant hindleg muscles are also developed by the extra weight carried by the hindlegs and the more anterior steps. The net torque of the hamstrings arises from three major attachment sites: the caudal aspect of the hip (extensor torque), stifle (flexor torque) and hock (extensor torque), so variations in thrust probably arise from variations in the contributions of different components of the hamstrings (Clayton, 2007, personal communication). In addition, the sub-spinal and sub-lumbar muscles, the *psoas* and the *iliacus*, are also likely to make a large contribution to collection. This may be one reason that collection must be trained gradually: the symphony of muscles used in its expression differs from typical propulsion and must, therefore, be gradually strengthened.

As collection develops, a quality known as cadence also develops. The concept of cadence is

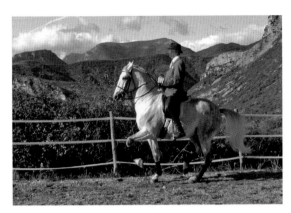

Figure 11.19 Cadence is the term ascribed to the accentuated suspension phase in the collected trot and its derivations (piaffe, passage). (Photo courtesy of Cadmos Verlag and Philippe Karl.)

derived from music, where it identifies a rhythmical motion accentuated by a pause. The period of suspension is at its greatest during the progressive development of collection leading ultimately to passage and piaffe. This suspension makes for a clear pause of the horse's legs in the swing phase, which is known as *cadence* (see Figure 11.19). The current debate surrounding the dressage training style called hyperflexion (where the horse is induced to hyperflex the cervical vertebrae to the point where its nose almost touches its chest) includes some criticism of the less fluid cadence of horses trained in this way (see Chapter 12, Unorthodox techniques). Classical dressage purists claim that it is an artefact of tension. More research is needed to fully understand such novel training styles (e.g. to test if physiological and behavioural stress levels differ between the two different styles of cadence).

Muscular development effects of horse sports

Collection is a result of the physical development of particular muscles, including the dorsal (topline) muscles; it is not a quality that can be quickly produced by forcing a particular neck outline. Because of the weight of the horse's forequarters including the head and neck, significant muscular effort is required to support them. The nuchal ligament and the muscles at the base of the neck, such as the *trapezius*, are attached to the muscles of the back (*latissimus dorsi*). The withers act as a fulcrum. When the horse moves, there is increased tension on the back as well as the topline of the neck and this tension is exacerbated during transitions. During downward transitions, the effects of deceleration and gravity on the horse's descending head and neck place excessive pressure on the muscles of the back. With repetitions, these transitions strengthen and have an anabolic (muscle-building) effect on the topline muscles of the back. On the other hand, as a result of inertia during upward transitions, the back muscles exert extra pressure on the associated neck muscles, which contributes to their development also.

As velocity increases, the effects of transitions are greater in the development of the topline. In fact, with every doubling of speed, the tension on the topline and limbs quadruples. This is expressed by $E = \frac{1}{2}\ mv^2$, where the energy involved (E) is equal to half the mass multiplied by the velocity (v) squared. This equation has profound effects for the dressage horse in terms of muscular tension and subsequent development. Because the increase in muscular effort has an anabolic effect, the anabolic requirements for the increased physical development of the dressage horse are proportional to the various speed loads it has been subjected to during training. Thus, it is the transitions at higher speeds (for example, collected canter to extended canter and vice versa) that have the most anabolic effects compared with transitions at walk or trot. For these reasons, the development of the collected physique is a gradual process, beginning with increments in impulsion. The risks of conflict behaviours and subsequent wastage are high if the young horse is forced to adopt such an outline in its early development.

As the correctly trained dressage horse develops, the limb muscles for collection increase in tone and this is likely to have an effect of bringing the hindhooves closer to the fronthooves, where the horse now shows the more collected posture described as 'sitting'.

On the other hand, horses that are used in horse trials, racing, polo, games and reining predominantly rely on their hamstrings for speed, and these horses tend to show the stance known as 'camped out' where the hind hooves during immobility stand farther from the fore hooves.

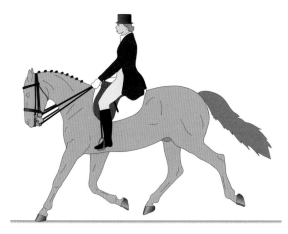

Figure 11.20 Negative DAP occurs when the foreleg begins its stance phase before its diagonal hindlimb. (Positive DAP is when the opposite situation occurs: the hindlimb begins its stance phase before the foreleg).

The shoulder muscle tone of the correctly trained reining horse also reveals greater muscle tone.

Diagonal advanced placement

The term diagonal advanced placement (DAP) is used to describe the interval between the diagonally paired foreleg and hindleg making contact with the ground. It has a positive value if the hindleg meets the ground before the foreleg, and negative if vice versa (see Figure 11.20). A DAP value of zero tells us that the diagonal pair contacts the ground simultaneously. A positive DAP arises when horses move with an elevated forehand and this is said to indicate good balance (Holmström *et al.*, 1995). In passage, diagonal pairs move with two well-defined suspensions in every stride, and large positive DAPs have been recorded. The DAP tends to be longest in the most successful contemporary dressage horses.

Interestingly, data from the Seoul Olympics showed that 15% of the extended trot strides analysed had a negative DAP (Deuel and Park, 1990). In the same event, the DAP for piaffe in several horses was negative (Argue, 1994; Holmström *et al.*, 1994) but the highest placed horses had a positive DAP (Clayton, 1997).

The existence of DAP has been central to arguments in the current hyperflexion debate.

Sometimes it has been implied that any DAP, positive or negative, signifies incorrect training and lack of self-carriage. Unfortunately, in the data collected so far there has been no quantitative rein tensiometry to test the veracity of the claims one way or the other. There is scope for more research on this topic.

Take-home messages

- The horse has four locomotory responses (acceleration, deceleration, turning with the forelimbs and turning with the hindlimbs) that are the basis for all movements in-hand and under-saddle.
- Achieving stimulus control of the forelegs in deceleration and turns automatically results in straightness. This directly contradicts the widely held but erroneous belief that straightness is a result of the hindhooves tracking into the foretracks.
- The thoracic and lumbar spine of the horse are much less flexible than generally believed.
- In optimal training, the horse should be in self-carriage, and the weight in the rider's hands should be the weight of the reins plus a light connection to the lips and tongue.

Ethical considerations

- Incorrect training methods that promote concurrent rein and leg pressures used to 'drive the horse onto the bit' result in false collection and compromise the welfare of the ridden horse. Such reduction in welfare may manifest as conflict behaviours and ultimately lead to wastage.

Areas for further research

- Characterisation of the transitions between gaits and how these are affected when the rider initiates the cue for a transition.
- Investigation into the relationship between stress levels and cadence, or lack thereof, especially in regard to reduced cadence that accompanies hyperflexion of the neck.
- Measurement of the relationship between DAP and training methods.

12 Unorthodox Techniques

Introduction

This chapter examines some potential sources of compromised welfare in ridden and non-ridden horses. The practices involved are unusual or radical, and some of the interventions we cover are popular but not orthodox.

Of the practices discussed here, the most confusing practices to horses are those that apply contradictory pressures (e.g. that send it forward while simultaneously halting it). Even without using mechanical devices, riders can coerce their horses to assume certain gaits and postural responses. In equestrian parlance, the horse is said to show lateral flexion, vertical flexion and longitudinal flexion (see Figure 12.1, noting that the term longitudinal flexion may confuse some veterinary readers since it describes what they would call extension). Some of the ways in which these types of flexion can be achieved can compromise horse welfare. This chapter is intended to demonstrate how, although such techniques may bring some short-term benefits to the rider, they are likely to have deleterious long-term side-effects (and, for that matter, short- and medium-term as well) for the horse.

Ridden Horses: Forcing the 'on the bit' head and neck position

Although over-bending does occur in nature, it lasts only for brief periods. Sustained over-bending, however, is becoming increasingly common for the ridden horse. A so-called broken neck (see Figure 12.2) is not a reference to a fractured vertebral column but a description of how horses with their necks flexed artificially by force appear to show the greatest amount of flexion at the junction of cervical vertebrae 4 and 5. An abrupt change in the longitudinal flexion can be seen in the crest of horses undergoing this intervention.

A horse is said to be over-bent when it carries (or is forced to carry) its nasal plane behind the vertical. At this point, minimal further flexion is possible. If the horse has been forced to show this flexion by rein tension or resistance in the rider's hands when it attempts to extend its neck, it can do nothing more to get relief from the pressure in its mouth. This leads to deficits in training (i.e. the quality of the slow/stop/step-back response declines) and subsequent conflict behaviours result from the confusion. This technique may

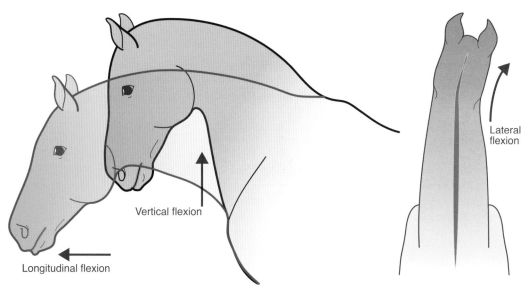

Figure 12.1   Longitudinal, vertical and lateral flexion as used in equestrian (rather than veterinary) parlance.

be carried out because riders are unaware of the correct neck outline that is required by the sport of dressage (nasal plane just in front of the vertical line). This posture is an emergent property of the correct shaping of the operant rein response of slowing. Instead, many contemporary riders use increasingly strong rein pressure until the horse brings its mouth towards the rider's hands and thus shortens its neck in an attempt to relieve the bit pressure. This neck-shortening is believed by

many to be an acceptable practice to achieve the required head and neck outline.

Hyperflexion (Rollkur)

Rollkur or, as it is known by the Fédération Equestre Internationale (FEI), hyperflexion, describes the technique where the horse's neck is dorsoventrally hyperflexed as a result of bit pressure to the point where the horse's chin may touch its pectoral region (see Figure 12.3). Proponents of this method claim that they shape this response

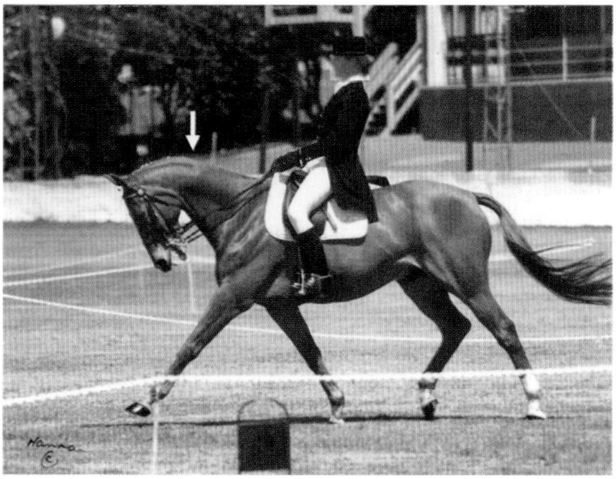

Figure 12.2   A horse with a so-called broken neck (arrow indicates the abrupt change in the positions of the cervical vertebrae relative to one another). (Photo courtesy of Sandy Hannan.)

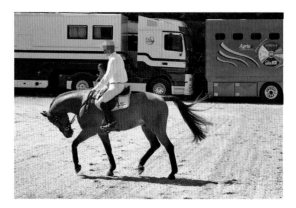

Figure 12.3   An example of a horse being hyperflexed under-saddle. (Photo courtesy of Julie Taylor/EponaTV.)

gradually and that the horse is ridden in this frame only for short periods of time. They attest to biomechanical benefits of this outline in inducing greater flexion of the hock joints. However, many observers have described longer durations, and the mechanisms by which this technique might achieve greater flexion of the hock joints are rather obscure.

The veterinary committee of the FEI has stated that hyperflexion of the neck is a degree of longitudinal flexion of the mid-region of the neck that cannot be self-maintained by the horse for a prolonged time without welfare implications. Furthermore, it has stated that hyperflexion as a training cue must be used correctly, as the technique can be an abuse when attempted by an inexperienced/unskilled rider/trainer.

Hyperflexion is believed to decrease stride length and increase elevation of the hindlimbs while also increasing the dorsoventral oscillation of the lumbar vertebrae (van Weeren *et al.*, 2006). Certainly, its current prevalence among elite dressage competitors strongly suggests that it lends some competitive advantage in that its use must help to produce a performance the judges wish to see. But, significantly, it is a practice that would detract considerably from scores if it were used in competition itself. Instead, it appears as part of the warm-up routine at many elite events.

There is opposition to sustained hyperflexion because it 'stiffens the horse', 'causes excessive flexion' and 'induces discomfort to the animal' while providing riders with 'complete domination' and control (FEI, 2006). Some dressage experts criticise the technique because they say it creates hollow loins and jerkiness of the hindlegs. There is also concern that the practice may create physical stress at the level of the intervertebral discs, in the nuchal ligament and in the withers, and that, although such extreme posturing may not necessarily cause primary lesions, it may cause pain in horses with pre-existing conditions (Denoix, 2006). In 2007, a high-profile trainer was subjected to disciplinary action by the FEI for inducing hyperflexion in a horse by lungeing for an extended period in side-reins that were considered too tight (Jenkins, 2007). A counterargument is that many top-class dressage horses known to have been trained using hyperflexion techniques have competed well into their twenties and that this would not be the case if they were in discomfort or if their welfare had been seriously jeopardised by any particular technique or practice.

The 2006 FEI workshop on hyperflexion also drew attention to the influence of head posture on the respiratory tract of healthy horses, and the effect on vision as well as a number of other issues that surround the use of horses in modern dressage. These include lameness in the dressage horse and the consequences of equestrianism generally on horse welfare (Racklyeft and Love, 1990; Petsche *et al.*, 1995; Harman *et al.*, 1999; Ödberg and Bouissou, 1999; Kold and Dyson, 2003; McGreevy, 2004).

It is worth considering whether there can be good and bad hyperflexion, and whether rein gauges or a test for self-carriage might be used to distinguish between them. From a behavioural perspective, the application of sustained pressure by the rider or relentless resistance from the horse amount to the same thing: pressure in the mouth, which can lead to habituation. Research is needed to remove emotiveness from the hyperflexion debate by establishing, for a range of equine athletes, how much contact is neutral, how much rein tension is too much, how discomfort and pain could be measured, and how learned helplessness manifests in horses (McGreevy and McLean, 2007).

Contraction

An illusion of collection can be created simply by shortening the neck (see Figure 12.4). Horses that

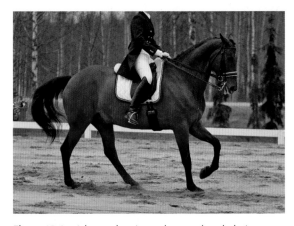

Figure 12.4   A horse showing a shortened neck during a flying change. If there are hyper-reactive associations with flying changes, tension can persist. (Photo courtesy of Minna Tallberg.)

have been trained to do this are likely to offer this response when they are subjected to pressure from the bit. The problem is that the same or dangerously similar pressure from the bit should be *slowing* the horse (a basic operant response typically trained during foundation training). The result can be a horse with habituation to rein signals (i.e. a hard-mouthed horse) that on occasions may be a bolter. False collection is said to occur when a comparison of the elevation of the withers relative to the hindquarters shows no significant differences.

Inducing confusion by using one signal for more than one response

When young horses undergo foundation training, they learn that increased pressure on a single rein is the signal for turning the forequarters by a process of abduction of the forelegs (in equestrian parlance this rein signal is known as the direct turn signal). It is an important early response because during challenging moments the reins, among an array of other classically conditioned signals such as seat or postural signals, provide the deepest signals that can induce the turn. So, maintaining the integrity of the basic operantly conditioned response is important for safety. However, it is now common for many trainers and coaches to use the single rein not for its original locomotory response, but simply to bend the horse's neck in an exaggerated fashion as a way of stopping the horse instead of using or re-training the operantly conditioned foundation response of equal pressure on both reins. Forcing the horse to bend its neck from rein pressure blurs the distinction between cues for an effective change of direction and simply bending the neck. This is because the signal is the same or similar while the response is different, with the result that the turn is detrained. The same can be said of using both reins to achieve the 'on the bit' head and neck posture at the expense of slowing.

Simultaneous, contradictory pressure

Perhaps the most insidious and widespread of all unorthodox techniques is the concurrent stimulation of two opposing operantly conditioned

signals, such as reins (the stop response) and legs (the go response). This concurrent signalling places the horse in a biomechanically impossible situation because the muscles it uses for go forward and stop are antagonistic, so, again, the result is a detraining effect. Detraining is not just a matter of losing the brakes or accelerator, the subsequent confusion can induce conflict-resolution behaviours in horses. Like all animals, horses seek to avoid pain. When they are prevented from doing so (e.g. when trapped between reins and legs) they become hyper-reactive, using *active* coping mechanisms. They are actively trying to escape, but escape is thwarted. Hyper-reactive escape behaviour switches to other active coping strategies such as hyper-reactive predator removal behaviours (e.g. bucking, rearing and shying). Active coping mechanisms share similar characteristics and brain pathways as cutaneous pain: in rats, they include hyper-reactivity, increased vigilance, raised heart rate and raised blood pressure (Keay and Bandler, 2008).

If the pain persists over a sufficiently long period and the horse cannot resolve the pain issue, hyper-reactive behaviour can spiral down into passive coping behaviours, where the horse is now hypo-reactive and seemingly gives up. Its bucking and shying may diminish, but the horse is heading down the slippery slope of learned helplessness where it is, on the surface at least, careless about pain.

Internally, the horse may show all the physiological signs of chronic stress. Passive coping states such as learned helplessness show similar characteristics and brain pathways as deep visceral pain: hypo-reactivity, apathy, decreased vigilance, lowered heart rate and lowered blood pressure (Keay and Bandler, 2008).

Non-ridden techniques

Rapping

Rapping (see also Chapter 9, Horses in sport and work) is the technique of hitting a horse's hindlegs as they pass over a rail during jumping (see Figure 12.5). The dorsally directed strike, often achieved by raising a whip or cane at the height of the horse's trajectory, punishes it for

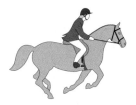

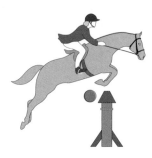

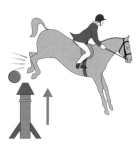

Figure 12.5   An illustration of the so-called 'rapping' technique banned by the Fédération Equestre Internationale. It involves hitting the horse's underside as it jumps a fence to make it allow greater clearance than each obstacle would seem to require.

jumping adequately and thus trains it to overcompensate when sizing-up fences. This is believed to make the horse more cautious when jumping and reduces the risk of it hitting a fence when pushed in competition (e.g. when forced to flatten its trajectory when jumping against the clock). The main argument against rapping is that it punishes horses for making any effort. It is forbidden both at events and during training, but the ban is extremely difficult to enforce during training. While it is appropriate that the FEI takes a dim view of this practice, many observers feel that practices known to accompany dressage training (such as forcing the mouth shut with crank nosebands) are even more of a priority because they are arguably harsher and certainly more relentless.

Gingering

Gingering is the use of irritants (traditionally, peeled ginger) *per rectum* with the aim of causing rectal discomfort. It is a practice known to occur in the show ring, especially where high postural tonus (e.g. a raised tail carriage) is considered desirable. For this reason, it is more likely to be found in shows for Arabians than for other breeds.

Considered a breech of the rules under most codes of showing, it is difficult to detect once the agent itself has been passed by defecation. Inarguably, any manipulations of horse's tail carriage or conformation (including, of course, docking) should be undertaken only when there is a veterinary reason (Lefebvre *et al.*, 2007).

Soring

Damaging the skin of the pasterns with caustic topical applications and then fitting chains or beads so that they lie on the damaged tissue can cause extravagant lifting of the lower limbs and flexion of the fetlocks. It is practised in show classes where high limb action is highly desired (e.g. for Tennessee Walkers). Practices such as this are more likely to be controlled if veterinarians remain aware of them and prioritise the welfare of the animals in their care. Legislation may have outlawed many such interventions, but policing the emergent rules relies on the cooperation of the profession. Detection depends on being able to correctly age any evidence of scarification in the horse's limbs; old lesions are not likely to cause current behavioural modifications and can easily be blamed on a previous owner, handler or groom.

Sedation and nerve blocks

Where a lack of reactivity in horses is highly prized in the show ring (e.g. in Western pleasure riding), a raised tail carriage may detract from the horse's score. So competitors may surreptitiously use nerve blocks or even neurectomy to reduce tail movement (Houpt, 2000). The tail may appear to be clamped between the hindlegs or suspiciously inactive, but detection is difficult and depends on the use of electromyography.

There are also numerous reports of competitors using psychopharmaceuticals (notably, sedatives) to make horses more tractable. One of the ironies of this practice is that the recipients of these treatments are often horses that have, just prior to the event, been overfed with concentrates and so are less likely to be manageable. Over-feeding horses so that they look in top show condition and confining them to contain their energy and reduce the need to groom them just increases their ebullience.

The practice of manipulating the behaviour of horses with pharmaceuticals (including fluphenazine, acepromazine and zuclophenthixol) is unethical and is rigorously monitored by the FEI. Nevertheless, even in local shows, competitors may be tempted to eliminate undesirable responses, usually ones that make the horse or pony difficult to control. Largely confined to the show ring, this intervention is also dangerous since it can affect the horse's ability to move safely and so is of particular concern when it arises in jumping competitions.

Electric shock-collars

Electric shock-collars, which can be triggered remotely to release a discharge, have received considerable attention from animal trainers. Undesirable long-term and short-term behavioural changes in dogs, notably those indicating distress (Schilder and van der Borg, 2004) and problems with the use of electric shock-collars in horse-training have been described (McGreevy and Boakes, 2007). Dogs that have received shocks (even remotely triggered shocks) begin to react fearfully to their owners (who become a predictor of the aversive stimuli).

These devices have also been used to punish crib-biting, but horses often moderate their stereotypic behaviour when wearing the collar only to resume it as soon as the collar is removed, sometimes with a transient increase in the response, possibly as the result of a post-inhibitory rebound (McGreevy and Nicol, 1998).

Horse-walkers

Although a mainstream means of exercising stabled horses, horse-walking machines have come under scrutiny over concern that they are dragging machines that force horses to undertake locomotion. The implication that they merely pull horses (tied up within them by their head-collars) seems to ignore the reality that these devices also feature rubber boarding that taps the horse's hindquarters should it begin to lag and that many people use walkers without tying the horse's head. Either way, coercion is certainly involved but, paradoxically, the coercive forces may be more consistent than many handlers and this may explain why accidents involving horse-walkers are rare.

Their use in foundation training for horses, especially during backing, has been reported recently (Murphy, 2007). Effectively, it is a form of overshadowing in that the pressure of the head-collar that evokes a leading response is used to overshadow the pressure of the rider on the horse's back. There are concerns about the dangers to both horse and rider should a flight response emerge within this sort of assembly, which is clearly not designed with foundation training (horse-breaking) in mind.

Water deprivation

It is believed by some that water deprivation makes horses appear more compliant. Certainly, clinical dehydration will compromise the ability of horses to show flight responses, many of which are seen in confused and poorly trained horses and few of which are desirable. Furthermore, as Xenophon (translated by Morgan, 1962) proposed, depriving a horse of water allows one to use water as a reward. For example, this is seen in methods that advocate the imposition of dehydration as a valid step for remediating horses that refuse to be led into a trailer. Horses may have the ability to adapt to considerable periods with little water but dehydration is highly questionable on ethical grounds and should never be advocated since it can cause irreversible renal damage.

Conclusion

There are numerous questionable practices in current equitation. It is usually, but not always, easy to see why they might work, but the ethics and sustainability of their use are subject to continuing debate.

Take-home messages

- Horses are so behaviourally flexible that they will give the appearance of tolerating relentless pressure.
- Some unorthodox techniques are popularised by elite riders and mimicked by less competent riders with disastrous effects on horse welfare.
- Pressure can be used to force a horse to adopt a given posture in a time-frame much shorter than is the case in conventional training.
- If techniques compromise horse welfare and future trainability for short-term gains, they can be considered neither sustainable nor ethical.

Areas for further research

- Investigation into learned helplessness as applied to the ridden horse.
- Establishment of the range of rein pressures on a range from neutral to aversive.

13 Fight and Flight Responses and Manifestations

Introduction

Fear is generally considered to be an intervening variable linked not only to a raft of noxious and dangerous stimuli that potentially compromise an animal's welfare, but also to a series of physiological and behavioural stress responses in the animal that afford appropriate responses to the noxious stimuli. It can be defined as the emotional reaction to a stimulus that the animal is motivated to terminate, escape from, or avoid (Gray, 1987). The goal of the fear reaction is critical to an animal's survival and for optimal exploitation of its environment. It is important to differentiate between stress and distress. *Prima facie*, the term distress seems anthropomorphic, but it is useful in distinguishing between a non-threatening stress response and a biological state where the animal's welfare is negatively affected by the stress response (Moberg and Mench, 2000). Fear and anxiety are two closely related emotions. Fear is generally defined as a reaction to the perception of actual danger, whereas anxiety is defined as the reaction to a potential danger that threatens the integrity of the individual (Boissy, 1998). Critical reviews of fear tests used in various domestic species are available (Forkman *et al.*, 2007).

An animal's fear reaction may be active or passive. Active coping mechanisms broadly comprise two categories, escape or attack, while passive coping strategies may be more subtle and include apparently ambivalent behaviours, displacement behaviours or freezing (Moberg and Mench, 2000; McLean, 2005b). Both active and passive mechanisms entail physiological changes such as alterations in heart rate and blood pressure. Nicol *et al.* (2005) showed that diet can have a modulatory effect on fearfulness. They found that foals fed after weaning on fat and fibre diets compared with foals fed on starch and sugar diets were more investigative and were more likely to approach unfamiliar people. In addition, they cantered about less, seemed calmer and were less distressed immediately after weaning.

Von Borell *et al.* (2007) describe active and passive coping mechanisms using the terms proactive (instead of active) and reactive (instead of passive). The notion of passive can lead to a misunderstanding that the animal is doing nothing, whereas, in the absence of control, its survival strategy may actually be to preserve energy as a 'last ditch' mechanism. Physiologically, the animal exhibits changes compared with the normal state. It is suggested that active coping may be termed proactive because such mechanisms as flight response are indeed proactive.

Stress has major biological consequences for all animals, but because horse-training involves aversive stimuli in the form of negative reinforcement and sometimes punishment, the risk for reducing

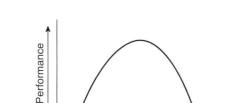

Figure 13.1   Yerkes–Dodson's law describes how stress can enhance learning performance to a point and then inhibit it (i.e. at low levels it can be beneficial for learning but at higher levels it is detrimental).

horse welfare is particularly high if stress is not kept to a minimum. Stress, however, is not entirely negative in terms of an animal's wellbeing. Low levels of stress are adaptive for survival, conferring optimal learning conditions as a result of raised attention and awareness (Moberg and Mench, 2000). Yerkes–Dodson's (1908) law neatly illustrates (Figure 13.1) how stress can be seen as neutral, negative or positive (de Graaf-Roelfsema, 2007). If stress can be seen as advantageous on the one hand and maladaptive at higher levels, then there must be intermediate levels where the effects are neutral. Optimal learning, therefore, requires a specific narrow range of stress. For example, when training a horse to step sideways from the rider's leg pressure, stress levels increase as the horse shows raised muscular tonus levels. When the response becomes habitual to a cue, stress levels decrease to the normal range.

More recently, it has been suggested that there is no simple division of stress into categories of 'good' and 'bad' stress. Any frequent stressor, including 'good' stresses (such as frequent mating), can have a detrimental effect on an animal's welfare (Ladewig, 2000). As prey animals, horses are generally more inclined to escape aversive stimuli where possible; aggression is mainly confined to situations where the animal is cornered or trapped or when defending foals from certain predators. Thus, horses generally have a strongly developed flight response and possess morphological characteristics for running away from danger, such as acute senses and fleet locomotory abilities. It is likely that selective breeding over the past few millennia to facilitate habituation to towing carts and having humans on their backs has dulled the flight

response of horses to some extent. In equestrian circles it is common to describe some breeds and individual horses as *hot* and some as *cold*, meaning that they are more or less sensitive and more or less prone to express a flight response when presented with an aversive stimulus. A mixture of hot and cold breeds is known as a Warmblood.

There is a great variation among breeds and individual horses with regard to their predisposition to express the flight response (Visser *et al.*, 2001; Hausberger *et al.*, 2004). Murphey *et al.* (1981) showed similar variation in flight response between *Bos indicus* and *Bos taurus* cattle. Fear responses show a great deal of variation both within individuals and among individuals, depending on the nature and intensity of the perceived stressor; they can also be modified by age, experience, genetics, physiological state and season (Moberg and Mench, 2000; Hausberger *et al.*, 2004).

Fearful behaviour in horses can have serious implications for both horse and rider safety, so it is not surprising that relaxation and low levels of fear and stress are ubiquitous goals in horse-training. Research has shown that many serious human injuries with horses occur as a result of unexpected fear reactions (Keeling *et al.*, 1999). Recently, anecdotal experiences have been substantiated with scientific evidence that a rider is able to induce nervousness in a horse that can potentially lead to dangerous fear reactions (Von Borstel *et al.*, 2007). The fear response can be the horse-trainer's greatest adversary, inversely correlating with learning and performance. Once the brain has perceived a fearful stimulus, alertness is raised and less salient stimuli are ignored. That is why a horse in a full-blown flight response can seem senseless, and can gallop into fences and cars or collide with trees and other obstacles.

The jumping response of an intensely fearful horse may be altered to the extent that it scrapes over fences and may drag its legs through the top wires of a fence. A flat hollow jump characterises the flight response and is not uncommonly seen in incorrectly trained eventing horses in horse trials where the performance appears to be semi-controlled bolting (Figure 13.2). It is likely that flight response is highly implicated in the high levels of rider falls and deaths in that sport. The greater the amount of flight response, the greater the acceleration tendency and the more the horse

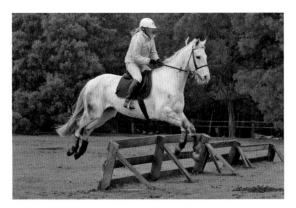

Figure 13.2 Flight response is strongly implicated in horses that jump hollow and flat.

is unresponsive to other stimuli, including the rider's signals. Such a horse invariably has what is known as a 'hard mouth'. In reality, the mouth is not insensitive, but the flight response outcompetes the rider's signals for salience.

The fear response

Fear responses manifest in various ways, including avoidance (running away), active defence (threat, attack), or the inhibition of movement, expressed as tonic immobility known as freezing (Christensen, 2007). Fear is also associated with increased vigilance and vocalisations such as alarm calls (Boissy, 1995). When a horse experiences conflicting motivations, fearful behaviours may be clearly expressed in some cases but less so in others. For example, a rider on a fearful (or confused) horse may restrain the horse with the reins and the horse's attempts to escape manifest as hyperreactive behaviour, such as jogging and increased muscular tonus. On the other hand, a cornered horse at liberty may find escape impossible and may actually approach its aggressor. Such a horse may not outwardly express fear. For such reasons it has been proposed that the most accurate assessments of fear should include both behavioural and physiological measures of stress (Manteca and Deag, 1993). When a horse encounters an intensely fearful stimulus, such as a predator, both neural and endocrine stress reactions occur.

The neural response

Fear responses activate the sympathetic nervous system. This in turn stimulates the spinal cord via the hypothalamus and reticular formation in the brain stem to prime the body for maximum physical action. Two systems are mobilised to facilitate escape or defence: the sympathetic-adrenal-medullary (SAM) and the hypothalamic–pituitary–adrenocortical (HPA) axes (Archer, 1973). This sympathetic stimulation raises blood pressure, heart rate and stroke force, as well as causing vasoconstriction of blood vessels surrounding the gut to facilitate maximum blood flow to the skeletal muscles and brain. In addition, glycolysis in the liver and muscles is accelerated, resulting in a rise in plasma sugar concentration. Sympathetic activation also causes the release of noradrenaline at the neuromuscular junctions to prepare the body for maximum physical exercise (Moberg and Mench, 2000).

The sympathetic reactions of both innate and learned fear stimuli are first intercepted by the thalamus, which has specialised parts for receiving visual, auditory and somatosensory stimuli. Messages are then sent to the amygdala, the tissue central to the rapid uptake of fear responses. From the thalamus, the amygdala is stimulated via two different pathways. The first path is direct, while the second connects to the amygdala via the brain's auditory, visual or somatosensory cortex (Figure 13.3). Emotions of fear that can outlast the physiological experience are a result of these dual routes of information leading to the amygdala (Kandel, 2006). This loop also plays a central role in the unique non-erasure features of fear responses. Both pathways terminate at the pyramidal cells of the amygdala's lateral nucleus. Connections from the lateral nucleus of the amygdala to its central nucleus enervate adaptive responses: the hypothalamus for activation of the fight-or-flight response and the cingulated cortex for the evaluation of the nature of the aversive stimulus.

The endocrine response

The secondary physiological fear reaction is endocrine and involves a cascade of events. The brain signals the adrenal medulla, via the SAM

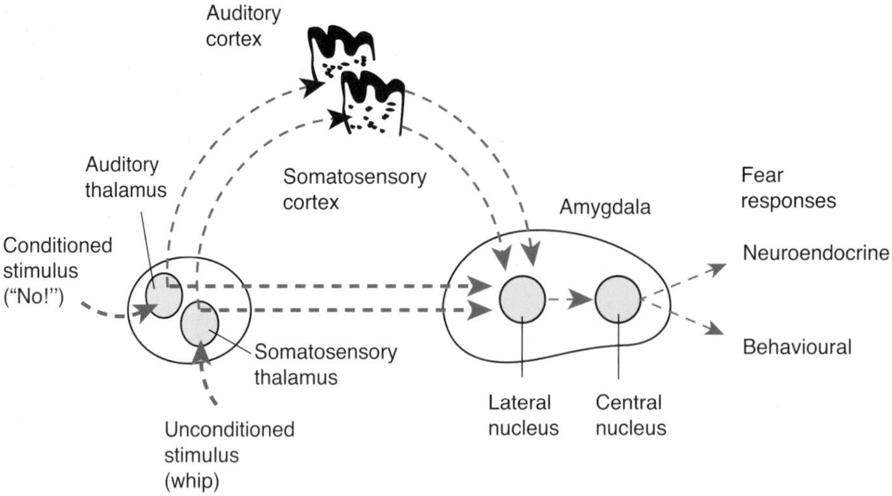

Figure 13.3 The neural pathways of fear using punishment as an example. In this case, a horse simultaneously hears the word 'No!' and feels the strike of the whip. The thalamus receives auditory and somatosensory inputs simultaneously, which converge in the amygdala via direct and indirect pathways, resulting in a fear response.

axis, to immediately release adrenaline in order to kick-start the flight response. The activation of the HPA is a little slower, beginning with the hypothalamus producing corticotrophin-releasing factor (CRF) and vasopressin (AVP). The CRF and AVP stimulate the pituitary gland and the release of corticosteroids, long-term stress hormones such as cortisol, which peaks minutes after the initial aversive stimulus. Cortisol provides for a sustained flight response, ensuring energy availability over a longer term (Korte, 2001). While the primary role of the HPA axis is to shift energy production during the stressful period, an unfortunate consequence is the disruption of critical events such as reproduction. Circulating cortisol concentrations have an inhibitory effect on preovulation secretion of luteinising hormone, and thus results in a failure to ovulate (Nangalama and Moberg, 1991). The adrenal glucocorticosteroids, such as cortisol and corticosterone, are also known to have a modulating effect on the release of other gonadotropins, such as follicle-stimulating hormone. In addition, prolactin and somatotropin (growth hormone) are also sensitive to glucocorticosteroids (Moberg and Mench, 2000). Blecha (2000) has also shown that the HPA axis negatively affects the immune system as a result of extreme environmental conditions or stress-

ful management practices. Chronically, socially isolated horses even show a depressed cortisol response on a CRF challenge test, suggesting a desensitisation of the HPA axis (Visser et al., 2008).

One-trial learning

While most things we try to train the horse to do require a number of repetitions, the flight response, unfortunately, can be learned in just one experience (see Chapter 7, Applying learning theory). It is adaptive for the animal to remember any response that enables it to survive a life-threatening experience. Patterns of escape that result in surviving a predatory attack are instantly recorded for later use (McLean, 2001), while trial-and-error learning may be redundant in such life-and-death situations. It was once believed that fear responses were like other behavioural responses – they could be learned and they could also be erased. However, Le Doux (1994) showed that fear is different. In experiments with rats, he showed that once a fear response is acquired, no matter how situations are altered, full-blown fear responses spontaneously can return with little provocation. This research has monumental implications for horse-trainers:

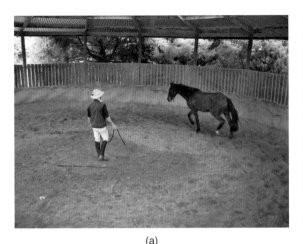

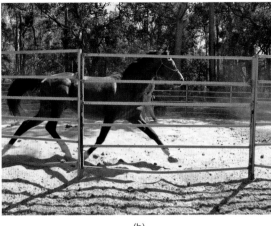

(a)   (b)

Figure 13.4   a and b. Round-pen training should be managed so that there is minimal or no flight response, otherwise it can make indelible associations between fearfulness in the horse and the presence of humans. Flight responses should be avoided at all costs in horse-training. (Photos courtesy of Amanda Warren-Smith and Carol Willcocks.)

avoid fearful reactions at all costs (Figure 13.4). If, during human interactions, the horse is showing hyper-reactive behaviours (high head, hollow back, short choppy strides), it may be acquiring associations between fear and humans. Chasing horses can be a recipe for further, and sometimes more severe expressions of, the fear response and for rifts in horse–human bonds. Krueger (2007) found in her experiments on the round-pen technique that 3 of 19 horses in her first set of trials had to be withdrawn on animal welfare grounds because of 'untypical immense sweating' and the problem that these horses 'did not respond to the experimenter anymore' (however, they did respond in subsequent trials).

Fear can also readily become associated with neutral stimuli and these neutral stimuli then become powerful triggers of the fear response. So chasing young horses to show off their movement, round-pen techniques, lungeing and long-reining fearful horses are all ill-advised and have negative welfare implications. There is no ethical justification for inducing fear during training.

Measuring fear

There is some conjecture surrounding the definition and measurement of fear and its consequent stress response (Hemsworth and Coleman, 1998). For example, questions arise as to what is measured, how biological manifestations are monitored and how intra-specific variation is dealt with. The vast difference between active and passive coping mechanisms (e.g. escape, aggression or freezing) cautions a single reductionist approach in measuring fear. Even the phenomenon of raised heart rate is an unreliable indicator of fear and stress and is therefore contraindicated in research. While an increase in heart rate may result from reduced vagal activity as well as from increased sympathetic activity or, in most cases, from a combination of concurrent changes in activity within both branches, the heart rate *variability* (HRV) allows a much more accurate and detailed determination of the functional regulatory characteristics of the autonomic nervous system. Thus, HRV has been found to be a particularly good indicator of the non-invasive assessment of autonomic nervous system activity in response to psychophysiological stress (see for review, Von Borell *et al.*, 2007). Typically, fearful horses tend to show low levels of HRV (i.e. they have relatively invariable heart rates; e.g. Visser, 2002). HRV has been used as an indicator of acute and chronic stress, mental challenges and emotional states in a number of farm animals and companion animal species. Thus, HRV is a useful indicator of an animal's level of fear (Sgoifo *et al.*, 1997). Measuring circulating glucocorticosteroids is also used – blood is taken from a catheterised horse or glucocorticosteroid concentrations in saliva samples are assessed.

Field tests may involve assessing the effect on the horse's behaviour of an immobile or approaching object or human, or of their sudden appearance. In horses, fear or anxiety is usually assessed with tests in which the horse is challenged with a potentially frightening stimulus, such as a suddenly lowered or opened umbrella or any other unknown obstacle in a familiar environment (e.g. Visser *et al.*, 2001; Christensen, 2007; Lansade *et al.*, 2007). If the stimulus is a human, horses are either approached or have the option to approach the human in their familiar environment within a limited time (e.g. Søndergaard and Halekoh, 2003; for review, see Waiblinger *et al.*, 2006). In both types of tests, horses' behavioural responses as well as some physiological measures (heart rate and blood measures) are taken to assess not only the level of fearfulness but also general activity and gregariousness. Currently, modifications of these types of tests are used in the selection of horses for mounted police work.

How close an animal allows something it finds aversive to approach is known as the animal's flight distance (Hediger, 1964). Flight distance differs for different stimuli: a well-handled horse familiar with people has a flight distance of zero. The concept of flight distance is important when droving animals and fundamental to round-pen techniques in horses. The concept of flight distance maintains that there is a minimum zone surrounding an animal and when this is penetrated the animal will attempt to escape. The animal ceases its escape attempts when the intruder retreats from the animal's flight zone. Entering and retreating from an animal's flight zone is an example of negative reinforcement and is the basis of techniques such as round-pen and advance retreat (see Chapter 8, Training). The retreat of the handler negatively reinforces the horse's fear reduction. For domestic free-ranging cattle, the flight distance is around 30 m on mountain ranges (Grandin, 1980). Flight distance shows both inter-specific and intra-specific variation. While actual figures in horses are unresearched, Brahman cattle show a larger flight distance than most English breeds (Grandin,

1978). It is likely that sensitive horse breeds, such as Arabians and Thoroughbreds, would show a greater flight distance than colder breeds, such as Shires and Welsh and Konik ponies.

Acute and chronic stress

In the domestic situation, horses may be subject to fearful experiences for various lengths of time. Horse-riding provides a common setting for short- or long-term stress because riders can directly enforce responses and, unlike other animal-training pursuits, can effectively prevent escape by trapping horses between rein and leg pain.

Active emotional coping is a characteristic of acute (short-term) stress. The animal becomes more engaged, vigilant and hyper-reactive when stress is escapable. Acute stress may appear disguised when it manifests as redirected aggression, displacement activities (Wiepkema, 1987) or passively as freezing or quiescence. However, it typically manifests hyper-reactively as conflict behaviours that range from increased muscle tonus and body tension to aggression, bolting, rearing, bucking, shying, leaping, flipping over, rushing backwards and freezing (McLean and McGreevy, 2004). Conflict behaviours are evolved anti-predator behaviours that arise from conflicting motivations when escape/avoidance responses are thwarted. They can be defined as 'a set of responses of varying duration that are usually characterised by hyper-reactivity and arise largely through confusion' (McGreevy *et al.*, 2005).

When stressful situations are regular, conflict behaviours may become ritualised as the effects of chronic stress accumulate (Ladewig, 2000). Passive emotional coping frequently characterises chronic stress resulting in disengagement, decreased vigilance, hypo-reactivity and quiescence. The heart rate and blood pressure may lower and the horse frequently appears dull. In such situations, trainers may mistakenly believe that the horse is now more accepting of current events, but the quiescence is actually a result of inescapable stress and lack of control.

Chronic stress results in physiological degradation such as raised corticosteroid concentration, immunological disturbances, gastric disorders and damage, development of stereotypies and injurious behaviours such as self-mutilation and increased aggression (Stolba *et al.*, 1983; Wiepkema, 1987; Moberg and Mench, 2000). Thus, chronic stress has profound welfare implications for horses.

Moberg and Mench (2000) observed that 'it is difficult to envisage a single chronic stressor in non-experimental animals, with the possible exception of unrelenting pain or prolonged exposure to an extreme environmental condition, such as severe cold'. However, unrelenting pain provided by continuous or simultaneous bit or spur pressure does provide such a scenario for the horse. Thus, conflicts in motivation are of great significance in any analysis of horse-training, because of the horse's inability to resolve the stressful situation. Currently, the accurate identification of chronic stress eludes us, and there are no specific tests for it (Ladewig, 2000), so there is a strong need for research on stress in domestic horses.

Positive domestic equine welfare can be defined by the absence of physiological and behavioural disorders (Ladewig, 2003). In a training regime where negative reinforcement is predominant and inherent, it follows that its correct use has positive welfare implications. Yet, studies have revealed that equestrian coaches are largely ignorant of learning theory. This deficit is at great odds with their responsibility to establish desirable learned responses in animals without causing conflict behaviours (McGreevy, 2007; Warren-Smith and McGreevy, 2008a). Peak equestrian coaching, training and regulatory bodies must legislate for the correct use of learning theory in equestrian activity as a matter of urgency.

The neural basis of chronic stress extends further from the central role of the amygdala. The basal ganglia are implicated not only in stress but also in stereotypic behaviour and alterations in learning. Inside the basal ganglia, the striatum filters and relays information to and from cortical structures and is integral in motivation, action and learning. Chronic stress alters dopaminergic modulation of the striatum in rats and similar physiological changes appear to occur in the horse (Parker *et al.*, 2008). For example, crib-biting horses have been reported with significantly higher receptor subtypes in regions of the basal ganglia associated with reward (the nucleus accumbens) and significantly lower number of receptors in

the basal ganglia region known as the caudatus, the tissue involved in determining action and outcome (Parker *et al.*, 2008). In rats, inactivation of the dorsomedial striatum impairs both reversal learning and strategy switching and is thus implicated in the perseverance of behaviours, including stereotypies (Ragozzino, 2007).

Pain

Pain is also interrelated with fear and stress. While pain is generally thought of as a sensation, there is justification for it to be described as a 'need' state in that it has more in common with primary reinforcers, such as hunger and thirst, than it has with the senses (Keay and Bandler, 2008). There are qualitative differences in pain of different origins. Cutaneous pain provides a different experience from the deep pain that arises from internal organs or muscles. While skin pain is associated with hyper-reactivity, hyper-vigilance and rising of pulse and blood pressure, deep pain is associated with quiescence, slowing of the pulse, fall in blood pressure sweating and nausea (Keay and Bandler, 2008). These different expressions of pain bear striking similarities with active and passive emotional coping strategies.

Active emotional coping is characterised by engagement with the environment (fight or flight) when pain is escapable (Figure 13.5). There is increased vigilance, hyper-reactivity, increased somatomotor activity and increased sympathetic activity. Passive emotional coping is the opposite: it involves disengagement (conservation and withdrawal), decreased vigilance, hypo-reactivity, quiescence, lowering in blood pressure and heart rate. Passive coping is a response to inescapable pain, pain of a deep origin, such as persistent and chronic visceral or muscular pain (Keay and Bandler, 2008).

These two strategies have a different neural basis. They are localised in different areas of the midbrain periaqueductal grey (PAG) longitudinal columns: the lateral PAG and the dorsolateral PAG are integral in active coping; the dorsolateral PAG has connections from the prefrontal cortex and hypothalamus, accounting for increased attention and vigilance. The ventrolateral PAG is involved in passive coping and has spinal cord and

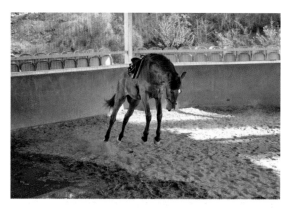

Figure 13.5   All hyper-reactive states (attempts to run away, bucking, bolting, shying and rearing) are active coping mechanisms. (Photo courtesy of Rob Duncan.)

brainstem connections that are implicit in inattention and withdrawal. Before undertaking any behaviour modification, such as proposed in this book, veterinary examination should be used to rule out pain as a cause of unwelcome responses.

Umwelt controllability

Fear can be thought of as a homeostatic mechanism designed to enhance the level of control an animal has of its umwelt. The animal assesses the situation and compares its perception with what it is motivated to do. A perceived mismatch between what is (known as *istwerte*) and what is wanted (*sollwerte*) results in the activations of behavioural and/or physiological responses (Wiepkema, 1987). Learning signals that couple with consistent responses have an important function in terms of umwelt predictability and controllability. While high levels of predictability and controllability are adaptive, low levels are stressful and maladaptive, and result in conflict behaviours. Dickinson (1980) summarised this in a general form in terms of probabilities (P) of outcome, whereby animals learn that a specific response (E1) produces a specific outcome (E2). Wiepkema (1987) extrapolated that in any given situation for an animal when $P(E2/E1) = 1$ there is no conflict for the animal about that particular stimulus response entity. When $P(E2/E1)$ is greater than zero, but less than one, it becomes a source of stress. In nature, an animal can generally flee (or fight) a stressful situation, thus resolving the conflict. However, when escape is thwarted, stress may accumulate. In training, the horse is mostly unable to flee from confusion because it is prevented from doing so by the reins. Ridden animals thus present a unique potential for acquiring stress. The amount of stress or conflict behaviour a trained horse exhibits can be seen as a summary of all of its E1/E2 entities. Using this model, all horses have unique profiles of their E2/E1 entities, so the probability of a consistent outcome from a signal positively correlates with relaxation, and inversely correlates with conflict behaviours.

The notion of conflict behaviours as a product of umwelt predictability and controllability is extremely important for our understanding of horse welfare. Consider that not only are horses unable to flee most stressful situations, but the instruments used to train them can also be highly aversive. For most domestic horses, the most aversive events that occur on a regular basis are not in their paddock (see Figure 13.6) or stable. Horses have some control over their lives in these situations: they are able to escape an aggressive conspecific or attack one; food is provided regularly; and shelter is largely available via housing or horse rugs (blankets and covers). Yet, very few riders indeed would contemplate that the most regular aversive events for a horse occur during handling and riding. Steel bits are placed in the horse's sensitive mouth, and strong pressures, and in many cases relentless pressures, may be applied there. The rider may also kick the horse in the thorax constantly, believing that the horse is

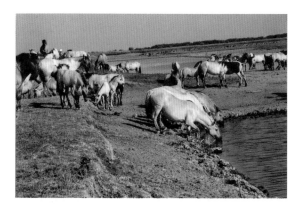

Figure 13.6   Horses at liberty have control of the environment to the extent that they can retreat or attack.

lazy. The so-called lazy horse, having no means of ameliorating the situation, may then be invaded with spurs or whips instantly and haphazardly. Even a well-trained horse may still have to endure the least obtrusive of pressure from apparatus to induce acceleration or deceleration. In-hand, also, various apparatus may be used to control an animal that is deemed unruly or lazy. The tragedy of such welfare issues is that horsepeople do not wilfully intend to injure horses and most would be aghast that there is another way of interpreting such issues.

When they are not trained to respond to the lightest of signals, often invisible to the onlooker, and when they are not consistently in self-carriage, many ridden and led horses endure pain on a regular basis. They show this in a variety of ways, sometimes as direct responses to the extant aversive stimuli, and at other times as neurotic manifestations of chronic invasions of pain (McLean, 2003, 2004, 2005a, 2005b, 2008; McLean and McGreevy, 2004; McGreevy and McLean, 2007; McLean and McLean, 2008).

The following tables describe manifestations of fear in domestic horses and emphasise not only that the problems have strong links with dysfunctions in various stimulus–response entities trained by negative reinforcement, but also that the reinstallation of associated responses by negative reinforcement provides the key to rehabilitation. While it is important to stress that many of these behaviours may have associated age, breed, sex and genetic predispositions, it is also important to recognise that, by and large, learning and experience confirms or denies these tendencies. These behaviours, therefore, stand as testimony to humanity's collective misunderstanding of horse cognition and learning processes.

Manifestations of fear

From the standpoint of behaviour, fear has many guises. Typically, and throughout the centuries, fear responses in horses have been described in anthropomorphic ways (see Table 2.3 and Chapter 3, Anthropomorphism). Usually, these behavioural descriptors categorise them as resistances and evasions and sometimes as vices. Fearful behaviours that result from training interventions are numerous and diverse. They may show up overtly as a direct result of the horse's interaction with apparatus used in training, handling and riding (as shown in Table 13.1). Some of these reactions to apparatus are a result of the variation in hypersensitivities among individual horses. Some horses show variations in their sensitivity to being touched on the head, body and legs and some are especially reactive to girth pressure.

Head-shyness is a progressive hypersensitivity in the head/ears region, where the horse has learned to rapidly withdraw its head to escape human touch. It is learned by negative reinforcement: the horse learns rapidly that raising its head results in removal of the handler's hand. Gradual habituation (desensitisation) can be successful but may be less so if the horse has learned to show escape behaviour. Then, the next technique may involve overshadowing (outcompeting) the head-shyness with sequences of step-back and forward until they become more salient than the head contact (McLean, 2008). Horses are quick to develop aversions to specific stimuli. So, typically, a horse that is fearful of the human hand has fewer problems with a hand inside a towel. The towel can be rubbed around the horse's head and, if necessary, gradually brought closer to the more sensitive areas (see Figure 13.7). As the horse habituates to the towel, the fingers can gradually be allowed to protrude from the towel until the horse has lost its hypersensitivity to the human touch. The towel may be dampened to add a further variation in tactile stimulus that will assist in habituation. Similarly with *bit-shyness*, the avoidance behaviour is reinforced by freedom from contact. This interpretation informs the remedy: gradual habituation or overshadowing until the horse habituates to the approach, touch and insertion of fingers and bit into its mouth. Counter-conditioning provides further depth to the remedy in that the approach of the bit or, with head-shyness, touching the head can be trained as a secondary reinforcer that is antecedent to the delivery of food or tactile contact such as wither caressing. Correct skills are necessary in handling horses' heads and especially in inserting things into their mouths. Sometimes horses may raise their heads when the bridle is removed and the bit can become caught for a moment in the diastema of the lower jaw. As the horse raises its head, the

Table 13.1 Hypersensitivities and dysfunctional responses to apparatus

Problem	Mechanism	Category of response	Increase in reactivity	At liberty in stable or enclosure	Under-saddle	In-hand	Ethological relevance	Role of pain	Training flaws that lead to conflict	Training remedy
Head-shy	Horse suddenly removes handler's hand from head when handled	Apparatus-induced hyper-sensitivity	++	−	−	+	+	Possible	Insufficient habituation, incorrect application of negative reinforcement	Gradual habituation towards horse's ears with a soft towel where hand is removed when horse's head is immobile
Bit-shy	Horse raises head and won't allow bit to be inserted into mouth	Apparatus-induced hyper-sensitivity	+	−	−	+	−	Possible	Insufficient habituation, incorrect application of negative reinforcement	Progressive habituation of touching lips, inserting fingers into mouth may require some overshadowing or counter conditioning
Leg-shy	Horse suddenly removes handler's hand from leg when handled	Limb hyper-sensitivity	++	−	−	+	+	Possible	Insufficient habituation, incorrect application of negative reinforcement	Progressive habituation with handler's hand where hand is removed from leg when it is immobile
Aerosol-shy	Horse shows hyper-reactive and avoidance behaviour when sprayed with aerosols	Aural hyper-sensitivity	++	−	−	+	++	Unlikely	Insufficient habituation, incorrect application of negative reinforcement	Progressive habituation with aerosols or hose spray where aerosol is removed when horse is immobile

Pulling back from tether	Horse rushes backwards when tethered, usually breaking tether or halter	Head hyper-sensitivity	++	−	−	+	+	Possible	Inconsistent responses to operant acceleration signals, incorrect application of negative reinforcement	Re-install operant responses from forward signals so that the horse can go, quicken and lengthen its stride and go sideways from light forward or sideways signals
Cold back (including girth-shy, cinch-bound)	Horse becomes hyper-reactive, usually bucks or bolts forward when girth is tightened around thorax	Apparatus-induced hyper-sensitivity	++	−	+	+	+	Possible	Insufficient habituation and possible inconsistent responses to operant deceleration signals	Habituate to touch in girth region. Re-install operant responses from rein signals so that the horse can stop, slow, step-back and shorten its stride from the lightest of rein signals and overshadow hypersensitive reaction by eliciting step-back response during girthing
Shoeing difficulties	Horse moves its legs during shoeing, kicks out or strikes	Limb hyper-sensitivity	++	−	−	+	0/+	Possible	Insufficient habituation to feet handling and incorrect application of negative reinforcement	Habituate to feet being handled. Re-install operant responses from rein signals so that the horse can stop, slow, step-back and shorten its stride from the lightest of rein signals and overshadow kicking out

(Continued)

Table 13.1 (Continued)

Problem	Mechanism	Category of response	Increase in reactivity	At liberty in stable or enclosure	Under-saddle	In-hand	Ethological relevance	Role of pain	Training flaws that lead to conflict	Training remedy
Refusing to load into floats (trailers)	Horse baulks when led towards float	Apparatus-induced fear response	+++	–	–	+	+	Unlikely	Inconsistent responses to operant acceleration signals, incorrect application of negative reinforcement	Re-install operant responses from forward signals so that the horse can go, quicken and lengthen its stride and go sideways from light forward or sideways signals and repeat at the float/trailer
Rushing out of floats (trailers)	Escapes from float fast backwards	Apparatus-induced fear response	+++	N/A	–	+	+	Unlikely	Inconsistent responses to operant acceleration signals, incorrect application of negative reinforcement	Re-install operant responses from forward signals so that the horse can go, quicken and lengthen its stride and go sideways from light forward or sideways signals and repeat at the float/trailer
Barrier/starting stall problems	Won't enter starting stalls	Apparatus-induced fear response	++	N/A	+	+	+	Unlikely	Inconsistent responses to operant acceleration signals, incorrect application of negative reinforcement	Re-install operant responses from forward signals so that the horse can go, quicken and lengthen its stride and go sideways from light forward or sideways signals and repeat at the starting stalls

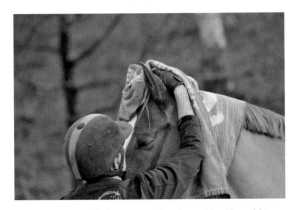

Figure 13.7   Head-shyness may be desensitised by rubbing the horse's head with a towel or other novel or innocuous stimulus, which may be further elaborated by moistening it and then gradually reintroducing human fingers.

mouth pressure may increase and the increasing pain can result in fearfulness of the bit.

Leg-shyness describes the condition where the horse's legs show hypersensitivity to touch. Gradual habituation is a typical approach, but the danger of touching the horse's hindlegs cautions handlers to stand in a safe position and to use a soft long-whip that can touch the legs safely and remain in contact until the instant the hyper-reactivity subsides. The moment of removal is crucial. One of the most successful approaches here is to hose the leg (McLean and McLean, 2008), because the handler can stand at a safe distance and can vary the intensity of the hose spray so that the habituation process can be more thorough as a result of this variation. It is usually easier to touch the horse's legs during hosing and then the spray can be applied and removed randomly during this touching. When horses are *fearful of aerosols* the same hosing method can be used and, during the hosing, the aerosol can usually be applied with no adverse reaction. The hose spray is then varied and switched off from time to time so that the aerosol and hose are randomly applied and intermingled at first. It is not surprising that horses develop aversion to sprays because the hissing sound is probably ethologically relevant as an indicator of events that may be dangerous.

Just as horses show large variations in their initial reactions to the rider's leg pressure (see Chapter 6, Learning III: Associative (aversive)), they may also show similar variations to pressure on their heads. While some horses may trial stepping forward in response to pressure on their halters or bridles, others react strongly by *pulling back from the tether*. If this backwards reaction results in removal of pressure, either by the handler releasing the pressure or by the tether breaking, the backwards reaction is reinforced. Again, this analysis informs the remedy. The horse should be trained to lead forward correctly and it is significant to observe that horses that pull back tend to raise their heads as their first reaction to anterior lead pressure. So repetitions of lead forward from pressure are efficacious. Because horses that resist leading forward can easily rear, it is safer to apply the lead forward pressure sideways at about 45 degrees. This is repeated until the horse leads forward immediately from a light lead signal and without raising its head. However, many problems are context-specific, so when the horse that has had such effective treatment is tethered, it may still attempt to pull back. It is safer to tether the animal to a car inner tube attached to a safe strong post. This way, the horse learns that the pressure remains until it steps forward.

Girthing the horse is perhaps the most challenging habituation event. Some horses find it highly aversive to have their thoraxes compressed and become *cold-backed (or girth-shy, or cinch-bound)*. In affected horses, this compression generally elicits a running forward response with a simultaneous or subsequent bucking reflex. Driving the horse forward under such circumstances is futile as it assists the already activated forward flight response. The best solution is to overshadow the hypersensitive reaction with well-established sequences of step-back reactions and then, when calm, sequences of forward steps followed by step-backs (see Figure 13.8).

When horses show problem behaviour with the farrier and are *difficult to shoe*, it is generally associated with fast forward reactions. The worst scenario involves kicking out and this can be interpreted as synonymous with running forward because both the kick and running forward consist of hyper-reactive retractions of the hindleg, the major difference being that one is in the swing phase, the other in the stance phase. Because some horses find having the feet handled offensive and hammering especially so, these problems may involve considerably high levels of hyper-reactivity

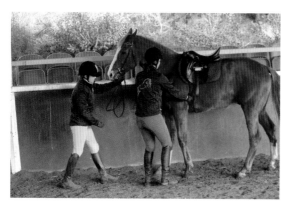

Figure 13.8 The girth-shy response can be successfully overshadowed by simultaneously stepping the horse forward and back.

horse ceases kicking but simply moves its leg, the handler can vibrate the stallion bit more mildly to negatively reinforce complete immobility. If the horse is trained to lower its head from downward pressure on the halter or stallion bit, this can overshadow any attempts to move its leg, but because this head lowering stimulus is unlikely to outcompete a hyper-reactive state, it is best left until after the step-back sequences are completed.

Horses are ethologically compelled to avoid dark, narrow and confined places, so it is not surprising that *loading onto horse floats and trailers* presents considerable difficulty for many horses (see Figure 13.9). Those that refuse to load onto trailers show deficits in their leading forward responses (McLean, 2005b), which may either contribute to the loading problem or be exacerbated by it. The first step in rehabilitating such a horse is to re-train its acceleration and deceleration responses in-hand. When it is then brought to the float, it is important to maintain the pressure forward until the horse steps a single step forward in the direction of the float/trailer. This step should be repeated until the horse steps forward from a light lead signal. Then the next step is attempted, repeating until the horse steps forward from a light signal. Repetitions continue until the horse

and are therefore difficult to arrest. Using a stallion bit is the best option provided the horse is well trained to step-back and forward with it. The farrier or leg handler should be well informed that the horse will be strongly signalled to step-back when it kicks out, so the handler should be ready to drop the foot when tension shows up. The amount of step-back stimulus should be proportional to the hyper-reactivity so that the kicking out is not reinforced. When the

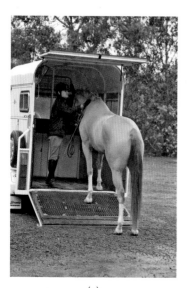

(a)

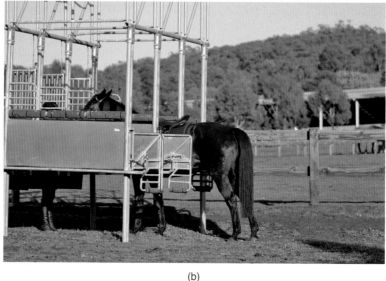

(b)

Figure 13.9 Training or re-training the horse to load onto the (a) float/trailer or (b) into racecourse starting gates is a matter of reinforcing the correct response and shaping it so that the smallest correct attempts and all improvements are rewarded.

steps easily all the way into the float without further signalling after the initial signal for forward. Forward signals may be fortified by tapping the horse on the ribcage with the long-whip in association with the light forward lead signal. The tapping should stop as soon as the horse steps forward. Secondary reinforcement when the horse successfully loads into the float, and target training the steps on the way into the float can have some success, but these do not address deficits in forward-leading responses. The best use of secondary positive reinforcements is to reward the horse for entering the float from light signals following completion of lead-forward training (McLean and McLean, 2008).

Similarly, the horse that **rushes backwards** out of the float shows deficits in leading forward because, when it rushes backwards, it pulls on the lead-rein held by the handler in the forward direction. The horse should be trained to step forward from lead pressure so that it does so immediately and from light signals. When it rushes out of the float, care should be taken not to raise the lead-rein pressure too much for forward as the horse may raise its head and connect with the roof of the float, creating more problems. The best solution is to train the horse to go forward from whip-taps on his ribcage with the long-whip to step forward in association with light forward lead pressure so that when it rushes out of the float, the handler can tap the ribcage rhythmically during rushing backwards, ceasing only when the horse steps forward (McLean, 2003).

Problems with starting stalls (starting gates, starting barriers) show up as either refusing to load into the stalls or hyper-reactive behaviours once inside. There are a number of problems that confront the horse when loading into starting stalls. The first is their appearance: they are closed spaces with low overhead frames (except for New Zealand starting gates). In addition, the space is narrow so the horse's body may easily connect with the opened back gates and with the foot platforms. All these are aversive to some horses and as soon as they feel the foot platforms on their sides they may rush out backwards, which only serves to reinforce the aversiveness of the gates. Future starting gate design should take these aversive aspects into account. Remedying loading problems follows the same principles as described above for

loading into floats. It is important that the horse is trained to stand still (without being held) inside the starting gates through equally thorough training of stop and go responses.

While the goal of all equestrian disciplines is to gain control over the horse's speed and direction, this is not necessarily the aim of the horse. So, it is not surprising that most problems are associated with speed and direction issues as shown in Table 13.2. Furthermore, when riders attenuate the acceleration and deceleration responses by concurrent signalling (simultaneous reins and leg pressures), horses may show conflict behaviours that manifest largely as dysfunctions of speed and line.

In many cases the deceleration responses are unintentionally overshadowed, so the conflict behaviours manifest as attempts to escape and run away. **Bolting, rushing, running away, jogging, pulling** and **above the bit** are all manifestations of poor deceleration responses (see Figure 13.10). They are all remedied by re-installing deceleration responses so that the horse is able to stop, slow, step-back and shorten its stride from light rein signals. This involves retuning to the earlier parts of the shaping scale and reinforcing single strides of stop or step-back responses. For example, the horse is signalled to step-back with the reins only for two steps of the forelegs (one complete stride of all four legs) and the reins are released on completion of the second step of the forelegs. Downward inter-gait and intra-gait transitions are repeated, releasing the reins pressure immediately after the transition is complete.

Rushing at jumping obstacles generally begins when the horse either hurts its legs on a pole or the rider pulls it in the mouth over the fence and the pain causes the horse to run away. Soon, the obstacle itself is associated with the pain and it now elicits a running response *towards* the fence. Jumping low cross-rails and gradually training the horse to stop from rein pressure 6 m before the cross-rail soon results in the horse losing its acceleration response towards the fence (McLean, 2003). This may need to be repeated at various obstacles. When horses are above the bit, the hyper-reactive behaviour and rein heaviness are not always apparent to the rider, but the above-the-bit reaction is a defensive head-carriage suggesting painful bit invasions, which, in turn, suggest slowing deficits. **Reefing** and **head tossing**

Table 13.2 Direct dysfunctions of speed and line conflicts

Problem	Mechanism	Category of response	Increase in reactivity	At liberty in stable or enclosure	Under-saddle	In-hand	Ethological relevance	Role of pain	Training flaws that lead to conflict	Training remedy
Bolting	Horse accelerates out of stimulus control	Escape/avoidance behaviour	+++	–	+	+	0/+	Unlikely	Inconsistent responses to operant deceleration signals, incorrect application of negative reinforcement	Re-install operant responses from rein signals so that the horse can stop, slow, step-back and shorten its stride from the lightest of rein signals
Rushing	Horse accelerates partly or completely beyond stimulus control	Escape/avoidance behaviour	+++	–	+	+	0/+	Possible	Inconsistent responses to operant deceleration signals, incorrect application of negative reinforcement	Re-install operant responses from rein signals so that the horse can stop, slow, step-back and shorten its stride from the lightest of rein signals
Running away	Horse accelerates partly or completely beyond stimulus control	Escape/avoidance behaviour	+++	–	+	+	0/+	Possible	Inconsistent responses to operant deceleration signals, incorrect application of negative reinforcement	Re-install operant responses from rein signals so that the horse can stop, slow, step-back and shorten its stride from the lightest of rein signals
Jogging	Horse accelerates partly beyond stimulus control	Escape/avoidance behaviour	++	–	+	+	0/+	Possible	Inconsistent responses to operant deceleration signals, incorrect application of negative reinforcement	Re-install operant responses from rein signals so that the horse can stop, slow, step-back and shorten its stride from the lightest of rein signals

Pulling	Horse accelerates partly beyond stimulus control, making reins feel heavy	Escape/ avoidance behaviour	++	–	+	+	0/+	Possible	Inconsistent responses to operant deceleration signals, incorrect application of negative reinforcement	Re-install operant responses from rein signals so that the horse can stop, slow, step-back and shorten its stride from the lightest of rein signals
Above the bit	Horse holds head high; usually associated with accelerating partly beyond stimulus control	Escape/ avoidance behaviour	++	–	+	+	0/+	Possible	Inconsistent responses to operant deceleration signals, incorrect application of negative reinforcement	Re-install operant responses from rein signals so that the horse can stop, slow, step-back and shorten its stride from the lightest of rein signals
Reefing	Horse reefs forward or down with the bit	Escape/ avoidance behaviour	++	–	+	+	0/+	Possible	Inconsistent responses to operant deceleration and sometimes acceleration signals, incorrect application of negative reinforcement	Re-install operant responses from acceleration and deceleration signals so that the horse can stop, slow, step-back and shorten its stride from the lightest of rein signals and it can go, quicken and lengthen its stride and go sideways from light forward or sideways signals

(Continued)

Table 13.2 (Continued)

Problem	Mechanism	Category of response	Increase in reactivity	At liberty in stable or enclosure	Under-saddle	In-hand	Ethological relevance	Role of pain	Training flaws that lead to conflict	Training remedy
Head tossing	Horse flicks head forward and up creating inconsistent pressure on the bit	Escape/avoidance behaviour	++	−	+	+	0/+	Possible	Inconsistent responses to operant deceleration and sometimes acceleration signals, incorrect application of negative reinforcement	Re-install operant responses from acceleration and deceleration signals so that the horse can stop, slow, step-back and shorten its stride from the lightest of rein signals and it can go, quicken and lengthen its stride and go sideways from light forward or sideways signals
Bucking (including pig-rooting)	Anti-predator bounding and pronking movements	Escape/avoidance behaviour	+++	+	+	+	0/+	Possible	Inconsistent responses to operant acceleration and deceleration signals, incorrect application of negative reinforcement	Re-install operant responses from acceleration and deceleration signals so that the horse can stop, slow, step-back and shorten its stride from the lightest of rein signals and it can go, quicken and lengthen its stride and go sideways from light forward or sideways signals

Rearing	Standing on hindlegs not under stimulus control	Escape/avoidance behaviour	++++	+	+	+	0/+	Possible	Inconsistent responses to operant acceleration, deceleration and turn of the forelegs signals, incorrect application of negative reinforcement	Re-install operant responses from acceleration and deceleration signals so that the horse can stop, slow, step-back and shorten its stride from the lightest of rein signals and it can go, quicken and lengthen its stride and go sideways from light forward or sideways signals and that it can turn right and left equally well from light turn signals
Freezing	Sudden immobility not under stimulus control	Escape/avoidance behaviour	+	−	+	+	0/+	Possible	Inconsistent responses to operant acceleration and deceleration signals, incorrect application of negative reinforcement	Re-install operant responses from acceleration and deceleration signals so that the horse can stop, slow, step-back and shorten its stride from the lightest of rein signals and it can go, quicken and lengthen its stride and go sideways from light forward or sideways signals

(Continued)

Table 13.2 (*Continued*)

Problem	Mechanism	Category of response	Increase in reactivity	At liberty in stable or enclosure	Under-saddle	In-hand	Ethological relevance	Role of pain	Training flaws that lead to conflict	Training remedy
Jibbing	Horse slows and stops beyond stimulus control	Escape/ avoidance behaviour	+	–	+	+	0/+	Possible	Inconsistent responses to operant acceleration signals, incorrect application of negative reinforcement	Re-install operant responses from forward signals so that the horse can go, quicken and lengthen its stride and go sideways from light forward or sideways signals
Napping	Horse stops and turns beyond stimulus control	Escape/ avoidance behaviour	0/+	–	+	+	0/+	Possible	Inconsistent responses to operant acceleration and turn signals, incorrect application of negative reinforcement	Re-install operant responses from forward signals so that the horse can go, quicken and lengthen its stride from light forward signals and it can turn from light signals
Baulking	Horse suddenly stops beyond stimulus control	Escape/ avoidance behaviour	0/+	–	+	+	0/+	Possible	Inconsistent responses to operant acceleration signals, incorrect application of negative reinforcement	Re-install operant responses from forward signals so that the horse can go, quicken and lengthen its stride and go sideways from light forward or sideways signals
Refusing	Horse suddenly stops in front of jumping obstacle beyond stimulus control	Escape/ avoidance behaviour	0/+	-	+	+	0/+	Possible	Inconsistent responses to operant acceleration signals, incorrect application of negative reinforcement	Re-install operant responses from forward signals so that the horse can go, quicken and lengthen its stride and go sideways from light forward or sideways signals

Shying	Sudden abduction of foreleg in stance phase resulting in swerving	Escape/ avoidance behaviour	+++	−	+	+	0/+	Possible	Inconsistent responses to operant acceleration and deceleration signals, incorrect application of negative reinforcement	Re-install operant responses from acceleration and deceleration signals so that the horse can stop, slow, step-back and shorten its stride from the lightest of rein signals and it can go, quicken and lengthen its stride and go sideways from light forward or sideways signals
Spinning	Horse suddenly changes direction	Escape/ avoidance behaviour	+++	−	+	+	0/+	Possible	Inconsistent responses to operant acceleration and deceleration signals, incorrect application of negative reinforcement	Re-install operant responses from acceleration and deceleration signals so that the horse can stop, slow, step-back and shorten its stride from the lightest of rein signals and it can go, quicken and lengthen its stride and go sideways from light forward or sideways signals
Lugging (hanging)	Horse holds one side of the bit more strongly than the other	Bilateral asymmetry in propulsion	++	−	+	+	0/+	Possible	Inconsistent responses to operant acceleration signals, incorrect application of negative reinforcement	Re-install operant responses from forward signals so that the horse can go, quicken and lengthen its stride and go sideways from light forward or sideways signals

(Continued)

Table 13.2 (Continued)

Problem	Mechanism	Category of response	Increase in reactivity	At liberty in stable or enclosure	Under-saddle	In-hand	Ethological relevance	Role of pain	Training flaws that lead to conflict	Training remedy
Falling in and falling out	Horse drifts in or out during riding on a designated line	Bilateral asymmetry in propulsion	0	−	+	+	0/+	Possible	Inconsistent responses to operant acceleration and deceleration signals, incorrect application of negative reinforcement	Re-install operant responses from acceleration and deceleration signals so that the horse can stop, slow, step-back and shorten its stride from the lightest of rein signals and it can go, quicken and lengthen its stride and go sideways from light forward or sideways signals
Dropping the shoulder	Horse becomes unlevel in shoulders during riding, usually accompanied by mild drifting	Bilateral asymmetry in propulsion	0	−	+	+	0/+	Possible	Inconsistent responses to operant acceleration and deceleration signals, incorrect application of negative reinforcement	Re-install operant responses from acceleration and deceleration signals so that the horse can stop, slow, step-back and shorten its stride from the lightest of rein signals and it can go, quicken and lengthen its stride and go sideways from light forward or sideways signals

Unlevelness	As above but without drifting	Bilateral asymmetry in propulsion	0	−	+	−	0/+	Possible	Inconsistent responses to operant acceleration and deceleration signals, incorrect application of negative reinforcement	Re-install operant responses from acceleration and deceleration signals so that the horse can stop, slow, step-back and shorten its stride from the lightest of rein signals and it can go, quicken and lengthen its stride and go sideways from light forward or sideways signals
Bridle lameness	Horse limps with foreleg during riding	Rider-induced rein contact issue	0	−	+	+	0/+	Possible	Inconsistent responses to operant acceleration and deceleration signals, incorrect application of negative reinforcement	Re-install operant responses from acceleration and deceleration signals so that the horse can stop, slow, step-back and shorten its stride from the lightest of rein signals and it can go, quicken and lengthen its stride and go sideways from light forward or sideways signals
Barging	Horse drifts sideways during leading towards handler	Bilateral asymmetry in propulsion	++	−	−	+	0/+	Unlikely	Inconsistent responses to operant deceleration signals, incorrect application of negative reinforcement	Re-install operant responses from rein signals so that the horse can stop, slow, step-back and shorten its stride from the lightest of rein signals

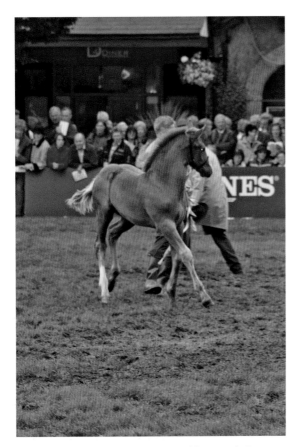

Figure 13.10 Rushing and jogging problems (including bolting) in-hand and under-saddle are largely associated with inadequately trained stop/slow responses.

learned in just a few trials and are not subject to erasure, the remedy is not to ride forward but to slow the legs. When horses buck under-saddle, most riders attempt to use the reins not to stop but to maintain balance. The bucking horse does not respond to the slowing effect of the reins but continues to buck, so training effective stop and slowing responses provides a means of arresting this behaviour. Training horses that buck under-saddle to have better stop responses is best undertaken in-hand, focussing on powerful transitions, such as those from trot to halt in two beats of the forelegs, releasing as soon as the legs are still (McLean and McLean, 2008).

Rearing is another problem characterised by dysfunctions in both acceleration and deceleration responses. Like bucking, it is often a result of concurrent signalling of both stop and go signals. While rearing is part of the typical social ethogram of horses (McDonnell, 2003), it is also an anti-predator behaviour and can also be dangerous to riders, although riding a rear may be less challenging than riding a buck (see Figure 13.11). Skilled jumping riders are usually capable of riding rears because of the similarity between rearing and riding tall vertical obstacles. Rearing generally begins with stalling and jibbing and then progresses to spins and finally rearing emerges. Most horses rear to some extent to the left and the result is further dysfunction in the right turn response. Thus, rearing results in deficits of acceleration, deceleration and turn

are generally also associated with running away behaviours but they may be associated with problems in acceleration (McLean and McLean, 2008), so upward inter-gait and intra-gait transitions involving reinforcement of single strides of each gait provide the remedy for these also.

Bucking is an anti-predator behaviour (evolved for feline predators) that presents perhaps the most dangerous and challenging hyper-reactive events a horse can offer. While bucking is well known to be associated with forward problems, it is also associated with dysfunctions in stop responses (McLean, 2005b). Here, it is important to consider that because bucking involves random acceleration responses or acceleration responses not under stimulus control of the rider (or handler), and because flight responses can be

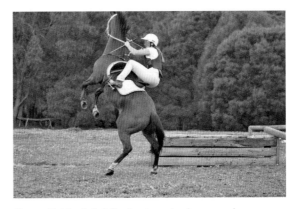

Figure 13.11 Rehabilitating a rearing horse can be very dangerous to attempt as the horse can easily be pulled off balance by the rider's efforts to stay aboard.

responses. Rearing is reinforced by the release of the effort of going forward, as well as release of the rider's reins and leg pressures. Rehabilitating a rearing horse is a matter of re-training deceleration, acceleration and turn responses and is a job for skilled riders as it involves removing the reinforcement from (i.e. behavioural extinction of) the rearing response. Remedying rearing in-hand typically involves using a stallion bit, which is vibrated in the opposite direction to the rear during the rear and released as soon as the horse lands.

Freezing is the final dual dysfunction of deceleration and acceleration responses and is characterised by tonic immobility where the horse refuses to move altogether in spite of strong signalling. When the horse eventually does move, it is likely to be explosive and uncontrollable. This behaviour is most likely to be a 'last-ditch' anti-predator reaction. Because freezing is often followed by a sudden explosive reaction, it can be very dangerous for riders and the horse may lose any sense of self-preservation in its panic. Freezing is less common than rearing or bucking and is typically a conflict behaviour that is a consequence of inconsistent acceleration and deceleration responses and concurrent signalling of stop and go signals. Because of the degree of dysfunction of pressure-based signals, freezing may have significant links with learned helplessness.

Jibbing, napping, baulking and *refusing* are behaviours that manifest as deficits in acceleration responses. In general, these behaviours are not dangerous to personnel as they are usually not as hyper-reactive as behaviours that involve acceleration. Jibbing and baulking involve random slowing outside the rider's or handler's stimulus control. The rider or handler may inadvertently reinforce these behaviours by relenting on the pressures for forward at the wrong moment and thus negatively reinforcing these behaviours. Rehabilitating these problems involves re-training the acceleration responses so that these are immediately initiated by the horse and from light signals. This involves negatively reinforcing either a single step forward or, if that is easily elicited, reinforcing a single stride forward. It may be necessary to increase the motivating level of pressure so the horse is more motivated to move off (e.g. by using whip-taps that increase in frequency). It is important that the whip is not

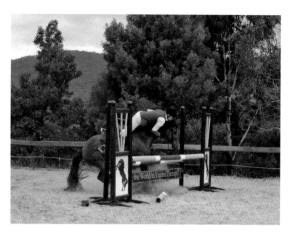

Figure 13.12 Horses can learn to refuse jumping obstacles if riders reward losses of effort and turning away. Once horses have learned to refuse and run out to the left, approaching at greater speeds will generally result in faster swerving.

used to deliver sharp punitive pain, but that it instead conforms to the optimal use of negative reinforcement by gradually increasing in speed of whip-taps. Re-training napping also involves re-training acceleration responses as well as turns due to the losses of line. Refusing at jumping obstacles is reinforced by two factors: losses of effort and turning away from the obstacle (see Figure 13.12). Thus, successful rehabilitation of refusing at jumps can be obtained by lowering the fence (i.e. using show-jumping obstacles for rehabilitation) and jumping the lowered fence from a standstill or by stepping back so that the obstacle does not depart (is not removed) from the horse's field of vision (McLean and McLean, 2008).

Losses of the designated line intended by a rider manifest as various behaviours all characterised by greater or lesser amounts of propulsion asymmetry. In all of these behaviours there is some tendency on the horse's part to drift sideways with varying degrees of hyper-reactivity. The most hyper-reactive loss of line is seen in *shying*, where the horse suddenly veers sideways. Shying has ethological relevance in escaping predators and is conferred by a rapid abduction in the stance phase of the foreleg proximate to the aversive object, followed usually by an acceleration forward and away from the aversive object. The abduction and subsequent acceleration, like many conflict behaviours, are out of the stimulus control of the rider (or handler). Remedying shying thus involves regaining stimulus control over the abducting stance-phase foreleg, which means re-training turn and stop responses. Because the individual reins provide the fundamental signals through negative reinforcement of turning, and the two reins provide the means of stopping, the reins are instrumental in re-training the turn. When the horse shies, the rider should immediately implement a downward transition and then return the forelegs to the designated line. It is often useful in re-training shying to steer the horse's forelegs in a specific line, such as the extreme edge of the manège. Typically, shying horses have considerably more difficulty with this exercise than non-shying horses. *Spinning* is synonymous with shying, except that in spinning the horse continues turning for more than one or two steps. Spinning horses require similar re-training as shying horses due to the losses of line involved.

Lugging (or *hanging*) is where the horse maintains contact on one side of the bit more strongly than on the other, and in doing so it drifts or attempts to drift (see Figure 13.13). Sometimes riders hold the reins with stronger contact on one side than the other, thus preventing the losses of line that normally accompany such inequalities in contact. Lugging is typically seen in racehorses, and this is usually remedied by using a lugging bit – a ring bit that encircles the entire lower mandible and enables the jockey to pull the horse back on line or hold it on a line. This, however, does not cure the horse. The most effective cure is to re-train the uneven turns associated with

lugging. If the horse lugs to the right, then more time is spent on training left turns, reinforcing single strides of turn until the left turn arises from a single light signal. Riding shallow serpentine shapes on the racetrack assists in re-training these turns (McLean and McLean, 2008).

Falling-in and *falling-out* are similar behaviours characterised by drifting in on the circle (falling-in) or drifting out of the circle (falling-out). They result from insufficient training of turns, confused turns and uneven rein contacts by riders. Falling-in and falling-out thus involve losses of line through uneven propulsion of the forelegs where one foreleg abducts in the stance phase more than the other. This uneven propulsion is conferred by bending the horse's neck so that the head and neck, which weigh around 10% of its body mass, place more weight on one foreleg than on the other, causing it to abduct more powerfully in the stance phase. Thus, the horse falls-in or out, away from the side on which its head is carried. Again, these are dysfunctions of turning, and are appropriately corrected and re-trained using the reins (because these are errors of the forelegs). This is the role of the indirect turn where the horse can be neck reined (rein firmly against the neck until the neck straightens and the forelegs shift sideways) to some extent to straighten the neck and bring the forelegs back on the designated line. Again, a single stride of the correct turn should be elicited and reinforced. *Dropping the shoulder* and *unlevelness* are synonymous and also involve losses of line, except that these are more minor deviations and differ from falling-in and falling-out in that they do not involve bending the neck.

Bridle lameness refers to an apparent lameness as a result of rein contact. Such horses are usually not lame in-hand, but are clearly lame under-saddle. Because it arises from uneven rein contact that is too strong, bridle lameness causes uneven propulsion that becomes habitual under-saddle. Bridle-lame horses require re-training of deceleration and turn responses under-saddle where single correct strides are reinforced. *Barging* refers to in-hand problems where horses drift during leading, sometimes stepping on the feet of the handler (see Figure 13.14). These deviations of line also result from uneven propulsion and incorrect leading training where straightness is not reinforced. Downward inter-gait transitions to halt, followed by upward ones where the handler's

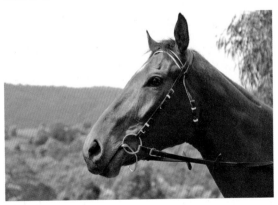

Figure 13.13 Lugging bits are typically used on racehorses to hold them onto their designated line and prevent drifting out. This drifting tendency involves losses of speed. A more sensible approach is to train the horse to maintain its designated line.

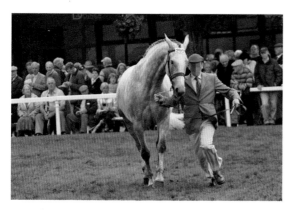

Figure 13.14 Horses that barge into the handler's space are frequently described as having no respect. However, the simplest explanation that shifts blame from the horse is that the horse has not been trained to maintain its designated line in-hand: it does not lead straight.

hand pushes the horse away from the handler's body whenever the horse shows a deviation of line, provide the corrections for this behaviour.

Conflict behaviours resulting from confusions of speed and line signals do not always manifest as alterations of speed or line. Sometimes they may show up as other behaviours (see Table 13.3). For example, **tension problems involving increased muscle tonus** are usually the result of confusions primarily with deceleration responses (see Figure 13.15). Whereas confusions with acceleration responses may still result in poor welfare, confusions involving the mouth are generally more hyper-reactive, most likely because the horse's mouth is so sensitive and not adapted to carrying and being pressured by steel bits. Thus, increased muscle tonus is indicative of poor deceleration responses, where the horse leans on the bit and slows inconsistently from it. Therefore, the rehabilitation of tense horses involves reinforcing single strides of downward transitions. Further relaxation is most easily effected by lengthening the stride until the horse stretches its neck forward (longitudinal flexion) and then shortening the stride with the reins so that the horse learns not only to slow but also to shorten its stride from light rein signals.

Similarly, **teeth grinding, pawing** and **champing the bit** have strong associations with deficits in deceleration responses though are not necessarily accompanied by obvious accelerations. As with increased muscle tension, these problems typically result in the ridden horse from inconsistent

reinforcement of deceleration responses or concurrent signalling of deceleration and acceleration responses (simultaneous rein and leg pressures). The rehabilitation of these involves the same methodology as above for tension: re-training stop responses so that the horse can stop and slow from light signals, achieving relaxation in a longer body frame (McLean and McLean, 2008).

Tail swishing, on the other hand, is typically associated with losses of self-carriage and subsequent dysfunctions in the acceleration responses. It may also result from hypersensitive body reactions. When associated with poor acceleration responses, the cause is usually inconsistent negative reinforcement of the acceleration responses, but again, these may also have associations with confusions arising from concurrent signalling of both acceleration and deceleration responses. The remedy for tail swishing is to re-install acceleration responses so that a single stride is reinforced to arise immediately and from a light signal. Therefore, upward transitions are integral in this process.

Horses may develop chronic behaviour disorders if their attempts to cope with fearful events regularly fail. These disorders may show up as aggressive or defensive behaviours or as insecurities (see Table 13.4). Such behaviours may be influenced by testosterone in that stallions are more inclined to become aggressive than geldings or mares. These behaviours are unique in that they manifest out of the original conflicting situation: the horse may simply show aggression whenever it comes into contact with people. Such horses are usually kept in protective custody where they are less exposed to people, which might exacerbate their neuroses. **Biting, kicking, striking** and **threatening** can become habitual and, furthermore (and quite understandably), can be reinforced by the retreat of people during these attacks (see Figure 13.16). Horses showing these behaviours should be treated with caution and handled only by experienced personnel. Their rehabilitation may be a lengthy process, owing to the chronic nature of their condition. The rehabilitation of these horses requires thorough in-hand re-training of acceleration and deceleration responses, reinforcing single strides of correct behaviour through the release of pressure until the responses emerge from light signals.

Separation anxiety is common in horses and may have age-related associations: horses

Table 13.3 Indirect dysfunctions of speed and line signal conflicts

Problem	Mechanism	Category of response	Increase in reactivity	At liberty in stable or enclosure	Under-saddle	In-hand	Ethological relevance	Role of pain	Training flaws that lead to conflict	Training remedy
Tension: increase in muscle tonus	Hyper-reactive body posture	Conflict behaviour	++	*/−	+++	+++	0/+	Possible	Inconsistent stop/slow/step-back responses from bit signals, incorrect application of negative reinforcement	Re-install operant responses from rein signals so that the horse can stop, slow, step-back and shorten its stride from the lightest of rein signals
Teeth grinding	Grinding of upper and lower mandibular surfaces	Conflict behaviour	++	−	+	+	+	Possible	Inconsistent stop/slow/step-back responses from bit signals, incorrect application of negative reinforcement	Re-install operant responses from rein signals so that the horse can stop, slow, step-back and shorten its stride from the lightest of rein signals
Pawing	Vigorous pawing on ground with one or alternate forelegs	Displacement	++	+	+	+	0	Unlikely	Inconsistent stop/slow/step-back responses from bit signals, incorrect application of negative reinforcement	Re-install operant responses from rein signals so that the horse can stop, slow, step-back and shorten its stride from the lightest of rein signals

Champing the bit	Biting the bit with inconsistent and alternating pressures	Ambivalent	++	−	+	++	0/+	Possible	Inconsistent stop/slow/step-back responses from bit signals, incorrect application of negative reinforcement	Re-install operant responses from rein signals so that the horse can stop, slow, step-back and shorten its stride from light rein signals
Tail swishing	Tail swishes hyper-reactively	Conflict behaviour	++	−	+	+	0/+	Possible	Inconsistent responses to operant acceleration and deceleration signals, incorrect application of negative reinforcement	Re-install operant responses from forward and rein signals

Table 13.4 Fearful, defensive and agonistic responses

Problem	Mechanism	Category of response	Increase in reactivity	At liberty in stable or enclosure	Under-saddle	In-hand	Ethological relevance	Role of pain	Training flaws that lead to conflict	Training remedy
Biting	Biting into a person or thing by closing upper and lower incisors	Possible insecurity arising from confusion	++	+	–	+	0/+	Possible	Inconsistent responses to operant deceleration signals, incorrect application of negative reinforcement	Re-install operant responses from rein signals so that the horse can stop, slow, step-back and shorten its stride from the lightest of rein signals
Kicking	Kicking out with hindleg	Possible insecurity arising from confusion	++	+	+	+	0/+	Possible	Likely dysfunctions in operant acceleration and deceleration responses, incorrect application of negative reinforcement	Re-install operant responses from acceleration and deceleration signals so that the horse can stop, slow, step-back and shorten its stride from the lightest of rein signals and it can go, quicken and lengthen its stride and go sideways from light forward or sideways signals

Striking	Striking forward with foreleg	Possible insecurity arising from confusion	++	+		+	0/+	Possible	Inconsistent responses to operant deceleration signals, incorrect application of negative reinforcement	Re-install operant responses from rein signals so that the horse can stop, slow, step-back and shorten its stride from the lightest of rein signals
Threatening	Using threat gestures such as ears back	Possible insecurity arising from confusion	++	+	−	+	0/+	Possible	Likely dysfunctions in operant acceleration and deceleration responses, incorrect application of negative reinforcement	Re-install operant responses from acceleration and deceleration signals so that the horse can stop, slow, step-back and shorten its stride from the lightest of rein signals and it can go, quicken and lengthen its stride and go sideways from light forward or sideways signals

(Continued)

Table 13.4 (Continued)

Problem	Mechanism	Category of response	Increase in reactivity	At liberty in stable or enclosure	Under-saddle	In-hand	Ethological relevance	Role of pain	Training flaws that lead to conflict	Training remedy
Horse-shy	Swerving violently during approach of another horse	Conflict behaviour	++	++	+	+	+	Possible	Inconsistent responses to operant acceleration and deceleration signals, incorrect application of negative reinforcement	Re-install operant responses from acceleration and deceleration signals so that the horse can stop, slow, step-back and shorten its stride from the lightest of rein signals and it can go, quicken and lengthen its stride and go sideways from light forward or sideways signals
Separation anxiety	Vocalisation and distress when alone or separated from affiliate, usually a conspecific	Conflict behaviour	++	++	+	+	0/+	Possible	Inconsistent responses to operant acceleration and deceleration signals, incorrect application of negative reinforcement	Re-install operant responses from acceleration and deceleration signals so that the horse can stop, slow, step-back and shorten its stride from the lightest of rein signals and it can go, quicken and lengthen its stride and go sideways from light forward or sideways signals

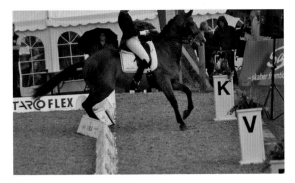

Figure 13.15   Tension is a hyper-reactive state of running away that is thwarted by the reins. When escape is thwarted, anxiety escalates. (Photo courtesy of Julie Taylor/EponaTV.)

younger than five are more inclined to show these behaviours, possibly because their social bonds and status are not yet mature. However, separation anxiety also seems to have greater expression in horses that are confused and subject to inconsistent reinforcement of responses. The insecurity is a result of a motivational conflict (the drive to be with conspecifics is successfully competing with the handler's signals). Inconsistent reinforcement of correct responses renders horses more motivated to seek conspecifics, in the same way as meeting a predator might make a horse similarly motivated. The increased predictability conferred by consistent reinforcement and light, less obtrusive signals lowers the horse's motivation to seek conspecifics. Similarly, horses that show *horse-shy* behaviour (being fearful of

approaching other horses) may be motivated in part by deficits in pressure-based signals. The rehabilitation of these horses, therefore, involves consistent reinforcement of correct responses (McLean and McLean, 2008).

Take-home messages

The following principles apply to horse-training with regard to managing fear:

- Identify and diminish all expressions of the flight response. When a horse shows fearful behaviours beyond the requirements of the gait, slow the horse's legs with downward transitions.
- Reduce the pressure required to elicit responses trained by negative reinforcement to the least obtrusive cues (light cues).
- Train only one consistent response from one specific cue and avoid asking for opposing responses at the same time.
- Shape the qualities of responses progressively, beginning with the smallest elements of each learned response.
- Aim to achieve self-carriage at every stage of training.

Ethical implications

- Equestrian coaches are largely ignorant of learning theory. Regulatory bodies for equestrian coaching must legislate for the correct use of learning theory in all equestrian coaching activity as a matter of urgency.
- Many ridden and led horses endure pain on a regular basis.
- Chronic stress has profound welfare implications for horses.

Areas for further research

- An accurate description of, and specific tests for, distress in the ridden horse is needed.
- A horse-friendly design for starting barriers that takes into account equine ethology should be developed.

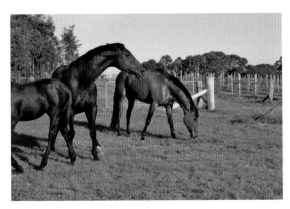

Figure 13.16   Aggression can arise from age, temperament or sex-related issues, but it also frequently correlates with dysfunctions in stop responses in-hand and under-saddle.

14 Ethical Equitation

Introduction

In principle, our use of the horse differs little from our use of other animals for food, fibre, transport, traction, entertainment, and so on (Midgley, 1983; Regan, 1983). However, equitation offers a novel motivation for the use of animals, namely, the drive of some people to use horses in pursuit of a particular psychological satisfaction: 'winning'. The desire to win appears to go beyond the notion of pleasure or even success because it requires that we outperform other people. Does this make it the ultimate exercise in human pride, vanity and individualism? And if so, does this provide a justifiable motivation for the use of animals even when pain and suffering may be involved? This line of thinking has prompted cynicism about the use of terms such as the 'equine athlete', as if horses can be willing participants in the heavy slog and self-sacrifice we generally associate with human athletes (Cathy Schuller, personal communication, 2008).

People can be very clever at finding the means to justify practices they might secretly have misgivings about. Critics may say that until we can prove that horses read scoreboards there is no evidence at all that they share an interest in winning. They would go on to urge that we dispense with anthropomorphic rhetoric that spuriously suggests such a shared interest in winning, and review some of the common practices that can compromise equine welfare.

Generally speaking, ethical arguments are based on cost/benefits analysis. Do the costs for the working horse outweigh the benefits for humans? If we acknowledge that horses will always be required to work for us, how can we refine their use so that it is morally justified. The debate about what defines ethical horse use and, in particular, ethical equitation, has yet to be heard. A frank appraisal of horse-riding as an ethical pursuit may seem absurd to many riders, but we believe that the issue of ethical equitation is a fascinating and largely unexplored one. Just because we *can* do something to a horse does not make it an ethically sound practice. Horses may appear extremely tolerant, seeming to put up with interventions even when these are broadly aversive. However, this could simply be a manifestation of their outstanding abilities in habituation and associative learning.

If horses were truly able to comprehend their environment, then perhaps they would not be so trainable and rideable and maybe it would be unethical to ride them. After all, if horses *were* capable of reflection, they would be suffering as a result of comprehending their own enslavement and the ubiquity of pressure during ridden work, of having to jump clearly avoidable obstacles, and of having to carry another being. The horse would be consumed by his longing for freedom to simply be a horse: to eat grass, be with affiliates and be free of human exploitation. That said, there is reason to believe that the correctly and humanely trained horse is not distressed by his interactions with humans. Indeed, ethical training and riding can be seen as environmental and behavioural enrichment (O'Brien *et al.*, 2008). This is a valid proposition because the horse has evolved to discriminate and respond to multiple stimuli in a complex landscape covering hundreds of hectares. For the modern horse kept in a comparatively uneventful few square metres, clear, consistent learning outcomes that arise during their interactions with humans most likely fulfil the behavioural need to learn how best to interact with the environment.

This book emphasises the reliance on pressure and release in horse-riding, and how the use of pressure of any sort distinguishes equitation from training in most other species. Given that negative reinforcement is the critical control mechanism, horses cannot be safely ridden without some degree of pressure. Ethical equitation demands that minimal pressure and immediate release is used for both contact (if relevant for the sport) and signalling at all times. If horsemanship relies on consistency (and therefore clarity in training), what are the long-term consequences of inconsistent training techniques? Can poor training affect aspects of the horse's ethogram that do not seem to be directly related to the trained responses? For example, this may explain the anecdotal finding that training flaws confined to human–horse interactions seem to lead to social dysfunctions in horse–horse interactions (McLean, 2005b).

As in other sports, many horse-owners, trainers and riders will arrive at a choice between doing something 'bad' that may increase their chances of winning, or not doing it and relinquishing the possibility of a first place. It may be a decision about using a gadget or a drug, withholding food or water, or hurting the horse.

The extent to which sport horses are coerced to perform is often the focus of welfare debates. The roads-and-tracks and steeplechase elements have disappeared from the sport of horse-trials. It is also possible that steeplechasing and the use of the whip in racing may be moderated as a result of pressure from outside the racing industry. The horse-welfare lobby has begun to voice its con-

cerns about other elite equestrian events – some people find the dressage movement called piaffe unacceptable.

Equitation Science will be able to play a vital role in deciding the outcome of these debates. In particular, in dressage competition, emergent technology will remove objectivity from judging and will underpin the development of high-welfare dressage. Science may be able to help us value training of any manoeuvre that is dependent on and achieved through lightness of pressure (i.e. attesting to self-carriage and the horse's self-maintenance of rhythm, straightness and outline; McGreevy *et al.*, 2005). Imagine dressage scores being awarded for the most humane training techniques. Despite its anthropomorphic connotations, the introduction of the concept of the happy equine athlete by the Fédération Equestre Internationale (FEI) to its rules governing dressage competition may be seen as a step toward better welfare in that sport. Although problematic to judge, the introduction of the happiest horse prize to the Olympics and World championships for dressage may yield positive effects.

Whips and welfare

Across the various sports and equestrian codes, any real consensus on equine welfare indicators is superficial at best. Prime examples of this are regulations governing the use of the whip. Compare these with the FEI's general regulations. The British Horseracing Authority (BHA) has the world's most exhaustive instructions on the use of the whip in racing (BHA, 2009). These dictate that the whip should be used for 'safety, correction and encouragement only'. The ways in which the whip may and should not be used are described in Table 14.1.

The BHA's disciplinary enquiries usually relate to how the horse ran, for example, a failure to run a horse on its merits; interference with other runners; excessive use of the whip. The first and last of these imply use of the whip that appears, at first glance, to be contradictory. To be convinced that a jockey has run a horse on its merits ('ridden a horse out'), many punters would need to see him use the whip. So, what constitutes excessive use of the whip? This is poorly described, not

Table 14.1 Verbatim instructions on acceptable and unacceptable use of the whip according to the BHA rules

Acceptable use of the whip	Unacceptable
Showing the horse the whip and giving it time to respond before using it	Hitting: • To the extent of injury • With the whip arm above shoulder height • Rapidly without regard for their (the horse's) stride • With excessive force • With excessive frequency • Without giving the horse time to respond
Using the whip in the backhand* position for a reminder	Hitting horses that are: • Showing no response • Out of contention • Clearly winning • Past the winning post
Having used the whip, giving the horse a chance to respond to it before using it again	Hitting horses in any place except: • On the quarters (hindquarters) with the whip in either the backhand or forehand position • Down the shoulder with the whip in the backhand position unless exceptional circumstances prevail
Keeping both hands on the reins when using the whip down the shoulder in the backhand position	
Using the whip in rhythm with the horse's stride and close to its side	
Swinging the whip or actually using it to keep the horse straight	

Adapted with permission from BHA (2008).
*Backhand position means a rotation that is clockwise from the jockey's perspective.

least because both pressure and frequency must be assessed. Fundamentally, it is difficult to make a visual appraisal of the amount of force being used – although breakable whips might be a useful means of placing an upper limit on this variable. Instead, jockeys may be accused of hitting the horse on multiple occasions without giving it time to respond.

This point is critical because jockeys and trainers know that the response of the horse to the whip cannot be assumed. In other words, to some extent the use of the whip, if only as a test of whether the horse has the energy to respond, becomes obligatory. Some horses speed up; others slow down. For example, in a study of Quarterhorses at the gallop, the use of a whip on the shoulder of the leading forelimb, in rhythm with the stride, did not increase speed but reduced stride length and increased stride frequency (Deuel and Lawrence, 1987). To learning theorists, this report might suggest a flawed understanding of negative reinforcement since the stimulus to run faster was withdrawn following the wrong response (slowing). An analysis of racetrack patrol videos has shown that 38% of breakdown injuries occur after use of the whip (Ueda *et al.*, 1993). This may reflect the rider's response when a horse begins to pull up with an acute lameness.

Racing stewards' judgments commonly focus on the frequency of whip use. They base their judgments on whether the number of hits was reasonable and necessary over the distance they were given, taking into account the horse's experience and whether it was continuing to respond. Clearly, this is subjective. It is blurred further by the stewards' need to factor in the degree of force used: 'the more times a horse has been hit, the stricter will be the view taken over the degree of force which is reasonable' (BHA, 2009).

As identified already, these rules are subjective. For instance, the definition of a 'reminder' is questionable (see Table 14.1) in terms of learning theory and one might question whether keeping both hands on the reins while using the whip (down the shoulder) constitutes a good riding technique.

In current best practice, the whip is swung by the jockey in a clockwise rotation and may not even make contact with the horse; each iteration coincides with suspension of the gallop (see Chapter 11, Biomechanics) and any contact coincides with the beginning of the stance phases of each stride.

In performance sports, the whip should be held like a ski pole (see Figure 14.1(a)), not like a tennis racquet (see Figure 14.1(b)). To align with learning

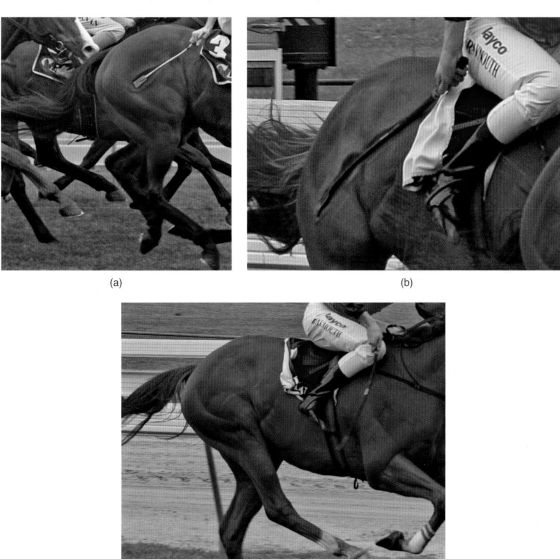

(a)

(b)

(c)

Figure 14.1   The whip can exert different forces on impact, depending on how it is held. Both regular whips (a) and padded whips (b) can leave welt marks (c).

theory, the whip must be applied with very light pressure at first, so it becomes a discriminative signal (see Chapter 7, Applying learning theory). This can be followed by contiguous evenly spaced rhythm of increasing or maintained pressure that is removed when the horse offers the correct response. The FEI's General Regulations (2007) stipulate that no person may abuse a horse at *any* time (i.e. not only during an official event). They define abuse as any actions or omissions that cause or are likely to cause pain or unnecessary discomfort. These include:

- whipping or beating a horse excessively;
- subjecting a horse to any kind of electric shock device;
- using spurs excessively or persistently;
- jabbing the horse in the mouth with the bit or any other device;
- competing using an exhausted, lame or injured horse;
- 'rapping' a horse (see Chapter 12, Unorthodox techniques);
- abnormally sensitising or desensitising any part of a horse (see Chapter 12, Unorthodox techniques);
- leaving a horse without adequate food, drink or exercise (interestingly, Xenophon would have been barred, on the strength of his proposal that horses should be kept for periods without food and water so that eventually they associate the human carer with the arrival of these resources);
- using any device or equipment that causes excessive pain to the horse if it knocks down an obstacle.

How are FEI stewards to decide whether a beating has been excessive? Is it excessive for that particular horse, its particular perceived crime or the combination of these in light of its 'prior form'? Fundamentally, the term 'excessive' implies that a certain amount of whipping is indeed appropriate or even required. This is of concern since it presumes that an onlooker (in this case, the steward or judge) can calculate a prescribed dose of pain without even having ridden the horse or known its history, let alone the principles of learning theory as they apply to aversive stimuli in equitation. Fundamentally, it is difficult to make a visual ap-

praisal of the amount of force being used. There are sound arguments for banning the use of the whip altogether in horse racing. Apart from welfare benefits, this would encourage trainers and jockeys to use more enlightened training methods and of course there would still be winners. Perhaps too, the horses would be easier to re-home at the end of their careers if they were not subject to punishment in racing.

It could be argued that the welfare of the UK racing horse has better safeguards than the horse competing under the protection of the FEI, since at least the ways in which it cannot be whipped are stipulated. The recent ban by the Danish Equestrian Federation on the use of whips and spurs in punishment has raised the possibility of a global move to forbid the use of aversive stimuli for non-performance.

Ethical considerations and Equitation Science

Equitation Science can help to inform the decisions we make as equestrians. For example, there is a need for debate around some of the central tenets of horse-training, such as contact and half halts, which are too loosely interpreted to be universally understood. These issues are currently the source of too much data-free and, therefore, largely semantic, debate among coaches, confusion among riders and conflict in horses.

Perhaps Equitation Science will permit the rules of equestrian sport to be revisited in the light of more scientific rigour. For example, the FEI rules stipulate that in passage the toe of the forehoof should be elevated to the middle of the contralateral cannon (whereas the toe of the hindhoof should be raised slightly above the contralateral fetlock joint; FEI 2008). In the individual medal finals at the Barcelona Olympics, none of the horses performing passage achieved this amount of elevation in the forelimbs (Argue, 1994). It may be that Equitation Science will help to show why this height is difficult to achieve in contemporary training.

Ethical equitation may help us to answer the question: 'Can happiness ever be measured in an equine athlete?' Can we ever be sure of happiness in a horse beyond satiation or absence of pain? Some might say that happiness is an emergent property of higher mental abilities, while others feel that happiness *in horses* occurs simply when they are in a familiar but fresh pasture, with clement weather, familiar conspecific company, no flies and no evidence of predators. There is a growing body of literature on the conscious life of animals, and this may be relevant when trying to determine what 'matters' to them (e.g. McMillan, 2005).

Ethical equitation could also lead to calls for better matching of horses and humans. For example, should certain humans be allowed to ride horses with which they are poorly matched? Are novice riders a potential threat to the welfare of the horses they learn on? Should sentient beings be exposed to complete novices who are not simply learning to ride but are learning to balance? Perhaps, before allowing them to balance and provide negative reinforcement humanely on a horse, we should teach novice riders (including children) the principles of associative learning and negative reinforcement.

Now is the right moment for those bodies that govern horse sports to identify the types of scientific evidence they require when considering the welfare implications of novel techniques and technological advances. The governing bodies of horse sports should encourage research into the most

humane application of pressure and alternative means of communicating with horses and reinforcing them.

Horses that are of no further use have low monetary value and are therefore more likely to be neglected. Thus, we can see a direct relationship between welfare and usefulness and so should look forward to a time when more emphasis is placed on ensuring that sport horses are under stimulus control and not exposed to motivational conflict and thus remain useful after their competitive careers have ended.

It is even possible to look to a time when competitions that use horses (and therefore aversive stimuli under a negative reinforcement framework) reward welfare above all else. This would be especially important if we ever see the emergence of technological advances (such as rein-tension meters) that facilitate restraint with due regard for welfare. The emphasis on lightness that is receiving increased attention in some sections of the dressage world is likely to prove critical here. At the same time, the rules concerning the mandatory use of the double bridle and spurs in higher levels of dressage will come under close scrutiny.

Ethical horse-use also demands ethical horse-breeding and this raises some interesting questions. For example, if laterality studies and temperament tests identify foals that are likely to

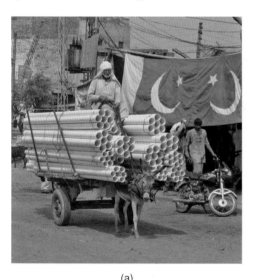
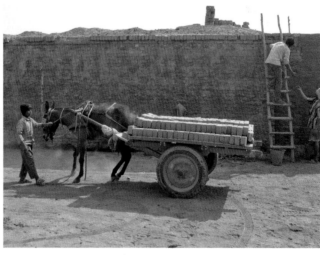

(a)   (b)

Figure 14.2 In less developed countries, donkeys and mules remain an important source of power. Their health and ability to work can directly affect a family's livelihood. (Photos courtesy of Becky Whay.)

prove difficult to train, how will this affect those foals' commercial value and ultimately their welfare. Will horses' tolerance of poor riding be a quality that we value and therefore select for? Have we in fact been doing this for some time? Biotechnologies (and ultimately cloning) may allow horses of extraordinary ability or tolerance to become more predictably available, meaning that riders and trainers do not have to modify or moderate their own behaviour as much as they currently do.

However, these debates must be considered in light of the fact that, despite the growth of horse numbers used in sport and leisure, these are easily eclipsed by those in working contexts. There are an estimated 90 million equids in the developing world (FAO statistical database, 2003). Indeed, more than 95% of all donkeys and mules and 60% of all horses are found in developing countries (Fielding, 1991), the majority being used for work (see Figure 14.2). Working and competition horses all thrive on the appropriate application of learning theory even though the responses expected of them often seem worlds apart. Just as the military use of horses foreshadowed competitive dressage, perhaps we can look forward to a time when skills refined in competition find a place in working contexts. So, while best practice in training allows riders to get the best out of the horse in competition, the same principles could ensure that the working equid is spared from abuse and the catabolic effects of chronic stress (Moberg and Mench, 2000). The lot of the working horse in the western context was the primary focus of the first piece of UK anti-cruelty legislation (in 1822) and was highlighted by Sewell (1877), whose popular novel is credited with fuelling the UK animal welfare movements by making people consider an animal perspective. It is worth reflecting that, despite the passage of time and the wholesale improvement of awareness, much remains to be done.

Take-home messages

- The concept of the happy equine athlete may influence our decisions about how far horses can be pushed to perform for human glory.
- Ethical equitation demands that minimal pressure and immediate release are used for both contact (if relevant to the sport) and signalling at all times.
- Whipping horses to ensure they perform may one day be considered abuse, regardless of the context.

15 The Future of Equitation Science

Introduction

Equitation Science is as yet in its infancy and appropriately embraces a broad portfolio. To give some idea of the breadth of enquiry that defines Equitation Science, the areas covered by the first four international Equitation Science symposia (in Melbourne, Milan, Michigan and Dublin) are listed in Table 15.1.

The anticipated limitations on further research relate chiefly to the crudeness of the tools we use to measure small changes such as the cues from the rider's seat or elusive qualities such as the horse's mood. Though we currently lack the wherewithal to make these measurements, we can look forward to the day when it will be possible. Then, we will have the knowledge to be able to refine our understanding of individual differences between horses, and truly match horses with riders, while retaining a focus on the need for rider improvement.

Areas and anticipated limitations for further research

New technologies

Technology has marked advances in equitation since the invention of the bridle, so it is logical to assume that the twenty-first century's technologi-cal advances will enable equitation to take a great stride forward. That said, the quest for the next great technological advance must be matched by a quantum leap in good horsemanship.

The development of tensiometers (for the reins) and pressure pads (for the seat, legs, spurs and whips) will address the need for measurement of rider interventions that may compromise horse welfare. The right equipment will allow us to measure, analyse and describe the correct and humane use of devices and practices in equitation, without which the good public image of equitation in general is potentially jeopardised. The sustainability of the industry can be assured only if the appeal of horse-riding as a sporting and leisure activity for animal-lovers is retained (Endenburg, 1999).

Technological advances such as applied tension and pressure-detecting technologies (see Figure 15.1) will also help to educate riders of all levels in how best to apply the core principles of learning theory. By reducing confusion among riders and therefore conflict in horses, such technology forms a foundation for continuing advances in training practices and the design of equipment that will allow Equitation Science to make horse-riding safer (Waran *et al.*, 2002; McGreevy and McLean, 2005). In an apparent paradox, electronic devices are the most impartial means of establishing the effectiveness of less orthodox coaching and riding tools, such as imaging techniques. These

Table 15.1 Some of the topics addressed in the first four international Equitation Science symposia. All the topics have practical importance but they are grouped here in terms of their focus on either measurement, practice or theory. For details, see www.equitationscience.com

Emphasis	Topic
Measurement and evaluation	• A low-cost device for measuring the pressures exerted on horses by riders and handlers
	• Breed differences in equine retinae
	• The use of head lowering in horses as a method of inducing calmness
	• A preliminary investigation into verbal cue/colour association learning in horses
	• Do horses exhibit motor bias when their balance is tested?
	• Visuomotor influences on jump stride kinematics in show-jumping horses
	• Optimising the biomechanics of the equine athlete: background and perspectives
	• Assessment of ethological methods as a diagnostic tool to determine early overtraining in horses
	• Fear reactions in dressage versus show-jumping horses may be linked to genetics but not training
	• Behaviour of horses during habituation to a novel object
	• Poll-flexion does not induce hypoxia in unridden ponies while trotting
	• Horse temperament and riding performances
	• Impact of riding in rollkur-posture on welfare and fear of performance horses
	• The prevalence of ridden behaviour problems in the UK leisure horse population and associated risk factors
	• Investigating horse–human interactions
	• Does the provision of creep feed post-weaning affect the development of oral stereotypies in foals?
	• Changes in heart rate during the initial training period of 3-year-old Warmblood sport horse stallions
	• The effect of two different training methods on the behaviour, heart rate and performance of horses
	• Effects on behaviour and rein tension in horses ridden with/without martingales and rein inserts
	• The effects of a treeless and treed saddle on stride length, neck length and shoulder range of motion in the horse
	• Building a scale of behavioural indicators of stress in domestic horses
	• Keeping riding horses in groups – a descriptive study on the common procedure of separating a horse from the group for riding or training purposes
	• Can standardised behaviour tests predict suitability for use in horses?
	• Behavioural reactions of horses ridden by beginner riders
	• Consequences of fluctuations in density and group composition on social behaviour of group-housed horses
	• The influence of filler pole layout on jumping technique of horses
	• The effects of gender on learning ability in the horse
	• The effects of prior handling experiences on the stress responses of semi-feral foals presented at auction
	• An evaluation of a trickle feeding system for horses
	• Association of facial hair whorl direction and motor laterality during grazing in the domestic horse
	• Detection of emotionality in horses during physical activity
	• Horse trials: fence design and cross-country falls
	• Equestrian participation: a case study of the Irish Sport Horse Industry
	• Are there advantages to a cantilevered saddle over traditional English and western type saddles?
Practice	• An approach to stress induced by a rider in show-jumping horses
	• Relations between subjectively assessed dressage performances and objective welfare parameters
	• Training from an earlier age
	• Training methods for modifying fear in horses
	• How can we use learning theory to help train horses: habituation and positive reinforcement
	• The addition of positive reinforcement enhances the ability to learn a frightening task (but only for frightened horses)
	• An innovative approach to equitation foundation training (backing the horse) within an automated horse walker may reduce conflict behaviour in the horse
	• Group housing with automatic feeding systems: implications for behaviour and horse welfare
	• Transfer of nervousness from competition rider to horse

Table 15.1 (*Continued*)

Emphasis	Topic
	• Assessing the rider's seat and horse's behaviour: difficulties and perspectives
	• Tight tendon/brushing boots: lower limb protection or innovative lower limb sensitisation training technique in the show-jumping horse
	• Preliminary investigations of horses' responses to bitted and bitless bridles during foundation training
	• A preliminary investigation into the effectiveness of different halter types used on horses
	• Effects of diet on learning and responsive behaviour of young foals
	• Factors influencing gastric ulceration in Irish racehorses
	• The contribution of craniosacral therapy to the rehabilitation of problem horses
	• The effect of forage nonstructural carbohydrate on glycemic response
	• Merits of an automated system in determining and implementing optimal feeding schedules for the stabled horse
	• Rider asymmetry within equitation: preliminary observations
	• Stretching regime effects on stride length and range of motion in equine trot
Theory	• The evolution of training principles and their influence on the horse's welfare
	• Defining the terms and processes associated with equitation
	• Equestrianism and horse welfare: the need for an equine-centred approach to training
	• Epidemiology of horses leaving the Thoroughbred and standardbred racing industries
	• Ethological challenges for working horses and the limitations of ethological solutions in training
	• The application of the principles of Equitation Science by qualified equestrian instructors
	• Reducing wastage in the trained horse: training principles that arise from learning theory
	• Horse-show ethics: survey results from a US adult extension workshop
	• Assessment of the behaviour of unhandled horses: influence of three different training methods
	• HorseConnexion: improving horse welfare through knowledge transfer
	• Is there evidence of 'learned helplessness' in horses?
	• Overshadowing: a silver lining for a dark cloud in horse-training
	• Welfare implications for the competition horse away from the training arena
	• Investigating cribbing and weaving behaviour in horses in Michigan
	• Different expectations between producers (vendors) and purchasers may lead to wastage and welfare concerns for the horse
	• Paedomorphosis: a novel explanation of physical and behavioural differences in horses
	• Preliminary investigations into the ethological relevance of round-pen training with horses
	• Horse sense: social status of horses affects their likelihood of copying other horses' behaviour
	• Evaluating learning theory in horses and donkeys when presented with a novel task
	• The additive effect of stress and genotype on learning systems; implications for equine training
	• SMART: Sensitivity Models for Animals in Response to Training
	• Estimating actual and minimum trajectories of the performance horse when jumping fences of given dimensions
	• Weighted boots alter the jump stride kinematics in the performance horse
	• The horse–human dyad: Does physical training of horses have to be attritional and can we ever resolve performance and welfare?
	• Visual memory and rider experience in a show-jumping context
	• The horse–human dyad: improving rider stability and biomechanics through coaching with sensory-specific language
	• Horsemanship: Conventional, Natural and Equitation Science
	• Habituation and object generalisation in horses
	• Equine Chronobiology – an emerging scientific field with implications for health and performance in the horse
	• Can we improve short-term memory in the horse?
	• The horse–human dyad: Can we align horse-training and handling activities with the equid ethogram?
	• Are there 'optimal timeframes' for handling the foal?
	• Goal-related educational staircase in show-jumping
	• Changing attitudes towards horses' defensive aggression body language communication

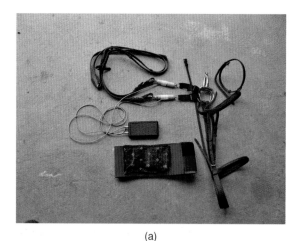

(a)

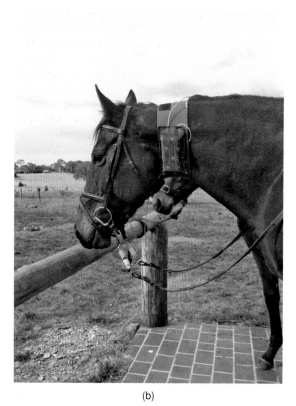

(b)

Figure 15.1 Tensiometers will play an increasing role in Equitation Science, coaching and possibly even competition.

new technologies may also prove to be the best means of elucidating the behavioural qualities that characterise humans who are said to have 'horse sense'. By helping to upskill humans who lack this sense, improvements in coaching and

equipment will also reduce the rate of euthanasia because of unacceptable horse behaviour – the so-called behavioural wastage (Hayek *et al.*, 2005).

Tension and pressure detecting technologies could be used to measure the qualities of effective coaching, not just effective signalling to the horse. They may also provide objective information for riders who are geographically isolated. For example, because Australia is removed geographically from Europe, its elite competition riders struggle to readily access higher levels of coaching. The validation of novel measuring and feedback technology will be the first step towards elite riders accessing real-time feedback from remote coaches.

Mathematical models may allow equitation scientists to compare horses and, over time, the efficacy of training systems (McGreevy et al., 2009b; see Figure 15.2). This will assist the development of empirically sound coaching plans. Such models also have the potential to expose individual and breed differences in reactivity levels and identify sensory lateralisation in particular horses (McGreevy and Rogers, 2005) that may counter asymmetries in certain riders. Traditional adherence to leather, PVC and elastic may be limiting our ability to work and compete with horses. The emergence of new polymers and so-called smart materials could possibly enhance the effectiveness of traditional items of saddlery.

One domain that merits particularly close scrutiny is the development of materials to be placed in the mouths of horses. Since the discovery of the bit as a means of restraint and control, a plethora of bits, bridles and devices have been used to deliver discomfort and pain to horses. However, devising a novel source of stimuli aversive to the horse is not an adequate response to a training deficit. Horses that do not trial conflict behaviours (and thus successfully resolve the escalated discomfort of such devices) usually habituate rapidly. The new bit is then less effective in producing a desired response and once more the rider is driven to pull on the reins. Thus begins an unhappy escalation.

The minimal space in which a bit can be placed inside the mouth may catalyse the search for novel means of head control. So, instead of using bits, we may explore the use of other means of applying pressure to the head. For example, the current range of bitless bridles may germinate innovations

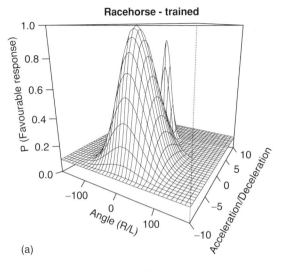

Racehorse - trained

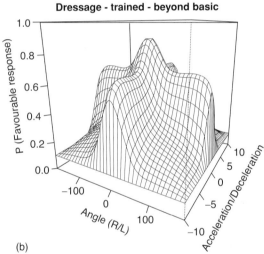

Dressage - trained - beyond basic

Figure 15.2 (a) An example of a response surface for a racehorse with only rudimentary foundation training and a highly probable high-speed forward response shown as a peak in sensitivity to acceleration cues. (b) An example of a response surface for a highly trained dressage horse, showing multiple peaks for given speeds and high responsiveness to slow, stop and step-back signals.

that allow riders to communicate clearly with their horses while being as humane as possible. Whatever devices emerge, the pressure from them will be applied fairly low down the head so that some leverage along the axis of the nose can effect a turn. One can imagine how bland and therefore ineffective any pressure would be if it were applied,

say, near the ears. Equitation Science will be able to measure and evaluate the effectiveness of such bitless bridles and identify which horses are the best candidates for various pieces of traditional and novel gear. It will eventually explore inherent breed and individual differences in head and mouth sensitivity, so that conflict can be avoided from the outset.

Animal welfare science must address the possibility of learned helplessness in horses used in sport, leisure and as a consequence of any radical restraining technique. This will provide physiological measures of the stress that accompanies passive coping. In addition, horse welfare will improve if we can identify horses that are simply not capable of a response. For example, an 'on-board' device that measures fatigue and exhaustion may one day allow riders to know when to quit before inducing a cycle of over-training. The same approach may allow judges and veterinarians to monitor the welfare of horses in competition. This sort of advance has the potential to ensure that fatigued horses are not pushed or beaten in the name of sport. Of course, competitive endurance riding already provides a model of such a system, which is meant to ensure that fatigued horses are not pushed beyond certain limits. This means that endurance competitors are relatively advanced in their knowledge of diet, farriery, welfare and physiology.

Ethology

The ethological aspects of Equitation Science will continue as rich seams for research into defining the enhanced relationship some people have with their horses, and the ways in which this connection may go beyond learning theory alone. Once we have established the variability and consistency of cues used in inter-specific communication and know exactly how classical conditioning can replace one cue with another, we can coach those less blessed with horse sense. Looking for ethological salience as we unravel the complexities and jargon of various coaching systems will allow as many stakeholders as possible to access the most critical information for the benefit of the horse.

As we have seen (in Chapter 2, Cognitive etholgy), there is still much to discover about the way in which horses learn from the environment, from each other and from human interactions (Murphy and Arkins, 2007). For example, context-specific learning needs further investigation (e.g. the effect on performance of a novel environment or the direction in which a horse approaches an obstacle). Furthermore, it is suggested that horses somehow percolate training and come back to work after a break with evidence of having made great leaps in their learning, almost as if the training needs to be interrupted to fully mature as a result of neuronal change, growth and vascularisation. It would be interesting to investigate more fully how training contingencies mature or decline with gaps in training. For example, individual horse progress could be plotted on a weekly basis to see how much learning is retained from one week to the next.

Learning theory too is far from complete when we consider the context of the ridden horse. Since one cannot ride a rat, the lessons from the rodent model of avoidance learning are of only limited use when explaining equestrians' application of negative reinforcement. There are also many questions remaining about positive reinforcement and how it can be administered to horses. Apart from the importance of timing, the quality of delivered rewards in horse-training has yet to be fully explored, especially for in-hand work. We should never assume that the results to date are in any way the full story. There may be practical ways of delivering jackpots to ridden horses that do not slow them down or prompt them to wait for more rewards.

It is becoming clear that ethological considerations may collide with learning theory to explain deficits in trainability. Training and performance differences between stereotypers such as crib-biters and weavers and other horses merit a thorough longitudinal investigation so that the long-term effects of stereotypy on learning can be evaluated. This may help to create further incentives for breeders and trainers to avoid management styles that trigger the emergence of stereotypies in predisposed horses. While ongoing research efforts are likely to identify specific risk factors for all equine stereotypies, they should be used to refine stable management rather than to select horses that tolerate existing practices.

When developing their stereotypies, crib-biters and weavers can be regarded as useful sentinels of sub-optimal husbandry, sentinels that should alert us to problems that are being encountered by all resident horses, not just those that produce a stereotypic response to the challenge.

As clinical equine behavioral medicine matures, we will become better at identifying individuals that are high risk for certain disorders and managing them accordingly. We should also become more skilled at identifying horses that have true learning deficits rendering them likely to show dangerous or sustained fight and flight responses. The impact of such advances on human safety will be significant.

Eventually, the racing industry may become more involved in Equitation Science as the physiology of the horse at exercise becomes less mysterious and trainers are left asking, 'What is the will to win?' The significance of mood, trust, stoicism and even attitude may then vie with cardiac output and gaseous exchange as behavioural qualities to be measured and selected for. And we may also see more scrutiny of the evidence of communication among horses competing as a group.

Nutrition

The deleterious effects of low-forage diets on the time-budgeting and health of horses have been recognised for many years (Kiley-Worthington 1987; McGreevy et al., 1995a, 1995b). More recently, the effects of increased starch loads on restlessness (Freire et al., 2009), gastric ulceration (Nadeau et al., 2000) and behaviour (Nicol et al., 2005) have been highlighted. It appears that we still have some way to go in delivering appropriate nutrition to stabled horses, animals that often have the most pent-up and potentially dangerous energy. The composition of any concentrate content of a ration certainly warrants a mention in the context of behaviour and riding safety since so-called heating foods (such as oats given to ponies) are anecdotally regarded as an important cause of unwelcome hyper-reactivity. Research into the mechanisms underpinning this relationship is urgently needed. It may show that such diets have a negative impact on horse welfare.

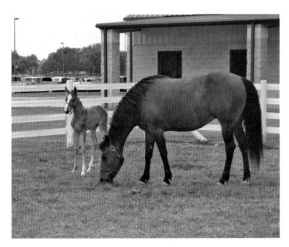

Figure 15.3 Paris Texas, one of the world's first cloned horses. (Photo courtesy of Eric Palmer, Texas A&M University, March 2005.)

Genetics

Temperament characteristics of elite horses should be measured and characterised more fully. This will promote our understanding of breed traits that favour certain equestrian activities and selection for these where desirable and possible. An on-going exploration of temperament and laterality tests as predictors of reactivity and suitability for certain sports and work may reduce behavioural wastage. The emergence of equine clones (e.g. see Figure 15.3) will allow us to dissect the influences of nature and nurture on performance. However, a long-term perspective should be retained in any breeding program that is based on any suite of tests for reactivity or temperament so that the effects of selection for one set of traits can be tested in case it brings along any unwanted baggage (i.e. undesirable, unexpected traits).

Conclusion

Much of our traditional riding and stable management practices are at odds with the physical and behavioural adaptations of the horse; some horses cope, some do not. Equitation presents significant ethological challenges and, in many cases, training fails to adequately reflect the physical abilities and learning capacity of the horse. Riders often run into difficulties when they assume that the horse knows what the rider wants to achieve. All too often discord between horse and human emerges from the rider's inability to identify or accept his or her role in confusing the horse by issuing conflicting signals. Against this backdrop, we recognise that most horses are extremely tolerant – but just because we *can* do something to a horse does not make it an ethically sound practice. Just as dogs can be trained to salivate in response to electric shocks, we should not assume that just because a horse can be trained to offer a particular response, it enjoys giving that response.

Despite the enormous variety in horse sports and equine work, only four basic responses are required for them all: stop, go, turn the forequarters and turn the hindquarters. Foundation training these basic responses allows horses to be trained with a customised plan that is specific to the discipline they are intended for, but it also means that they can be re-trained for a second job when their first career is over.

Training relies on timing and consistency and so, by deduction, detraining soon arises when there is inconsistency and variable timing. Clear trainers are consistent in their signals and the way in which they set up puzzles for animal to solve (i.e. the way in which they pose questions). Good technique that reflects these qualities is more sustainable than a handler's size or strength or, indeed, any device that allows a handler to use more force.

Equitation Science improves performance in sport horses because of more accurate operant conditioning, classical conditioning and shaping. But our greatest responsibility is never to forget that the horse's welfare is paramount: it is a privilege to ride horses and remarkable that the possibility exists. Therefore, every horse-trainer should maintain an open mind about possible limitations in horse learning and confusion arising from training methods. This is especially important when the vast range of required responses in the trained horse is compared with the limited number of sites on the animal's body for eliciting those responses. Given that we are dealing with an animal that, so far at least, appears unable to extrapolate, we must always be mindful of the potentially confusing effects of applying pressure signals in common or overlapping sites on its body to elicit different responses. It is critical that we acknowledge how much of the global behavioural wastage tragedy is a result of our unclear interactions and the impossible expectations humans place on horses. What is needed, therefore, is a reappraisal and restructuring of contemporary horse-training within the framework of established and empirically tested principles of learning. And that is the purpose of Equitation Science.

Glossary of the Terms and Definitions and of Processes Associated with Equitation

Many of the glossary definitions offered below were presented at the First International Equitation Science Symposium as a collaboration by Natalie Waran, Amanda Warren-Smith and Debbie Goodwin. Underlined words have separate entries in this glossary.

Above the bit: A posture characteristic of a hyper-reactive ridden horse exhibiting conflict behaviour in which the horse attempts to escape the aversive situation by raising its head, quickening its pace, shortening its neck and stride and bracing its back, which becomes dorsally concave. The horse thus assumes a posture appropriate for running and therefore does not show impulsion.

Accepting the bit: The way a horse responds to the bit in particular and to cues in general. During locomotion and transitions, the horse's mouth remains closed, soft in the jaw and with relaxed lips. A horse that accepts the bit does not shorten or lengthen its neck or alter its head position during travelling and transitions. Accepting the bit is generally accompanied by relaxation of the neck and body.

Activity: The rhythmical speed of movement of the horse's legs within any gait. *See* Tempo.

Against the hand: When a horse does not stop/slow/step-back from the bit correctly. Consequently, the rein contact feels heavy to the rider. This is usually accompanied by a hyper-reactive (hollow) posture in which the neck shortens or lengthens during locomotion or transitions. There may be an element of learned helplessness in this behaviour. A horse may also be described as being against one of the rider's hands, in which case it is heavy on one rein only (lugging), demonstrating a diminished response to the turn signal of that rein.

Against the leg: A description of a horse that is not straight in its body and is continually flexing its thorax (*see* Flexion) against one of the rider's legs. Such a horse drifts or attempts to drift sideways. In addition, the horse may be against both legs (i.e. not going forward).

Agonistic behaviour: Pertaining to behaviour associated with conflict between individuals.

Aid: A stimulus that elicits a learned response in horses. We prefer the terms cues or signals.

Artificial aids: Equipment used to alter a horse's behaviour under-saddle or in-hand (e.g. whips and spurs). When employed correctly, these are generally used to negatively reinforce various locomotory responses and are most commonly used to fortify the light or natural cue to achieve the desired response. By convention, these are distinct from the natural cues since they do not involve direct use of parts of the rider's body.

Asking with the rein: Cues sent by the rider through the rein to signal the horse to respond in a specific way.

Associative learning: This involves the relationship between at least two events that are paired. There are two types of associative learning: classical and operant. Classical conditioning is the process whereby a response, either conditioned or unconditioned, becomes elicited from a conditioned stimulus.

Balanced seat: The position of a mounted rider that requires the minimum of muscular effort to remain in the saddle and which interferes least with the horse's movements and equilibrium. It is generally understood that the balanced seat allows delivery of the cues in the most effective manner. The rider has equal weight on both seat bones and feet. *See* Independent seat.

Bars of the mouth (diastema): Area of the horse's mandible between the incisors and the molars that is free of teeth and in which the bit lies.

Baulk: Refuse to move forward, usually because of the presence of an aversive object or obstacle (as in jumping). *See* Napping.

Behind the bit: A head and neck posture that is generally described as an evasion and which involves the horse persistently drawing its nose toward its chest, sometimes allowing the reins to become slack. This occurs in training because of mistakes made in negative reinforcement or due to the use of restraining devices (such as draw reins) that force the neck to be shortened. In this situation the horse gives two different and independent responses to one signal (i.e. slowing or dorsoventral flexion) and thus frequently develops conflict behaviour. This posture thwarts the development of impulsion.

Behind the leg: A horse that lacks self-maintained speed and rhythm requires the rider to continually deliver leg cues with each stride or each alternate stride.

Behind the vertical: The appearance of a horse with a shortened neck posture. As a result, it positions its nasal planum behind the vertical line (the horse's chin becomes closer to its chest). Such a horse is generally heavy in the feel of the reins or has no contact during locomotion and transitions and, when this occurs, its stop/slow/step-back response is diminished. As the horse offers two independent

responses (shortening neck or slowing) to one signal, it often exhibits conflict behaviours.

Bend (lateral bend): The lateral curvature of the body that arises principally by the flexing at four sites on the horse's vertebral column: the cervical region in general, and the thoracic (tenth thoracic vertebra), lumbar (first lumbar vertebra) and sacral (third sacral vertebra) regions (Faber *et al.*, 2000, 2001a, 2001b). Bend allows the horse to step into its foretracks with its hindfeet on a curved line or circle that is greater than 6 m in diameter. Bend is usually accompanied by flexion, lateral, longitudinal and vertical and is an accepted correct feature of all work on curved lines and all lateral movements.

Bit: An apparatus usually consisting of metal or other hard substances or a combination of both. It is positioned in the diastema of the horse's mouth and connected to the reins. As a result of tension in the reins, this apparatus places pressure on the lips, tongue and bars of the horse's mouth and results in the horse learning to stop/slow/step-back and turn, through the processes of negative reinforcement and classical conditioning.

Bitting: Accustoming a horse to having a bit in its mouth or the selection of the most appropriate bit for a horse.

Blocking: (a) Preventing a horse from performing appropriately in any given gait by the application of simultaneous rein and leg pressure. This can result in conflict behaviour. (b) The deleterious effects of the simultaneous application of two intense cues such that neither will be learned (Hull, 1943).

Blow-up: When a ridden or handled horse becomes hyper-reactive during training and exhibits behaviours ranging from mild tension to bucking or breaks from the gait in which it is meant to be travelling. It is most common in early training and exposure to novel environments as in 'showing'. It is generally a symptom of conflict behaviour.

Bolting: (a) Accelerating, usually to a gallop out of stimulus control (*see* Running (away)) and showing a lack of response to the stop/slow/step-back cues. Bolting reflects an extreme activation of the <u>HPA axis</u> (hypothalamic–pituitary–adrenal axis). This is a manifestation of <u>conflict behaviour</u>. Sometimes referred to as 'running blind'. (b) Eating (concentrated food) too rapidly.

Bounding: A hyper-reactive leaping movement where the horse springs from the hindlegs to the forelegs.

Break gait: The random change from one gait to another that is not under <u>stimulus control</u>.

Break in (gentle, start):   The basic foundation training of a young horse to respond to <u>cues</u> and <u>signals</u> that control its <u>rhythm</u> and <u>tempo</u>, direction and posture for whatever purpose it may be required.

Bridle lameness: An irregularity of gait <u>under-saddle</u> that has the appearance of lameness. Mostly seen in the trot, it arises as a result of a long-term training error in which the horse is unable to free itself of simultaneous and persistent <u>bit</u> and leg pressure during locomotion and <u>transitions</u>, or from persistent rising on the same or incorrect diagonal at trot. There is usually an associated crookedness to the longitudinal axis of the body.

Broken neck (over-bent):   The appearance of the neck of a horse in which there is (usually) a sudden change in angle (a break in the curve) in the vicinity of the third cervical vertebra. This is usually a result of persistent use of side reins that are too short, especially during early training, or draw reins that cause the neck to be too flexed and the nasal planum to be <u>behind the vertical</u>. It is believed that there is degeneration of the vertebrae and/or ligaments at the third cervical vertebra. Horses with broken necks generally exhibit <u>conflict behaviours</u> and tend to flex their necks to light rein pressure rather than give the <u>stop/slow/step-back</u> response.

Bronco: An unbroken or imperfectly broken wild horse, or one maintained in this state for rodeos.

Bucking: A sudden humping or arching of the back with the head and neck lowered, usually kicking out with the hindlegs or jumping/bounding forwards/sideways with an arched back and ears laid back (Waring, 2003). Bucking is a manoeuvre that evolved to dislodge predators. Persistent bucking is a man-

ifestation of <u>conflict behaviour</u> to the rein and leg cues (McLean, 2005b).

Cadence: The result of the combined effect of correct training that a horse shows when it moves with well-marked regularity, <u>impulsion</u>, balanced and rhythmic <u>strides</u>. There should be an enhanced period of suspension between steps that gives the horse the appearance of springing off the ground so the feet lift clear of the ground and float to the next step.

Catenary: The slight loop in a perfectly flexible and inextensible rope or chain of uniform cross-section and density as it hangs freely from two fixed points that are not in the same vertical line. The term is used in discussions of rein tension.

Champing (US):   *See* Mouthing.

Cinch bound (US):   *See* <u>Cold-back</u>.

Classical conditioning: The process whereby the unconditioned or conditioned response becomes elicited from a conditioned stimulus (Pavlov, 1927). In equitation it is the process where learned responses are elicited from more subtle versions of the same signal or to entirely new signals.

Clicker training: An application of secondary reinforcement where the secondary reinforcer is an auditory signal to the horse (or any other animal) that the correct response has been performed and that a primary reinforcer (usually food) is about to be delivered.

Cold-back (girth shy, US cinch bound):   <u>Hyper-reactive behaviour</u> (occasionally <u>bucking</u>) or instability, sometimes to the extent of collapse when the girth is tightened, or the saddle is placed on the back or the horse is mounted.

Cold-jawed (US tough-mouthed):   *See* <u>Hard-mouthed</u>.

Collected walk/trot/canter: Where each step of the <u>stride</u> of the gait is shorter and higher rather than longer. The horse should remain <u>on the bit</u>, the hindquarters should be <u>engaged</u> (lowered), with the horse showing <u>activity</u>, <u>impulsion</u> and <u>lightness</u>. Collected paces should develop from the correct training of the horse over time so that it is physically able to travel showing true <u>collection</u>.

Collection: The progressive development of increased carrying power in the hindquarters of the horse. The resultant transfer of weight from the forequarters to the hindquarters allows the poll and withers to be carried higher, the hindquarters to drop slightly and the hindfeet to step further forward and to carry more body-weight with higher and shorter steps. This confers more power to the hindquarters, enabling the horse to perform more collected movements. In classical equitation, collection develops from repeated gait and stride length transitions that occur in three beats of the rhythm. The combined effect of the transitions and the inertia of the animal is that over time the horse's physique changes. The propulsion of the body is then in a more upward and forward direction giving greater cadence to the strides and increased lightness of the forehand. Collection can occur in the walk, trot or canter. So, for example, in a collected canter, the strides are shorter and the horse's frame is short and compressed. *See also* False collection.

Conflict behaviour: A set of responses of varying duration that are usually characterised by hyper-reactivity and arise largely through confusion. In equitation, confusions that result in conflict behaviours may be caused by application of simultaneous opposing signals (such as go and stop/slow/step-back) such that the horse is unable to offer any learned responses sufficiently and is forced to endure discomfort from relentless rein and leg pressures. Attempts to flee the aversive situation result in hyper-reactivity. In addition, the desired response to one or both cues diminishes. Conflict behaviours may also result from one signal eliciting two or more responses independently, such as using the reins to achieve vertical flexion independently of the stop/slow/step-back response, or using a single rein to bend the neck of the horse independently of its previously conditioned turn response. Similarly, conflict behaviour may result from incorrect negative reinforcement, such as the reinforcement of inconsistent responses, incorrect responses, no removal of pressure or no shaping of responses. Often referred to as evasions and resistances.

Conformation: Features of the external morphology (i.e. the relative musculoskeletal di-

mensions) of a horse that interest breeders and exhibitors, not least because they can affect its performance (Loch, 1977).

Connection: The contact of the rein, seat and leg. This contact may be absent (no connection), correct (an easily habituated light connection) or too strong (unendurable pressure).

Contact: The connection of the rider's hands to the horse's mouth, of the legs to the horse's sides and of the seat to the horse's back via the saddle. The topic of contact with both hand and leg generates considerable confusion related to the pressure that the horse should endure if the contact is deemed to be correct. In classical equitation, contact to the rein and rider's leg involves a light pressure (approximately 200 g) to the horse's lips/tongue and body, respectively. Although a light contact is the aim, there are brief moments (seconds or parts of a second) when contact may need to be stronger, particularly at the start of training, or in retraining, to overcome resistances from the horse. Many contemporary horse-trainers insist that the contact should be much heavier than a light connection. This view may cause progressive habituation leading to learned helplessness to the rein and leg signals as a result of incorrect negative reinforcement and/or simultaneous application of the cues. Contact may therefore need to be the focus of discussion and debate.

Contiguous: Adjoining or touching. Stimuli that are closely associated by time and space with specific behaviours. For example, when a reinforcement (release of rein pressure) should immediately follow a response (step-back).

Contingent: Dependent upon; Contingent outcomes are those directly linked to a causal behaviour. For example, pressing a lever turns a light on.

Contralateral: That is on the opposite side, as opposed to ipsilateral.

Counter-bending,   counter-flexing,   counter-canter: The practice of bending or flexing the horse to the outside of the circle or away from the direction of the direct turn. Counter-canter arises when the horse is deliberately cued to canter with the contralateral canter lead (e.g. to canter to the left with the right fore leading).

Crabbing: A conflict behaviour in ridden and in-hand horses where the horse fails to go straight and the resistance manifests as a sideways and forward (frequently alternating the direction) crab-like motor behaviour. Crabbing may also be associated with a hyper-reactive horse under restraint.

Cue: An event that elicits a learned response. In equitation, cues are sometimes termed aids or signals. Rein, leg, whip and spur cues are initially learned through negative reinforcement and then transformed to light cues (light rein, light leg, voice, seat) via classical conditioning because of the temporal relation between the two. In traditional horsemanship, the cues are divided into two groups the natural cues and the artificial cues. This distinction is misleading as it neither identifies nor correlates with the two different learning modalities through which the horse acquires its responses to the cues. These are learned through classical conditioning when a response comes increasingly under stimulus control.

Deep and round (rollkur): A modern tendency to train the horse to carry its head low and its cervical vertebrae maximally flexed (chin closer to the chest) in the belief that the hindquarters are engaged and that the activity and power of the hindlegs is improved. To critics, the deep and round technique is seen as a form of false collection and it may also have welfare implications.

Detraining: Where a stimulus is applied without the learned response being performed. The result is reduction or extinction of the likelihood of the learned response arising from the stimulus.

Diagonal advanced placement (DAP): As a result of incorrect negative reinforcement and in particular the simultaneous application of forward and restraining pressures accompanied with maximal flexion of the cervical vertebrae (rollkur), it has been suggested that the diagonal pairing of legs during the trot and canter may be temporally split, with subsequent losses in the purity of the gaits and the possible emergence of conflict behaviours (*see* Rollkur).

Diagonal: (a) Refers to the forefoot moving in unison with the opposite hindfoot, as seen in the gaits of trot (two diagonal pairs) and canter (one diagonal pair). (b) Being on the correct diagonal refers to the rising and sitting of the rider being synchronised with the trotting horse's footfalls so that the rider sits when the outside foreleg and inside hindleg are on the ground and rises as they move forward.

Direct rein/indirect rein/turn: Using the rein to turn the horse's forequarters (abducting the forelegs) where the rider's hand shifts slightly (about 4 cm) towards the direction of turn. The direct rein is one held out wide away from the neck in an attempt to make the turn response clearer to the horse when increased pressure is applied to this rein relative to the closing rein. By contrast, an indirect rein is one that is parallel and closer to the horse's neck. The indirect turn is similar to neck reining where the indirect rein is the one with the greater pressure relative to the direct rein and motivates the horse to turn towards the direct rein. The indirect turn is used to gain lateral control over the forelegs and thus to improve the effect of the direct turn.

Disunited canter: An undesirable broken gait, most often seen in horses with a tendency to pace or horses that are not straight (*see* Straightness). It occurs when there is a shift from ipsilateral to contralateral coupling of fore and hindlegs.

Dominance/submission: Suites of behaviours in social interactions that signal rank or determine priority of access to resources (a dynamic process affected by motivation). A belief in horse-training that horse interactions are governed by dominance/submission implies that trainers need to be dominant over horses to train them effectively. The notion that a horse must respect a human to be effectively controlled may be at odds with learning theory. In equitation, the significance of dominance, submission and respect needs further investigation.

Dorsal: Pertaining to, or situated on, the back of an animal, as opposed to ventral.

Double-gaited: A horse that can both trot and pace.

Downhill: Conformational fault in a dressage horse, where the horse is noticeably higher at the point of the croup than at the withers. Such a horse may feel heavy on the forehand to the rider.

Driving: (a) Where either a horse or a team of horses pulls a vehicle. (b) *See* Long-reining. (c) Locomotion (*see* Engagement) in which the horse is pushing forward with its hocks underneath it at the moment of pushing. The moment of push should not continue beyond the point at which the fetlock is behind the vertical line of the hock.

Engagement/engaging the hocks (tarsal joints): Where the horse brings its hindfeet underneath its body so that proportionally more weight is placed on the hindlegs. Classically, this process is trained over time with concomitant physique changes; however, in contemporary training, it is sometimes produced by riders forcing the horse to shorten and raise its head and neck with rein pressure while simultaneously applying leg/forward pressure. Deep and round is frequently used as a precursor to this technique termed false collection. It should be clear that engagement is not the same as collection, but is a precursor to it.

Evading the bit: Oral behaviours (such as moving the tongue aborally) and neck postures (such as dorsoventral flexion) that enable horses to reduce the discomfort caused by bits or the extent to which riders can apply and maintain pressure. In training, these result from errors in negative reinforcement.

Evasions and resistances: Descriptive terms for conflict behaviours where evasions are similar to resistances, except that evasions refer to the more severe and violent behaviours. These terms arose because of the horse's natural tendency to avoid pressure/pain by learning through negative reinforcement to perform any attempted behaviour that results in lessening of pressure/pain. The problem with these terms is that they imply malevolent and calculated behaviour on the part of the horse whereas, in fact, these behaviours are more likely to be the result of errors in negative reinforcement.

Extension/extended strides: The longest stride within the rhythm of the particular gait. In equitation, extended paces arise only from collected paces. These strides involve straightened limbs at the end of the swing phase of the stride that allow the horse to cover as much ground as possible with each stride. For the average horse, in the extended walk and trot, the hindtrack should land approximately 20–30 cm in front of the foretracks and in extended canter the hindtracks land about 2 m in front of the foretracks.

Extinction: Omission of reinforcement following either classical or operant conditioning that results in the eventual weakening of the trained response.

Falling in/falling out: Losses of straightness associated with the horse drifting in or out of the circle. It is similar to lugging, but more apparent at the slower gaits.

False collection: Forcing a horse into an apparently collected outline through the simultaneous actions of the rein and leg or with the use of gadgets and pulleys rather than the progressive development of collection over time through training. False collection frequently results in conflict behaviour because concurrent stop and go signals cause confusion and pain.

Flexion: (a) Longitudinal: the dorsoventral lowering, lengthening and relaxing of the horse's neck and back. In reality, this is not a flexion but an extension and should be redefined as longitudinal extension. This is the most fundamental quality of being on the bit. Longitudinal flexion should not be confused with 'longitudinal bend' (*see* Impulsion). (b) Lateral: the lateral bending of the atlanto-occipital junction and including the first three cervical vertebrae of the horse's neck. This is primarily a shaped quality of correct turning and in the well-trained horse is thus involved whenever the turn, circles or the turn-position is required, such as in lateral movements. The extent of lateral flexion negatively correlates with the size of the circle. As lateral flexion is a shaped quality of the turn response, counter-flexing can result in conflict behaviour. Lateral flexion is a secondary precursor of being on the bit. Lateral flexion should not be confused with 'lateral bend' (*see* Bend). (c) Dorsoventral, vertical or direct: the dorsoventral flexion of the horse's cervical vertebrae so that the nasal plane is almost perpendicular to the ground (the nasal plane may be up to 6 degrees in front of the vertical). For a horse to be showing vertical flexion, it must be relaxed, straight, pushing forward from behind with its hocks underneath it, relaxed in its jaw and showing longitudinal flexion (Wallace, 1993). This is a precursor of the horse being on the bit. Dorsoventral flexion may be seen as a result of correct longitudinal flexion.

Forehand (forequarters): Those parts of the horse that lie in front of the rider (i.e. the head, neck, shoulders, withers and forelegs).

Freeze: The sudden alert motionless stance associated with a highly attentive reaction to an external stimulus (often visual) and typically resulting in conflict behaviours such as napping and spinning.

Gallop: A four-beat gait that provides maximum speed. Generally, the gallop is transverse where the leading hindleg and leading foreleg are on the same side of the body. A rotary gallop may also be seen when the horse is anxious under-saddle. In a rotary gallop, the leading foreleg and hindlegs are on opposite sides of the body.

Girth shy: *See* Cold-back.

Go: The acceleration response in horse-training that provides forward motion. The go response is trained via negative reinforcement using the rider's legs under-saddle and using anterior lead-rein pressure when working a horse in-hand. Through classical conditioning, these responses are converted first to light versions of the leg or lead-rein and then to the cues of seat, position and, perhaps, voice.

Good mouth: *See* Soft mouth.

Green: (a) An inexperienced horse with no training or one that has undergone foundation training but is not fully trained. (b) A racehorse that has yet to undergo a time trial.

Habit: When a learned response is consolidated as a result of long-term potentiation.

Habituation: The waning of a response to a repeated stimulus as a result of frequent exposure (not fatigue).

Half-halt: A subtle, sequential application of the seat, leg and rein cue that is separated in time by one beat of the rhythm of the gait. The half-halt is intended to increase the attention and balance of the ridden horse.

Halt: When the horse is stationary and, in dressage, this means that the horse needs to be standing with his weight evenly distributed, in other words, standing square.

Hanging: *See* Lugging.

Hard-mouthed (US cold-jawed, tough-mouthed): Habituation to rein pressure. This is generally a result of incorrect negative reinforcement and can result in learned helplessness and conflict behaviours in susceptible animals.

Heavy, heavy-mouthed: A term that describes a horse that has been trained with incorrect rein signals such that it will be accustomed to being ridden with a heavy tension in the reins at all times. When the reins are released, such horses accelerate, implying no persistence of the stop response (no self-carriage).

Hitch: (a) To tether a horse. (b) A defect in the gait noted in the hindlegs, which seem to skip at the trot.

Hollow: Undesirable contraction of the vertebral column, so that the head comes up and the neck and back become slightly concave. The strides of the horse generally become faster and shorter ('choppy'). Habitual hollowness is usually a result of incorrect negative reinforcement and is frequently associated with conflict behaviours. Because of its reported association with activation of the HPA axis, hollowness should be further researched.

Horse breaking: *See* Break in.

HPA axis (hypothalamic–pituitary–adrenal axis): The physiological response to arousal, involving the limbic system, which stimulates the hypothalamus to produce corticotrophin releasing factor, which, in turn, stimulates the anterior pituitary gland to produce adrenocorticotrophic hormone, which then stimulates the adrenal cortex to secrete glucocorticoids.

Hyperflexion (of the neck): This is a degree of dorsoventral flexion of the mid-region of the neck that cannot be self-maintained by the horse for a prolonged time without welfare implications (FEI, 2006).

Hyper-reactive behaviour: Behaviours characteristic of an activated HPA axis and associated with various levels of arousal. Such behaviours typically involve the horse having a hollow posture and leg movements with increased activity and tempo, yet shorter strides. Hyper-reactive behaviours are quickly learned and resistant to extinction because of their adaptiveness in the equid ethogram. Behavioural evidence of hyper-reactivity ranges from postural tonus to responses such as shying, bolting, bucking and rearing.

Hypersensitive: (a) The genetic tendency in an animal to be more sensitive than average. (b) A learned response where an animal has become sensitised to a stimulus.

Impulsion: The response of a horse that is correctly trained in its go/stop responses so that it moves forward energetically with a self-maintained rhythm, straightness and outline when signalled to do so. Impulsion is an early expression of the progressive development of collection, in which the animal progressively carries more weight on its hindquarters. Three types of impulsion have been described: (1) *Instinctive:* i.e. the inherited tendency to have more or less impulsion; (2) *mechanical:* it develops from instinctive impulsion and improves with work and gymnastic training; (3) *Transmitted:* that given to the horse by the rider in collecting the horse. True impulsion, in which the horse conveys itself calmly under a light rein and without constant pressure from the rider, is distinct from states of general excitement in which the horse pulls at the bit and requires forceful restraint to be controlled.

In front of the leg: A desirable quality in equitation describing a horse with a correctly trained go response, such that it is neither slowing nor accelerating of its own volition (i.e. it self-maintains its rhythm).

Independent seat: The ability of a rider to maintain a secure, firm and balanced position on a horse's back, without relying on the reins or stirrups; *see* Balanced seat.

Indirect rein: Using the rein to turn the horse's forequarters (abducting the forelegs) where the rider's hand shifts slightly (about 3.8 cm) towards the direction of turn. The active rein (i.e. with increased tension) is the one on the opposite side to which the horse is turning, while the other rein is passive (i.e. maintains contact only; McLean and McLean, 2008).

In-hand: In a routine of training in-hand, the trainer works from the ground rather than from the saddle, positioned beside and/or behind the horse and controlling it with rein, voice and training whip. In-hand work allows the horse to acquire signal response entities of go and stop as a prelude to foundation training, or during retraining or when training advanced movements.

Inside/outside: Identifies either side of the horse as it is being schooled. These require some clarification as to whether one is referring to the relative position in the arena, to the curvature of the path or to the bend of the horse (e.g. inside leg usually refers to the leg of the rider or horse nearest to the centre of the circle the horse is following, or on the bent side, which can be the outside of the arena as in renvers).

Ipsilateral: That is on the same side, as opposed to contralateral.

Jog: (a) A slow, short-striding trot, usually associated with heightened arousal and involving short choppy steps and constant tendencies to accelerate as the horse is attempting to flee the aversive situation. Habitual jogging can be associated with conflict behaviours and result in diminished responses to the slow/stop/step-back signals (McLean, 2005b). (b) In harness-racing, the term given to the exercise conducted on non-hopple days. (Hobble = restraint, hopple = harness). (c) A slow trot used mainly in Western pursuits.

Join-up: An element of round-pen training (popularised by US trainer Monty Roberts), in which the horse learns under some circumstances to remain close to the human.

Lateral: Towards the left or right side of the body, as opposed to medial.

Lateral movements: Any of the training exercises (such as leg-yield, shoulder-in, travers, renvers and half-pass) that involve the horse having longitudinal bend and travelling with the forelegs and hindlegs on two, three or four different tracks with the aim of improving its engagement and collection.

Leadership: According to one tenet of natural horsemanship, the horse must accept the human as a leader to respond correctly in training. This assumption may be contradicted by learning theory and, because of its inherent anthropomorphism, the significance of leadership in equitation calls for further study.

Leaning on the bit: A sign of habituation to bit pressure, which manifests with the horse persistently pressuring the rein(s) as though relying on the rider to support the weight of its head. This arises through incorrect negative reinforcement and can be associated with conflict behaviours and learned helplessness.

Learned helplessness: A state in which an animal has learned not to respond to pressure or pain. Arises from inappropriate application of negative reinforcement, which results in the horse not being able to obtain release from aversive stimuli. If this continues over a period of time, the horse will no longer make responses that were once appropriate. Learned helplessness has the following characteristics: a disinclination to trial behavioural responses to pressure, lowered levels of aggression, dullness, loss of appetite, physiological and immunological changes.

Leg-yield: The simplest of lateral movements in which the horse moves both forward and sideways from the rider's single leg signal. Leg-yield is usually trained before more complex lateral manoeuvres. In leg-yield, the horse is almost straight, except for slight lateral flexion away from the direction of travel.

Lightness: A desirable quality that reflects self-carriage and the horse's self-maintenance of rhythm, straightness and outline. Lightness involves the bringing into action by the rider and the use by the horse of only those muscles necessary for the intended movement. Activity in any other muscle groups can create resistance and thus detract from the lightness.

Long and low: Training the horse to go with its poll extended and lowered and its neck slightly dorsoventrally flexed while attempting to achieve more activity and impulsion. *See also* Hyperflexion (also known as rollkur, deep-and-round and long-deep-and-round).

Longitudinal flexion: A posture under-saddle that results from well-trained basic responses where the neck is lengthened, and the poll is carried at the level of the withers. In correct dressage training, it is the first prerequisite of a rounded outline. The lengthening of the neck suggests that a more correct term would be cervical extension.

Long-reining: A method of training the horse using two reins, each attached to the horse's bit and returning to the handler, who moves behind and/or beside the horse, as if driving it without being attached to any vehicle or load. Long-reining is sometimes used as a prelude to foundation training, retraining or in the training of advanced movements.

Long-term potentiation (LTP): The strengthening (or *potentiation*) of the connection between two nerve cells that lasts for an extended period; it is commonly regarded as the cellular basis of memory.

Loose training: Often used as an alternative to lungeing, long-reining or round-pen for exercise and training. The horse is typically loose schooled in the outer lane of an arena and frequently encounters grid exercises or series of fences for jumping on predetermined distances and stride patterns and so is said to learn independently.

Looseness: A term used in dressage when a horse is relaxed and has well-trained basic responses so that the locomotion of the horse is swinging and elastic.

Lope: The Western version of a very slow canter, this is a smooth, slow gait in which the head is carried low.

Lugging, pulling: A term, mostly used in horse-racing, that refers to a straightness problem where the horse drifts sideways, particularly at the gallop. In doing so, the horse becomes heavy on the rein on the side away from which it is drifting. A horse that habitually lugs does so as a result of incorrect negative reinforcement, because the rider holds the heavy rein tighter as he or she attempts to maintain a straight line; in other words, the horse is failing to respond to the turn cue.

Lunge (also longe): Exercising a horse in circles with the trainer in the middle of the circle using a long lead-rein or rope. Lungeing is used to habituate a horse to the saddle during foundation training, to train obedience, to warm up a horse and to tire a hyper-reactive horse.

Medial: Relating to the median plane or midline of the body; situated towards or nearer to the median plane, as opposed to lateral.

Medium walk/trot/canter: Stride length between that for the working and extended versions of those gaits. For example, in the medium canter, the stride length is between the working canter and extended canter.

Mouthing (US champing): (a) The process of habituating a horse to a bit in its mouth and learning to respond to the stop/slow/step-back and turn signals of the reins. (b) Champing is where the horse gently moves the bit. Mouthing is a response that is sometimes encouraged in bitting a young horse. Use of a bit with 'keys' attached to the mouthpiece facilitates saliva flow and keeps the mouth moist.

Napping, propping: When a horse fails to respond appropriately to the rider's signals, as in refusing to go forward, running sideways, spinning or running backwards. This conflict behaviour could also result in attempts at rearing.

Nasal: Pertaining to the nose. Sometimes used as an orientation term to locate a part of the head that lies more towards the nose than the dorsum.

Natural cues: The body, seat, hands (reins), legs, weight and voice, as used to signal to the horse. Some of these cues are acquired via negative reinforcement (e.g. leg and rein responses), while others are acquired by classical conditioning (e.g. weight and voice cues). The distinction, therefore, is not based on learning theory.

Natural horsemanship: A relatively modern system of horse-training that originated in Western training. It is based on an interpretation of the natural ethogram of the horse. Natural horsemanship focuses on concepts of dominance/submission, respect and leadership, which are currently controversial and may be at odds with learning theory.

Natural outline: Where the horse under-saddle or in-hand carries its head and neck freely without any force from the rider or handler (McLean and McLean, 2008).

Neck rein: To turn or steer a horse by pressure of the rein against the neck.

Negative punishment: The *removal* of a reinforcing stimulus (which makes a particular response less likely in the future).

Negative reinforcement: The *subtraction* of something aversive (such as pressure) to reward the desired response and thus lower the motivational drive (Skinner, 1953).

Non-associative learning: This involves repeated exposures to a single stimulus to cause the horse to become either habituated (i.e. to show a decrease in response) or sensitised (i.e. to show an increase in response).

Obedience: In traditional horsemanship, compliance to the cues. Perhaps a more objective definition is the horse's immediate initiation of the required response to a light cue (McLean, 2003).

Object permanence: The capacity to perceive that an object still exists even after it has been removed/obscured from the perceptual field.

Observational learning: Learning that emerges in an individual after watching another, rather than on the basis of direct experience.

Off the bit: The horse does not have contact or connection to the rider's hands through the reins. This is usually referred to as being above the bit or behind the bit (i.e. there is a lack of at least one of the three prerequisites for on the bit).

On the bit: The self-maintained neck and head position of the horse in correct training, where vertical flexion of the cervical vertebrae and atlanto-occipital joint (also known as poll flexion or roundness) results in the nasal planum being approximately 12 degrees in front of the vertical at walk or 6 degrees in other gaits. This posture is intended to improve the balance of the ridden horse (relocating extra weight to the hindquarters) and its willingness to respond to the signals transmitted by the rider through the reins. There are three precursors to the horse being on the bit. The first is longitudinal flexion, followed by lateral flexion and finally vertical flexion. To most people, 'on the bit' means that the horse travels with its neck arched and nose tucked in. However, a vertical nose does not necessarily mean that the horse is on the bit. On the bit is necessary in horse-training because, as a result of vertical flexion, the centre of gravity shifts posteriorly towards the rider's centre of gravity. There are various forms of false roundness where the horse is forced by the rider's hands or with the use of mechanical devices to flex his cervical vertebrae.

On the forehand: An undesirable form of locomotion that involves the horse carrying an inappropriate proportion of its weight on its forequarter, a posture that runs counter to impulsion, collection and self-carriage. Usually seen in young or poorly schooled horses where the withers appear lower than the croup of the horse during locomotion.

Opening/closing rein: *See* Direct/Indirect rein/turn.

Operant conditioning: Training the horse to respond consistently to signals through positive reinforcement and negative reinforcement (Skinner 1938; McLean, 2003).

Operant contingency: The three part series of events in response learning. It involves a cue, a response and a reinforcement.

Out behind: *See* Trailing hindquarters.

Outline (US shape, frame): An aspect of the horse's posture that refers to the curvature of the vertebral column and so encompasses the degree of flexion of the neck and poll and the associated flexion of the lumbosacral region. According to the ideals of equitation, the nasal planum should be no more than 12 degrees in front of the vertical at the walk and 6 degrees in other gaits and never behind the vertical, because such a departure results in loss of self-carriage and lightness. The back should be soft and relaxed and give the impression of being raised.

Outside: *See* Inside/outside.

Over-bent (broken-neck): Where the horse assumes a posture in which its nasal planum is described as being behind the vertical. Usually caused by faults in negative reinforcement, such as unrelenting pressure from the rider's hands on the bit.

Overface: Undertaking a task during riding or training that is beyond the horse's capacity or experience (where the trainer demands unachievable increments during shaping).

Over-shadowing: The effect of two signals of different intensity being applied together, such that only the most intense will result in a learned response (Hull, 1943).

Over-tracking: Associated with engagement of the hindlimbs to the point where the footfall of the hindlimb reaches forward and overlays or surpasses the print of the ipsilateral forelimb.

Pace: A two-time lateral gait in which the hindleg and the foreleg on the same side move together. Sometimes refers to a gait.

Pig-rooting: A conflict behaviour involving lowering the head and arching the back and with a kick out or bounding of the back legs (a minor form of bucking); it is often a prelude to bucking.

Positive punishment: The *addition* of an aversive stimulus (which makes a particular response less likely in the future).

Positive reinforcement: The *addition* of a pleasant stimulus (a reinforcer) to reward the desired response and thus make this response more likely in the future (Skinner, 1953; McLean, 2003).

Primary (unconditioned) reinforcer: A resource or stimulus that the animal is attracted to and that can serve to strengthen instrumental responding.

Progressive desensitisation: A step-by-step weakening of a fear response to a given stimulus or set of stimuli to the point of extinction (McGreevy, 2004).

Pulling: Reflects the resistance of a horse to bit pressure; this is seen when a horse pulls the reins and shows no deceleration.

Punishment: The presentation of an aversive stimulus that decreases the likelihood of a response or, in the case of negative punishment, the *removal* of a reinforcing stimulus. Punishment is often used incorrectly in horse-training (i.e. when not immediately contingent with the offending response). Incorrect use of punishment can lower an animal's motivation to trial new responses, desensitise the animal to the punishing stimulus and create fearful associations (Mills, 1998).

Purity of the gaits: The regular temporal sequence of the natural footfalls of the gaits of the horse. These are considered fundamental to the sport and practice of dressage (FEI, 2008). When these are not present due to incorrect negative reinforcement or the simultaneous application of go and stop/slow/step-back pressures, hyper-reactive behaviours may emerge and conflict behaviours may develop.

Rapping, touch up: Inappropriate strategy used to sensitise the legs in an attempt to improve jumping performance in the horse; various irritant substances are applied to the anterior aspects of the third metacarpal or cannon of the forelimbs such that the horse will try harder to avoid hitting a fence when jumping.

Rearing: A sudden postural change in a horse so that it stands only on its hindlegs. Rearing is both an innate anti-predator manoeuvre and an intra-specific social behaviour, usually between stallions or colts. Habitual rearing in horses usually accompanies other conflict behaviours.

Refusal: A conflict behaviour that is typically associated with the approach to jumping an obstacle during which the horse suddenly stops. A precursor to or a form of napping.

Rein back: A series of steps backwards with the legs in diagonal pairs. It is initially trained by the decelerating effects of the reins and later cued via classical conditioning by leg position of the rider.

Reinforcement schedule: The frequency of the reinforcers used in training the horse by the handler. The schedule may be continuous, intermittent or declining.

Reinforcement: The process in which a reinforcer follows a particular behaviour so that the frequency (or probability) of that behaviour increases (Wolpe, 1958; McGreevy, 2004).

Reinforcer: An environmental change that increases the likelihood that an animal will make a particular response, i.e. the *addition* of a reward (positive reinforcer), or *removal* of an aversive stimulus (negative reinforcer).

Resistance: *See* Conflict behaviour, Evasions and resistances.

Respect: A term used in general horsemanship and natural horsemanship that emphasises the significance and relevance of the hierarchy in horse–human interactions. The notion of respect may imply subjective mental states that the horse may not possess. Furthermore, in training and retraining, the concept of respect may encourage remedies for behaviour problems that are unrelated to the original behaviour problem. Thus, from the viewpoint of learning the-

ory, such a concept may be inappropriate and have negative welfare implications.

Response: A reaction to a stimulus.

Rhythm: The beat of the legs within a particular gait. In ideal equitation, rhythm is trained to be self-maintained.

Rollkur: *See* (Long or Low) Deep and round.

Round: Synonymous with on the bit.

Round-pen (round-yard) training: The practice of causing a horse to flee forward in a round-yard until it offers a desirable response (such as slowing), at which point the sending forward is instantly terminated. This can be interpreted as negative reinforcement. Critics of this technique question the accepted interpretation of the responses of the horse undergoing this process and, in particular, the allowance of fearful behaviour because of its obvious association with humans and the high risk of spontaneous recovery.

Running (away): A hyper-reactive state in the horse characterised by acceleration and, usually, heaviness in the reins. The horse is exhibiting conflict behaviour and attempting to flee the aversive situation. Such states are usually the result of incorrect negative reinforcement and can be associated with conflict behaviour. *See* Rushing.

Rushing: Seen in a horse that is not under the stimulus control of the cues to slow, usually in relation to approaching a jumping obstacle. Often anthropomorphically interpreted as 'keenness'.

Sagittal: A vertical plane passing through the standing body from front to back. The mid-sagittal or median plane splits the body into left and right halves.

School: (a) An enclosed area, either covered or open, in which a horse may be trained or exercised. (b) To train a horse for whatever purpose it may be required.

Scope: The range of both the stride patterns associated with the gaits and the ability to spring or jump.

Secondary reinforcement: Making a response more likely in the future by using a stimulus that has acquired reinforcing properties on the basis of its relationship to a primary (unconditioned) reinforcer.

Self-carriage: The way in which an educated horse deports itself. Because of the obtrusive and aversive potential of rein and leg pressures, it is important that the horse travels in-hand and under-saddle free of any constant rein or leg pressure for fear of habituation and/or conflict behaviour. Self-carriage refers to the self-maintenance of rhythm, tempo, direction, straightness and outline.

Shape, frame (US): See Outline.

Shaping: The successive approximation of a behaviour towards a targeted desirable behaviour through the consecutive training of one single quality of a response followed by the next. In horse-training, a shaping program is known as a training scale. Not paying due attention to shaping in horse-training has been associated with conflict behaviours (Morgan, 1974; McLean, 2003).

Shying: The sudden hyper-reactive sideways leaping of the horse either from an aversive object it encounters or as an expression of conflict behaviour that has arisen due to unresolved problems in negative reinforcement (e.g. when the contact is too strong). A shy begins with the horse turning away its forequarters followed by an acceleration response. Shying is frequently associated with other conflict behaviours and may be followed by bucking.

Signal: See Cue.

Slow gait: One of the gaits of the five-gaited breeds characterised by a prancing action in which each foot in turn is raised and then held momentarily in mid-air before descending.

Soft condition: Easily fatigued or unfit.

Soft mouth: Sensitive mouth, responsive to bit pressure.

Spinning: A sudden change in direction, akin to shying in origin and expression; it has associations with conflict behaviour.

Spooky: Shys or baulks readily/frequently.

Star-gazer: A horse that moves in-hand or under-saddle in an awkward position with its head elevated, as if looking upwards.

Step: The single complete movement of raising one foot and putting it down in another spot, as in walking, used in equitation parlance to describe the nature of the movement in an individual horse and often erroneously based on the observation of the forelimbs only.

Step-back: See Stop/slow/step-back.

Stereotypy: A repeated, relatively invariant sequence of movements that has no function obvious to the observer. A number of stereotypic behaviours seen in horses are erroneously referred to as stable vices.

Stimulus: See Cue.

Stimulus control: The process by which a response becomes consistently elicited by a signal or cue.

Stimulus generalisation: The reinforcement of a response in the presence of more than one stimulus.

Stop/slow/step-back: The decelerating response in the trained horse that results in it ceasing or decreasing its forward movement in-hand and under-saddle. The stop response is most commonly trained by negative reinforcement, using the bit in the horse's mouth, stimulated by the reins in the rider's hands. Classical conditioning converts the stop response to light cues and then to the bracing of the seat. Decelerating involves activation and emphasis of different musculature from that involved in forward motion. These muscles are isolated by the step-back response. Therefore, it is not surprising that training the step-back trains the stop response. Slowing the horse can occur through shortening the stride or slowing the activity or tempo of the legs.

Straightness: A fundamentally desirable trait in equitation such that the hindlegs move into the line of the foretracks on lines and circles and the longitudinal axis of the vertebral column is straight. Straightness is necessary in order to achieve maximal biomechanical and motor efficiency in the horse and consequently considered a tenet of basic training. When horses are not straight, they tend to drift towards the convex side. Thus, crookedness may be seen as a symptom; the deeper problem is that the horse is not following the rider's (or handler's) intended line.

Stress (acute and chronic): Stress, in its acute form, is a short-term dysfunction of the signal–response relationship presenting variously as raised tension levels, agonistic behaviours, redirected aggression and displacement activities. Chronic stress manifests as raised corticosteroid levels, physiological disturbances, gastric pathology, repetition and ritualisation of original conflict behaviours, redirected, ambivalent and displacement behaviours, development of stereotypies and injurious behaviours, such as self-mutilation and increased aggression (Wiepkema, 1987; Moberg and Mench, 2000).

Stress colic: Abdominal pain thought to be associated with inability to cope with aversive conditions (Hungerford, 1975).

Stride: (a) The set of changes occurring during a single complete locomotory cycle that includes the stance phase and the swing phase of a limb, from the one landing of a particular foot to the next. (b) Used in jumping to describe a rider's appreciation of the number of whole steps a horse takes between obstacles. (c) Medium walk/trot/canter: a descriptive term for strides that are longer than at working paces, but not as long as extended paces. Medium strides are therefore part of the development of longer strides in equitation. For the average horse in medium walk and trot, the hindtracks should land approximately 10–20 cm in front of the foretracks, whereas in medium canter the hindtracks land approximately 1.5 m in front of the foretracks.

Stubborn: A horse that appears unwilling to respond to cues, probably due to lack of motivation or habituation to signals as a result of incorrect negative reinforcement.

Submission: *See* Dominance/submission.

Swing, swinging the hindquarters: The lumbar musculature is described as swinging during collected movements. The hindquarters may move laterally and be said to swing out during lateral movements. Swinging out is also a term used to describe hindquarters that move laterally but not under stimulus control. This may indicate that the forelegs are not under the stimulus control of the reins. Thus, the forequarters also show deviations of line (McLean and McLean, 2008).

Switch off, tune out: A lack of response to any signal (altered attention and motivation levels) provided by a rider or handler when

a horse becomes hyper-reactive. This may be an expression of learned helplessness. Switching off and becoming 'dead to the cues' is likely to be accompanied by raised corticosteroid concentrations and may be partly caused by state-dependent learning (i.e. learning that takes place and is only retained when the internal milieu of the horse is in the particular state at the time of learning). When this state shifts, memory and learning may be reduced or absent. There are training implications associated with this concept if horses are trained only when they are calm.

Tail swishing: Lateral and dorsoventral movements of the tail symptomatic of conflict behaviour in hyper-reactive horses. In the absence of other irritants, tail swishing can be a clue to incorrect negative reinforcement of the go response or indicate a dislike of too-tight reins and unrelenting leg/spur pressure.

Teeth grinding: In the absence of dental or other health disorders, grinding the teeth is a response to unresolved stressors encountered during training, or a product of general management. It may be associated with incorrect negative reinforcement of the stop/slow/step-back response.

Tempo: The timing or rhythm of the horse's strides.

Temporal: (a) Anatomical term pertaining to the temple region of the head. The temporal lobe of the brain is located beneath the temple. (b) Also relating to time; lasting or existing only for a time; passing, temporary. From the Latin *tempus*, which means the temple of the head (and time).

Tension: In equitation, hyper-reactivity and, presumably, heightened HPA axis activity. Tense horses are frequently hollow and show various behavioural indicators of stress.

Tilting nose: A posture adopted by some horses during locomotion under-saddle such that the nose tilts to one side. It results from incorrect negative reinforcement, principally during the training of the turn response (no release for the correct response or pressuring for the turn when the inside leg is on the ground and unable to respond) but also in the training of the stop response (no release and contact too tight).

Tonic immobility, aka freezing: An aroused state in which the horse remains immobile, sometimes in spite of stimulation from the rider.

Tracking up: During locomotion, the horse's hindhooves land in the prints left by the ipsilateral forefeet.

Trailing hindquarters: In equitation, the action of the hindlegs such that, at the moment of thrust, the hindhooves are not underneath the hocks but behind them. The horse is said to be out behind and is usually also hollow. This prevents the horse from attaining impulsion and collection.

Training scale: A progressive order of training particular qualities of responses through the process of shaping. Shaping programs merit further research.

Transition: The change from one gait type to another, or from one stride length to another. A transition can be between gaits, within a gait or from one tempo to another as well as into and out of the halt.

Transverse: A horizontal plane passing through the standing body parallel to the ground.

Tune out: *See* Switch off.

Turn: A change in the line of locomotion by the horse. The turn is initiated by the forequarters with the hindfeet following the foretracks. Turning occurs through shifting the inside leg slightly to the side, decelerating it on contact with the ground, and accelerating the opposite foreleg in contact with the ground. The turn is trained by negative reinforcement using the stimulus of the single rein, which classically conditions to the light rein cue and then to cues of associated changes of the rider's position at the initiation of the turn. The turn cue should be applied when the turning leg is beginning to go forward.

Under-saddle: The situations in which horses are be ridden, rather than led or driven.

Under-tracking, stepping short: During locomotion, the horse's hindhooves land on the ground in front of the prints left by the ipsilateral forefeet.

Unlevel/uneven: A euphemism for abnormal action caused by either clinical lameness or a physical abnormality that changes the action of the horse.

Ventral: Pertaining to the underside of the horse, as opposed to dorsal.

Working trot/canter: A term that refers to the normal stride length within the gaits. In the working trot, the stride length is where the hindfeet land into the foretracks.

References

Adams, O.R. 1979. *Lameness in Horses*, 3rd edn. Lea & Febiger Publishing, Philadelphia.

AIHW National Injury Surveillance Unit. 2005. Mortality Data. Bulletin 24, Flinders University, http://www.nisu.flinders.edu.au/pubs/bulletin24/bulletin24-Mortalit.html. Accessed 9 December 2005.

Albert A., Bulcroft, K. 1988. Pets, families, and the life course. *Journal of Marriage and the Family*, 2, 543–552.

Albright, J.L., Arave, C.W. 1997. *The Behaviour of Cattle*. CABI Publishing, Wallingford, UK.

Appleby, M.C. 1997. Life in a variable world: behaviour, welfare and environmental design. *Applied Animal Behaviour Science*, 54(1), 1–19.

Archer, J. 1973. Tests for emotionality in rats and mice: a review. *Animal Behaviour*, 21, 205–235.

Archer, M. 1971. Preliminary studies on the palatability of grasses, legumes and herbs to horses. *Veterinary Record*, 89, 236.

Archer, J. 1997. Why do people love their pets? *Evolution and Human Behaviour*, 18, 237–259.

Argue, C.K. 1994. The kinematics of piaffe, passage and collected trot of dressage horses. MS Thesis, University of Saskatchewan, Saskatoon, Canada.

Argue, C.K., Clayton, H.M. 1993a. A preliminary study of transitions between the walk and trot in dressage horses. *Acta Anatomica*, 146, 179–182.

Argue, C.K., Clayton, H.M. 1993b. A study of transitions between the trot and canter in dressage horses. *Journal of Equine Veterinary Science*, 13, 171–174.

Back, W. 2001. Intra-limb co-ordination: the forelimb and the hindlimb. In: *Equine Locomotion*, pp. 95–153. Eds: W. Back and H.M. Clayton. W.B. Saunders, Edinburgh, UK.

Back, W., Clayton, H.M. 2001. *Equine Locomotion*. W.B. Saunders, Edinburgh, UK.

Baer, K.L., Potter, G.D., Friend, T.H., Beaver, B.V. 1983. Observation effects on learning in horses. *Applied Animal Ethology*, 11, 123–129.

Bagshaw, C.S., Ralston, S.L., Fisher, H. 1994. Behavioral and physiological effect of orally administered tryptophan on horses subjected to acute isolation stress. *Applied Animal Behaviour Science*, 40(1), 1–12.

Bailey, C.H., Chen, M. 1983. Morphological basis of long-term habituation and sensitization in Aplysia. *Science*, 220, 91–93.

Baker, A.E.M., Crawford, B.H. 1986. Observational learning in horses. *Applied Animal Behaviour Science*, 15, 7–13.

Ball, C., Ball, J., Kirkpatrick, A., Mulloy, R. 2007. Equestrian injuries: incidence, injury patterns, and risk factors for 10 years of major traumatic injuries. *The American Journal of Surgery*, 193(5), 636–640.

Barrey, E. 2001. Inter-limb Coordination. In: *Equine Locomotion*, p. 78. Eds: W. Back and H.M. Clayton. W.B. Saunders, Edinburgh, UK.

Baum, M. 1970. Extinction of avoidance responding through response prevention (flooding). *Psychological Bulletin*, 74, 276–284.

Beck, L., Madresh, E.A. 2008. Romantic partners and four-legged friends: an extension of attachment theory to relationships with pets. *Anthrozoös*, 21(1), 43–56.

Bekoff, M. 1995. Cognitive ethology, vigilance, information gathering, and representation: Who might know what and why? *Behavioural Processes*, 35, 225–237.

Bell, R.A., Nielsen, B.D., Waite, K., Rosenstein, D., Orth, M. 2001. Daily access to pasture turnout prevents loss of minerals in the third metacarpus of Arabian weanlings. *Journal of Animal Science*, 79(5), 1142–1150.

Bermond, B. 1997. The myth of animal suffering. In: *Animal Consciousness and Animal Ethics – Perspectives from the Netherlands*, pp. 125–143. Eds: M. Dol, S. Kasanmoentalib, S. Lijmbach, E. Rivas and R. Van Den Bos.

Animals in Philosophy and Science Series. Van Gorcum and Co., Assen, The Netherlands.

BHA 2008. Use of the whip in horseracing. British Horseracing Authority, London.

BHA 2009. Disciplinary: whip use. British Horseracing Authority, London. http://www.britishhorseracing.com/inside_horseracing/about/whatwedo/disciplinary/whipuse.asp. Accessed 18 July 2009.

Blackshaw, J.K., Kirk, D., Creiger, S.E. 1983. A different approach to horse handling, based on the Jeffrey method. *International Journal for the Study of Animal Problems*, 4(2), 117–123.

Blecha, F. 2000. Immune system in response to stress. In: *The Biology of Animal Stress. Basic Principles and Implications for Animal Welfare*, pp. 111–122. Eds: G.P. Moberg and J.A. Mench. CABI Publishing, Wallingford, UK.

Boissy, A. 1995. Fear and fearfulness in animals. *Quarterly Review of Biology*, 70(2), 165–191.

Boissy, A. 1998. Fear and fearfulness in determining behavior. In: *Genetics and the Behaviour of Domestic Animals*, pp. 67–111. Ed: T. Grandin. Academic Press, San Diego, USA.

Boyd, L., Bandi, N. 2002. Reintroduction of Takhi, *Equus ferus przewalskii*, to Hustai National Park, Mongolia: time budget and synchrony of activity pre- and post-release. *Applied Animal Behaviour Science*, 78(2–4), 87–102.

Brandt, K. 2004. A language of their own: an interactionist approach to horse–human communication. *Society and Animals*, 12(4), 299–316.

Breland, K., Breland, M. 1962. The misbehavior of organisms. *American Psychologist*, 16, 681–684.

Brown, D. 1984. Personality and gender influences in human relationships with horses and dogs. In: *The Pet Connection: Its Influence on Our Health and Quality of Life*, pp. 216–223. Eds: R.K. Anderson, B.L. Hart and L.A. Hart. Center to Study Human–Animal Relationships and Environments, University of Minnesota, Minneapolis, USA.

Buckley, P. 2007. Health and performance of Pony Club horses in Australia. PhD thesis. CSU, Wagga Wagga, NSW.

Cabib, S. 2006. The neurobiology of stereotypy II: the role of stress. In: *Stereotypic Animal Behaviour: Fundamentals and Applications to Welfare*, 2nd edn., pp. 227–255. Eds: G. Mason and J. Rushen. CABI Publishing, Wallingford, UK.

Caporael, L.R. 1986. Anthropomorphism and mechanomorphism: two faces of the human machine. *Computers in Human Behavior*, 2, 215–234.

Castellucci, V.F., Blumenfeld, H., Goelet, P., Kandel, E.R. 1989. Inhibitor of protein synthesis blocks long-term behavioral sensitization in the isolated gill-withdrawal reflex of Aplysia. *Journal of Neurobiology*, 20, 1–9.

Chamove, A.S., Crawley-Hartrick, O.J.E., Stafford, K.J. 2002. Horse reactions to human attitudes and behavior. *Anthrozoös*, 15, 323–331.

Chance, P. 1993. *Learning and Behaviour*. Brooks and Cole, Belmont, USA.

Chaya, L., Cowan, E., McGuire, B. 2006. A note on the relationship between time spent in turnout and behaviour during turnout in horses (*Equus caballus*). *Applied Animal Behaviour Science*, 98, 155–160.

Christensen, J.W. 2007. Fear in horses: social influence, generalisation and reactions to predator odour. PhD thesis, Faculties of Agriculture and Life Sciences, University of Copenhagen.

Christensen, J.W., Ladewig, J., Søndergaard, E., Malmkvist, J. 2002. Effects of individual versus group stabling on behaviour in domestic stallions. *Applied Animal Behaviour Science*, 75, 233–248.

Christensen, J.W., Rundgren, M., Olsson, K. 2006. Training methods for horses: habituation to a frightening stimulus. *Equine Veterinary Journal*, 38, 439–443.

Clarke, J., Nicol, C.J., Jones, R., McGreevy, P.D. 1996. Effects of observational learning on food selection in horses. *Applied Animal Behaviour Science*, 50, 177–184.

Clayton, H.M. 1989. Terminology for the description of equine jumping kinematics. *Journal of Equine Veterinary Science*, 9, 341–348.

Clayton, H.M. 1997. Classification of collected trot, passage and piaffe using stance phase temporal variables. *Equine Veterinary Journal Supplement*, 23, 54–57.

Clayton, H.M. 2004. The mysteries of self-carriage. *USDF Connection*, September, 14–17.

Clayton, H.M. 2005. Bitting: the inside story. *USDF Connection*, December, 28–32.

Clayton, H.M., Lanovaz, J.L., Schamhardt, H.C., van Wessum R. 1999. The effects of a rider's mass on ground reaction forces and fetlock kinematics at the trot. *Equine Veterinary Journal Supplement*, 30, 218–221.

Clayton, H.M., Singleton, W.H., Lanovaz, J.L., Cloud, G.L. 2003. Measurement of rein tension during horseback riding using strain-gauge transducers. *Experimental Techniques*, 27, 34–36.

Cooper, J., McGreevy, P. 2002. Stereotypic behaviour in the stabled horse: causes, effects and prevention without compromising horse welfare. In: *The Welfare of Horses*, pp. 99–124. Ed: N. Waran. Kluwer Academic Publishers, Dordrecht, The Netherlands.

Cooper, J.J., McDonald, L., Mills, D.S. 2000. The effect of increasing visual horizons on stereotypic weaving: implications for the social housing of stabled horses. *Applied Animal Behaviour Science*, 69(1), 67–83.

Cothran, E.G., MacCluer, J.W., Weitkamp, L.R., Bailey, E. 1987. Genetic differentiation associated with gait within American Standardbred horses. *Animal Genetics*, 18, 285–296.

Cregier, S. 1990. *Equine Behaviour* – The newsletter of the Equine Behaviour Study Circle. Issue 26. UK.

Creighton, E. 2007. Equine learning behaviour: limits of ability and ability limits of trainers. *Behavioural Processes*, 76, 43–44.

Darwin, C. 1872. *The Expression of Emotions in Man and Animals*. Republished 2002. Oxford University Press, New York.

Davies, H.M.S. 1996. The effects of different exercise conditions on metacarpal bone strains in Thoroughbred racehorses. *Pferdeheilkunde*, 12(4), 666–670.

de Cartier d'Yves, A., Ödberg, F.O. 2005. A preliminary study on the relation between subjectively assessing dressage performances and objective welfare parameters. In: Proceedings of the 1st International Equitation Science Symposium, Broadford, Victoria. Eds: P. McGreevy, A. McLean, N. Waran, D. Goodwin, A. and Warren-Smith. Post-Graduate Foundation in Veterinary Science, Sydney, pp. 89–110.

de Graaf-Roelfsema, E. 2007. Endocrinological and behavioural adaptations to experimentally induced physical stress in horses. PhD thesis, Faculty of Veterinary Medicine, Utrecht University, The Netherlands.

de la Guérinière, F.R. 1992. *Ecole de Cavalerie*. Xenophon Press, Ohio, USA. First imprinted 1733. J. Collombat, Paris.

Deacon, T.W. 1990. Fallacies of progression in theories of brain-size evolution. *International Journal of Primatology*, 11, 193–236.

Decarpentry, General, 1949. *Academic Equitation*. (Translated by N. Bartle, 1971) J.A. Allen, London.

Dennett, D.C. 1996. *Kinds of Minds*, p.13. Orion Books Ltd., London.

Denoix, J.-M. 2006. Functional anatomy and diagnostic imaging of the cervical spine. In: Report of the FEI Veterinary and Dressage Committee's Workshop. The use of over-bending ('Rollkur') in FEI Competition, 31 January, during the FEI Veterinary Committee meeting at the Olympic Museum, Lausanne.

Deuel, N.R., Lawrence, L.M. 1987. Effects of urging by the rider on equine gallop stride limb contacts. In: Proceedings of the Equine Nutrition and Physiology Symposium, 10, 487–494.

Deuel, N.R., Park, J-J. 1990. The gait patterns of Olympic dressage horses. *International Journal of Sport Biomechanics*, 6, 198–226.

Devenport, J.A., Patterson, M.R., Devenport, L.D. 2005. Dynamic averaging and foraging decisions in horses (*Equus caballus*). *Journal of Comparative Psychology*, 119(3), 352–358.

Dickinson, A. 1980. *Contemporary Animal Learning*. Cambridge University Press, Cambridge.

Diehl, K.D., Egan, B., Tozer, P. 2002. Intensive, early handling of neonatal foals: mare–foal interactions. In: Proceedings of the Havermeyer Foundation Horse Behavior and Welfare Workshop, Holar, Iceland, pp. 23–26.

Dougherty, D.M., Lewis, P. 1991. Stimulus-generalization, discrimination-learning, and peak shift in horses. *Journal of the Experimental Analysis of Behavior*, 56, 97–104.

Drevemo, S., Fredricson, I., Hjerten, G., McMiken, D. 1987. Early development of gait asymmetries in trotting Standardbred colts. *Equine Veterinary Journal*, 19, 189–191.

Dudink, S., Simonse, H., Marks, I., de Jonge, F.H., Spruijt, B.M. 2006. Announcing the arrival of enrichment increases play behavior and reduces weaning-stress-induced behaviors of piglets directly after weaning. *Applied Animal Behaviour Science*, 101, 86–101.

Duvall-Antonacopoulos, N.M., Pychyl, T.A. 2008. An examination of the relations between social support, anthropomorphism and stress among dog owners. *Anthrozoös*, 21(2), 139–142.

EFA. 2003. Endurance horse fatalities at the 2002 World Equestrian Games. www.efanational.com/default.asp?id=359. Accessed 11 January 2008.

Ehrenhofer, M.C.A., Deeg, C.A., Reese, S., Liebich, H-G., Stangassinger, M., Kaspers, B. 2002. Normal structure and age-related changes of the equine retina. *Veterinary Ophthalmology*, 5, 39–47.

Endenburg N. 1999. Perceptions and attitudes toward horses in European societies. The role of the horse in Europe. *Equine Veterinary Journal Supplement*, 28, 38–41.

Epley, N., Waytz, A., Cacioppo, J.T. 2007. On seeing human: a three-factor theory of anthropomorphism. *Psychological Review*, 114(4), 864–886.

Estes, R.D. 1991. *The Behavior Guide to African Mammals: Including Hoofed Mammals, Carnivores, Primates*. Wake Forest Studium Book, University of California Press, Berkeley and Los Angeles, California.

Evans, D., Jeffcott, L., Knight, P. 2006. Performance-related problems and exercise physiology. In: *The Equine Manual*, Vol. 2, pp. 1059–1104. Eds: A.J. Higgins and J.R. Snyder. W.B. Saunders, London.

Evans, K.E., McGreevy, P.D. 2005. Breed differences in equine retinae. In: Proceedings of the 1st International Equitation Science Symposium, Broadford, Victoria. Eds: P. McGreevy, A. McLean, N. Waran, D. Goodwin and A. Warren-Smith. Post-Graduate Foundation in Veterinary Science, Sydney, pp. 56–66.

Evans, K.E., McGreevy, P.D. 2006. The distribution of ganglion cells in the equine retina and its relationship to skull morphology. *Anatomia, Histologia, Embryologia*, 35, 1–6.

Ewers, J.C. 1955. The horse in Blackfoot Indian culture – with comparative material from other western tribes. Bureau of American Ethnology, Smithsonian

Institution, Bulletin 159, 62. Government Printing Office, Washington, DC.

Faber, M., Johnston, C., Schamhardt, H., van Weeren, R., Roepstorff, L., Barneveld, A. 2001a. Basic three-dimensional kinematics of the vertebral column of horses trotting on a treadmill. *American Journal of Veterinary Research*, 62(5), 757–764.

Faber, M., Johnston, C., Schamhardt, H.C., van Weeren, P.R., Roepstorff, L., Barneveld, A. 2001b. Three-dimensional kinematics of equine spine during canter. *Equine Veterinary Journal Supplement*, 33, 145–149.

Faber, M., Schamhardt, H.C., van Weeren, P.R. 1999. Determination of 3D spinal kinematics without defining a local vertebral coordinate system. *Journal of Biomechanics*, 32, 1355–1358.

Faber, M., Schamhardt, H.C., van Weeren, P.R., Johnston, C., Roepstorff, L., Barneveld, A. 2000. Basic three-dimensional kinematics of the vertebral column of horses walking on a treadmill. *American Journal Veterinary Research*, 61, 399–406.

Falewee, C., Gaultier, E., Lafont, C., Bougrat, L., Pageat, P. 2006. Effect of a synthetic equine maternal pheromone during a controlled fear-eliciting situation. *Applied Animal Behaviour Science*, 101, 144–153.

FAO. 2003. FAO Statistical Database Website. Food and Agriculture Organisation, Rome, Italy (FAOSTATS: http://apps.fao.org).

Farley, C.T., Taylor, C.R. 1991. A mechanical trigger for the trot–gallop transition in horses. *Science*, 253, 306–308.

Faverot de Kerbrech, F. 1891. The methodical training of the saddle horse after the last method of Baucher, recounted by one of his pupils. Jean-Michel Place, Paris.

Fédération Equestre International. 2006. Report of the FEI Veterinary and Dressage Committee's Workshop. The use of over-bending ('Rollkur') in FEI Competition, 31 January, during the FEI Veterinary Committee meeting at the Olympic Museum, Lausanne, Switzerland.

Fédération Equestre Internationale. 2007. Abuse of horses. In: *General Regulations*, 22nd edn. Lausanne, Switzerland.

Fédération Equestre Internationale, 2008. *Rules for Dressage Events*, 22nd edn. Lausanne, Switzerland.

Feh, C., de Mazières, J. 1993. Grooming at a preferred site reduces heart rate in horses. *Animal Behaviour*, 46, 1191–1194.

Fielding, D. 1991. The number and distribution of equines in the world. In *Donkeys, Mules and Horses in Tropical Agricultural Development*, pp. 62–66. Eds: D. Fielding and R.A. Pearson. Centre for Tropical Veterinary Medicine, University of Edinburgh, UK.

Fisher, J.A. 1990. The myth of anthropomorphism. In: *Interpretation and Explanation in the Study of Animal Behavior*. Eds: M. Bekoff and D. Jamieson, Vol. I, Interpretation, Intentionality, and Communication. Westview Press, Boulder, Colorado, USA.

Fiske, J.C., Potter, G.D. 1979. Discrimination reversal learning in yearling horses. *Journal of Animal Science*, 49, 583–588.

Flannery, B. 1997. Relational discrimination learning in horses. *Applied Animal Behaviour Science*, 54, 267–280.

Forkman, B., Boissy, A., Meunier-Salaün, M.-C., Canali, E., Jones, R.B. 2007. A critical review of fear tests used on cattle, pigs, sheep, poultry and horses. *Physiology & Behaviour*, 92, 340–374.

Francis-Smith, K., Wood-Gush, D.G.M. 1997. Coprophagia as seen in Thoroughbred foals. *Equine Veterinary Journal*, 9, 155–157.

Fraser, A.F. 1992. *The Behaviour of the Horse*. CABI Publishing, Wallingford, UK.

Fredricson, I., Dalin, G., Drevemo, S., Hjerten, G., Nilsson, G., Alm, L.O. 1975. Ergonomic aspects of poor racetrack design. *Equine Veterinary Journal*, 7, 63–65.

Freire, R., Clegg, H.A., Buckley, P., Friend, M.A., McGreevy, P.D. 2009. The effects of two different amounts of dietary grain on the digestibility of the diet and behaviour of intensively managed horses. *Applied Animal Behaviour Science*, 117(1–2), 69–73.

Freud, S. 1930. *Civilization and Its Discontents*. Republished 1989. Norton, New York.

Fukuzawa, M., Mills, D.S., Cooper, J.J. 2005. The effect of emotional content of verbal commands on the response of dogs. In: Proceedings of the 39th International Congress of the ISAE, ISAE, Japan. Eds: R. Kusunose and S. Sato, p. 45.

Gabriel, M. 1993. Discriminative avoidance learning: a model system. In: *Neurobiology of Cingulate Cortex and Limbic Thalamus*, pp. 478–523. Eds: M. Gabriel and B. Vogt. Birkhauser, Toronto.

Gardyn, R. 2002. Animal magnetism. *American demographics*, 24, 30–37.

Garner, J.P., Mason, G.J. 2002. Evidence for a relationship between cage stereotypies and behavioural disinhibition in laboratory rodents. *Behavioural Brain Research*, 136(1), 83–92.

Gehrke, E. 2007. Dr. Ellen Kaye Gehrke's Research Finding: Horse May be Key to Non-invasive Stress Detection. Alliant International University. http://www.alliant.edu. Accessed 9 December 2007.

German National Equestrian Federation. 1992. *The German Driving and Riding System: Book 2*. Kenilworth, UK.

German National Equestrian Federation. 1997. *The Principles of Riding – The Official Instruction Handbook of the German National Equestrian Federation*. Kenilworth, UK.

Gieling, E., Cox, M., van Dierendonck, M.C. 2007. Group housing with automatic feeding systems: implications for behavior and horse welfare. In: Proceedings of the 3rd International Equitation Science Symposium, Michigan. Eds: D. Goodwin, C. Heleski, P. McGreevy, A. McLean, H. Randle, C. Skelly, M. van Dierendonck and N. Waran. MSU, Michigan, USA, p. 16.

Gill, E.L. 1988. Factors affecting body condition in New Forest ponies. PhD Thesis, Department of Biology, University of Southampton.

Goodwin, D. 1999. The importance of ethology in understanding the behaviour of the horse. *Equine Veterinary Journal Supplement*, 28, 15–19.

Goodwin, D. 2002. Horse behaviour: evolution, domestication and feralisation. In: *The Welfare of Horses*, pp. 1–18. Ed: N. Waran. Kluwer Academic Publishers, The Netherlands.

Goodwin, D. 2007. Equine learning behaviour: what we know, what we don't and future research priorities. *Behavioural Processes*, 76(1), 17–19.

Goodwin, D., Bradshaw, J.W.S., Wickens, S.M. 1997. Paedomorphosis affects visual signals of domestic dogs. *Animal Behaviour*, 53, 297–304.

Goodwin, D., Davidson, H.P.B., Harris, P. 2002. Foraging enrichment for stabled horses: effects on behaviour and selection. *Equine Veterinary Journal*, 34(7), 686–691.

Goodwin, D., Davidson H.P.B., Harris, P. 2005. Sensory varieties in concentrate diets for stabled horses: effects on behaviour and selection. *Applied Animal Behaviour Science*, 90, 337–349.

Goodwin, D., Hughes, C.F. 2005. Equine play behaviour. In: *The Domestic Horse: The Evolution, Development and Management of Its Behaviour*, pp. 150–157. Eds: D. Mills and S. McDonnell. Cambridge University Press, Cambridge.

Goodwin, D., Levine, M., McGreevy, P.D. 2008. Preliminary investigation of morphological differences between ten breeds of horses suggests selection for Paedomorphosis. *Journal of Applied Animal Welfare Science*, 11, 204–212.

Gramsbergen, A. 2001. The neurobiology of locomotor development. In: *Equine Locomotion*, p. 37. Eds: W. Back and H.M. Clayton. W.B. Saunders, Edinburgh, UK.

Grandin, T. 1978. Observations of the spatial relationships between people and cattle during handling. *Proceedings, Western Section, American Society of Animal Science*, 29, 76–79.

Grandin, T. 1980. Observations of cattle behaviour applied to the design of cattle-handling facilities. *Applied Animal Ethology*, 6, 19–31.

Grandin, T. 2007. The Use of the Wheat Pressure Box on Horses (Equine Restraint System). http://www.grandin.com/behaviour/tips/equine.restraint.html. Accessed 18 September 2007.

Gray, J.A. 1987. *The Psychology of Fear and Stress*, 2nd edn. Cambridge University Press, Cambridge.

Greenebaum, J. 2004. It's a dog's life: elevating status from pet to 'fur baby' at yappy hour. *Society and Animals*, 12, 117–137.

Griffin, D.R. 1992. *Animal Minds*, pp. 24, 25, 53. The University of Chicago Press, Chicago.

Grzimek, B. 1952. Versuche uber das Farbsehen von Pflanzenessern. *Z. Tierpsychol.* 9, 23–39.

Haag, E.L., Rudman, R., Houpt, K.A. 1980. Avoidance, maze learning and social dominance in ponies. *Journal of Animal Science*, 50(2), 329–335.

Hahn, C. 2004. Behavior and the brain. In: *Equine Behaviour – A Guide for Veterinarians and Equine Scientists*, pp. 55–84. Ed: P.D. McGreevy. W.B. Saunders, Edinburgh, UK.

Hall, C.A. 2007. The impact of visual perception on equine learning. *Behavioural Processes*, 76, 29–33.

Hall, C.A., Cassaday, H.J., Derrington, A.M. 2003. The effect of stimulus height on visual discrimination in horses. *Journal of Animal Science*, 81, 1715–1720.

Hall, C.A., Cassaday, H.J., Vincent, C.J., Derrington, A.M. 2005. The selection of coloured stimuli by the horse. In: BSAS Conference (September 20–21): Applying Equine Science, Research into Business, Royal Agricultural College, Cirencester, UK, p. 1.

Hall, C.A., Goodwin, D., Heleski, C., Randle, H., Waran, N. 2007. Is there evidence of 'Learned Helplessness' in horses? In: Proceedings of the 3rd International Equitation Science Symposium, Michigan. Eds: D. Goodwin, C. Heleski, P. McGreevy, A. McLean, H. Randle, C. Skelly, M. van Dierendonck and N. Waran. MSU, Michigan, USA, p. 8.

Hamra, J.G., Kamerling, S.G., Wolfsheimer, K.J., Bagwell, C.A. 1993. Diurnal variation in plasma ir-beta-endorphin levels and experimental pain thresholds in the horse. *Life Sciences*, 53, 121–129.

Hanggi, E.B. 1999. Categorization learning in horses (*Equus caballus*). *Journal of Comparative Psychology*, 113, 243–252.

Hanggi, E.B. 2003. Discrimination learning based on relative size concepts in horses (*Equus caballus*). *Applied Animal Behaviour Science*, 83, 201–213.

Hannum, R.D., Rosellini, R.A., Seligman, M.E.P. 1976. Learned helplessness in the rat: retention and immunization. *Developmental Psychobiology*, 12 449–454.

Harman, A.M., Moore, S., Hoskins, R., Keller, P. 1999. Horse vision and the explanation of visual behaviour originally explained by the 'ramp retina'. *Equine Veterinary Journal*, 31(5), 384–390.

Hausberger, M., Bruderer, U., Le Scolan, N., Pierre, J.S. 2004. Interplay between environmental and genetic factors in temperament/personality traits in horses (*Equus caballus*). *Journal of Comparative Psychology*, 118(4), 434–446.

Hausberger, M., Muller, C., Gautier, E., Jego, P. 2007a. Lower learning abilities in stereotypic horses. *Applied Animal Behaviour Science*, 107(3–4), 299–306.

Hausberger, M., Roche, H., Henry, S., Visser, E.K. 2007b. A review of the human–horse relationship. *Applied Animal Behaviour Science*, 109, 1–24.

Haussler, K.K., Stover, S.M., Willits, N.H. 1999. Pathologic changes in the lumbosacral vertebrae and pelvis in Thoroughbred racehorses. *American Journal of Veterinary Research*, 60(2), 143–153.

Hayek, A.R., Jones, B., Evans, D.L., Thomson, P.C., McGreevy, P.D. 2005. Epidemiology of horses leaving the Thoroughbred and Standardbred racing industries. In: Proceedings of the 1st International Equitation Science Symposium, Broadford, Victoria. Eds: P. McGreevy, A. McLean, N. Waran, D. Goodwin and A. Warren-Smith. Post-Graduate Foundation in Veterinary Science, Sydney, pp. 84–89.

Hediger, H. 1964. *Wild Animals in Captivity*. Translated by G. Sircom, pp. 156–157. Dover Publications, New York, First published in 1950.

Heffner, H.E., Heffner, R.S. 1983. The hearing ability of horses. *Equine Practise*, 5, 27–32.

Heffner, H.E., Heffner, R.S. 1984. Sound localisation in large mammals: localisation of complex sounds by horses. *Behavioral Neuroscience*, 98, 541–555.

Heffner, H.E., Heffner, R.S. 1992. Auditory perception. In: *Farm Animal and the Environment*, pp. 159–184. Eds: C. Phillips and D. Piggens. CABI Publishing, Wallingford, UK.

Heffner, R.S., Heffner, H.E. 1986. Localisation of tones by horses: use of binaural cues and the superior olivary complex. *Behavioral Neuroscience*, 100, 93–103.

Heird, J., Lokey, C., Cogan, D. 1986a. Repeatability and comparison of two maze tests to measure learning ability in horses. *Applied Animal Behaviour Science*, 16, 103–119.

Heird, J.C., Whitaker, D.D., Bell, R.W., Ramsey, C.B., Lokey, C.E. 1986b. The effects of handling at different ages on the subsequent learning ability of 2-year-old horses. *Applied Animal Behaviour Science*, 15, 15–25.

Heitor, F., Vicente, L. 2007. Learning about horses: what is equine learning all about? *Behavioural Processes*, 76, 34–36.

Helton, W.S., Feltovich, P.J., Velkey, A.J. 2009. Skill and expertise in working dogs: a cognitive science perspective. In: *Canine Ergonomics: The Science of Working Dogs*, pp. 171–178. Ed.: W.S. Helton. CRC Press, Boca Raton, Florida, USA.

Hemmings, A., McBride, S.D., Hale, C.E. 2007. Perseverative responding and the aetiology of equine oral stereotypy. *Applied Animal Behaviour Science*, 104, 143–150.

Hemsworth, P.H., Coleman, G.J. 1998. *Human Livestock Interactions: The Stockperson and the Productivity and Welfare of Intensively Farmed Animals*. CABI Publishing, Wallingford, UK.

Hennessy, K., Quinn, K., Murphy, J. 2007. Different expectations between producers (vendors) and purchasers may lead to wastage and welfare concerns for the horse. In: Proceedings of the 3rd International Equitation Science Symposium, Michigan. Eds: D. Goodwin, C. Heleski, P. McGreevy, A. McLean, H. Randle, C. Skelly, M. van Dierendonck and N. Waran. MSU, Michigan, p. 20.

Henriquet, M. 2004. *Henriquet on Dressage*. Translated by Hilda Nelson. J.A. Allen and Co Ltd, London.

Henry, S., Hemery, D., Richard, M-A., Hausberger, M. 2005. Human–mare relationships and behaviour of foals toward humans. *Applied Animal Behaviour Science*, 93, 341–362.

Henry, S., Richard-Yris, M-A., Hausberger, M. 2006. Influence of various early human–foal interferences on subsequent human–foal relationship. *Developmental Psychobiology*, 48, 712–718.

Herbermann, E. 1980. *Dressage Formula*. J.A. Allen and Co Ltd, London.

Heuschmann, G. 2007. *Tug of War: Classical versus 'Modern' Dressage*. Trafalgar Square, Vermont, USA.

Higgins, A.J., Wright, I.M. 1995. *The Equine Manual*. Baillière Tindall, London.

Hiney, K.M., Nielsen, B.D., Rosenstein, D. 2004. Short-duration exercise and confinement alters bone mineral content and shape in weanling horses. *Journal of Animal Science*, 82, 2313–2320.

Hinnemann, J., van Baalen, C. 2003. *The Simplicity of Dressage*. J.A. Allen and Co Ltd, London.

Holmström, M., Fredricson, I., Drevemo, S. 1994. Biokinematic differences between riding horses judged as good and poor at the trot. *Equine Veterinary Journal Supplement*, 17, 51–56.

Holmström, M., Fredricson, I., Drevemo, S. 1995. Biokinematic effects of collection on the trotting gaits in the elite dressage horse. *Equine Veterinary Journal*, 27, 281–287.

Hölzel, W., Hölzel, P., Plewa, M. 1995. *Dressage Tips and Training Solutions*. Kenilworth Press, Addington, UK.

Hothersall, B., Nicol, C. 2007. Equine learning behaviour: accounting for ecological constraints and relationships with humans in experimental design. *Behavioural Processes*, 76, 45–48.

Houpt, K.A. 2000. Equine welfare. In: *Recent Advances in Companion Animal Behavior Problems*. Ithaca, NY: International Veterinary Information Services.

Houpt, K.A. 2007. Imprinting training and conditioned taste aversion. *Behavioural Processes*, 76, 14–16.

Houpt, K.A., Houpt, T.R. 1988. Social and illumination preferences of mares. *Journal of Animal Science*, 66, 2159–2164.

Houpt, K.A., Houpt, T.R., Johnson, J.L., Erb, H.N., Yeon, S.C. 2001. The effect of exercise deprivation on the behaviour and physiology of straight-stall confined pregnant mares. *Animal Welfare*, 10(3), 257–267.

Houpt, K.A., Keiper, R. 1982. The position of the stallion in the equine hierarchy of feral and domestic ponies. *Journal of Animal Science*, 54, 945–950.

Houpt, K.A., Marrow, M., Seeliger, M. 2000. A preliminary study of the effect of music on equine behaviour. *Journal of Equine Veterinary Science*, 20(11), 691–737.

Houpt, K.A., Parsons, M.S., Hintz, H.F. 1982. Learning ability of orphan foals, of normal foals and of their mothers. *Journal of Animal Science*, 55, 1027–1032.

Houpt, K.A., Wolski, T.R. 1982. *Domestic Animal Behavior for Veterinarians and Animal Scientists*. Ames University Press, Iowa, USA.

Howery, L.D., Bailey, D.W., Laca, E.A. 1999. Impact of spatial memory on habitat use. In: *Grazing Behavior of Livestock and Wildlife*, pp. 91–100. Eds: K.L. Lunchbaugh, K.D. Sanders and J.C. Mosley. University of Idaho, Moscow, ID, USA.

Hull, C.J. 1943. *Principles of Behavior*. Appleton-Century, New Haven, USA.

Hume, D. 1757. *The Natural History of Religion*. Republished 1956. Stanford University Press, Stanford, CA.

Hungerford, T.G. 1975. *Diseases of Livestock*, 8th edn. McGraw-Hill Book Company, Sydney, Australia.

Hutson, G.D. 2002. *Watching Racehorses: A Guide to Betting on Behavior*. Clifton Press, Melbourne, Australia.

Jeffcott, L.B., Dalin, G. 1980. Natural rigidity of the horse's backbone. *Equine Veterinary Journal*, 12, 101–108.

Jenkins, S. 2007. Dutch investigation into 'Rollkur' lunging. *Horse and Hound, 14 October*. http://www.horseandhound.co.uk/news/397/149313.html. *Accessed 26 February 2008.*

Jezierski, T., Jaworski, Z., Gorecka, A. 1999. Effects of handling on behaviour and heart rate in Konik horses: comparison of stable and forest reared young stock. *Applied Animal Behaviour Science*, 62, 1–11.

Jones, B. 1983. Just crazy about horses: the fact behind the fiction. In: *New Perspectives on Our Lives with Companion Animals*, pp. 87–111. Eds: A.H. Katcher and A.M. Beck. University of Philadelphia Press, Philadelphia, USA.

Jørgensen, G.H.M., Bøe K.E. 2007. A note on the effect of daily exercise and paddock size on the behaviour of domestic horses (*Equus caballus*). *Applied Animal Behaviour Science*, 107, 166–173.

Jung, C.G. 1968. *Man and His Symbols*. Dell Publishing Co., Laurel Edition, New York.

Kandel, E.R. 2006. *In Search of Memory: The Emergence of a New Science of Mind*. W.W. Norton and Co. New York, USA.

Kandel, E.R., Schwartz, J.H., Jessell, T.M. 2000. *Principles of Neural Science*, 4th edn. McGraw-Hill, New York.

Karl, P. 2006. *Twisted Truths of Modern Dressage: A Search for a Classical Alternative*. Cadmos Books, Glastonbury, UK.

Kawamura, S. 1959. The process of sub-culture propagation among Japanese macaques. *Primates*, 2, 43–60.

Keay, K., Bandler, R. 2008. Emotional and behavioural significance of the pain signal and the role of the midbrain periaqueductal gray (PAG). In: *The Senses: A Comprehensive Reference*. Eds: Allan I. Basbaum, Akimichi Kaneko, Gordon M. Shepherd and Gerald Westheimer. Volume 5, *Pain*, pp. 627–634. M. Catherine Busnell and Allan I. Basbaum. Academic Press, San Diego, USA.

Keeling, L.J., Blomberg, A., Ladewig J. 1999. Horse-riding accidents: when the human–animal relationship goes wrong! In: 33rd International Congress of the International Society for Applied Ethology, Lillehammer, Norway, p. 86.

Keeling, L.J., Jonare, L., Lanneborn. L. 2009. Investigating horse–human interactions: the effect of a nervous human. *The Veterinary Journal*, 181, 70–71.

Keiper, R.R., Sambraus, H.H. 1986. The stability of equine dominance hierarchies and the effects of kinship, proximity and foaling status on hierarchy status. *Applied Animal Behaviour Science*, 16, 121–130.

Kiley-Worthington, M. 1987. *The Behaviour of Horses in Relation to Management and Training*. J.A. Allen & Co Ltd, London.

King, S.R.B. 2002. Home range and habitat use of free-ranging Przewalski horses at Hustai National Park, Mongolia. *Applied Animal Behaviour Science*, 78(2–4), 103–113.

Kold, S.E., Dyson, S.J. 2003. *Lameness in the Dressage Horse. Diagnosis and Management of Lameness in the Horse*, pp. 975–983. Eds: Mike W. Ross and Sue J. Dyson. W.B. Saunders, Edinburgh, UK.

Korte, S.M. 2001. Corticosteroids in relation to fear, anxiety and psychopathology. *Neuroscience Biobehaviour Review*, 25, 117–142.

Kratzer, D.D., Netherland, W.M., Pulse, R.E., Baker, J.P. 1977. Maze learning in quarter horses. *Journal of Animal Science*, 46, 896–902.

Krueger, K. 2007. Behaviour of horses in the 'round-pen technique'. *Applied Animal Behaviour Science*, 104, 162–170.

Krueger, K., Flauger B. 2007. Social learning in horses from a novel perspective. *Behavioural Processes*, 76, 37–39.

Krueger, K., Heinze, J. 2008. Horse sense: social status of horses (*Equus caballus*) affects their likelihood of copying other horses' behaviour. *Animal Cognition*, DOI 10.1007/s10071–007–0133–0.

Kyrklund, K. 1998. *Dressage with Kyra: The Kyra Kyrklund Training Method*. Trafalgar Square Publishing, Vermont, USA.

Ladewig, J. 2000. Chronic intermittent stress: a model for the study of long-term stressors. In: *The Biology of Animal Stress. Basic Principles and Implications for Animal Welfare*, pp. 159–169. Eds: G.P. Moberg and J.A. Mench. CABI Publishing, Wallingford, UK.

Ladewig, J. 2003. Of mice and men: Improving welfare through clinical ethology. Wood-Gush memorial lecture, ISAE congress, Abano-terme, Italy.

Ladewig, J., Søndergaard, E., Christensen, J.W. 2005. Ontogeny: preparing the young horse for its adult life. In: *The Domestic Horse. The Origins, Development, and Management of Its Behaviour*, pp. 139–149. Eds: D.S. Mills and S.M. McDonnell. Cambridge University Press, Cambridge.

Lagerweij, E., Nelis, P.C., Wiegant, V.M., van Ree, J.M. 1984. The twitch in horses: a variant of acupuncture. *Science*, 225(4667), 1172–1174.

LaHoste, G.J., Mormede, P., Rivet, J-M., LeMoal, M. 1998. Differential sensitisation to amphetamine and stress responsivity as a function of inherent laterality. *Brain Research*, 453, 381–384.

Lansade, L., Bertrand, M., Boivin, X., Bouissou, M.-F. 2004. Effects of handling at weaning on manageability and reactivity of foals. *Applied Animal Behaviour Science*, 87, 131–149.

Lansade, L., Bertrand, M., Bouissou, M.-F. 2005. Effects of neonatal handling on subsequent manageability, reactivity and learning ability of foals. *Applied Animal Behaviour Science*, 92, 143–158.

Lansade, L., Bouissou, M.F., Boivin, X. 2007. Temperament in preweanling horses: development of reactions to humans and novelty, and startle responses. *Developmental Psychology*, 49(5), 501–513.

Le Doux, J.E. 1994. Emotion, memory and the brain. *Scientific American*, 270(6), 32–39.

Le Scolan, N., Hausberger, M., Wolff, A. 1997. Stability over situations in temperamental traits of horses as revealed by experimental and scoring approaches. *Behavioural Processes*, 41, 257–266.

Lea, S.E.G. 1984. In what sense do pigeons learn concepts? In: *Animal Cognition*, pp. 263–276. Eds: H.L. Roitblat, T.G. Bever and H.S. Terrace. Lawrence Erlbaum Associates, NJ, USA.

Lea, S.E.G., Kiley-Worthington, M. 1996. Can animals think? In: *Unsolved Mysteries of the Mind*, pp. 211–244. Ed: V. Bruce. Psychology Press Ltd., Hove, East Sussex.

Leach, D.H., Cymbaluk, N.F. 1986. Relationships between stride length, stride frequency, velocity and morphometrics of foals. *American Journal of Veterinary Research*, 47, 2090–2097.

Leblanc, M-A., Duncan, P. 2007. Can studies of cognitive abilities and of life in the wild really help us to understand equine learning? *Behavioural Processes*, 76, 49–52.

Lee, R., Coccaro, E. 2001. The neuropsychopharmacology of criminality and aggression. *Canadian Journal of Psychiatry*, 46(1), 35–44.

Lefebvre, D., Lips, D., Ödberg, F.O., Giffroy J.M. 2007. Tail docking in horses: a review of the issues. *Animal*, 1, 1167–1178.

Lefebvre, L., Helder, R. 1997. Scrounger numbers and the inhibition of social learning in pigeons. *Behavioural Processes*, 40, 201–207.

Leslie, J.C. 1996. *Principles of Behavioral Analysis*. Overseas Publishers Association, Amsterdam, the Netherlands.

Levine, M.A. 2005. Domestication and early history of the horse. In: *The Domestic Horse. The Origins, Development, and Management of its Behaviour*, pp. 5–22. Eds: D.S. Mills and S.M. McDonnell. Cambridge University Press, Cambridge, UK.

Lieberman, D.A. 1993. *Learning: Behaviour and Cognition*. Brooks/Cole Publishing, Pacific Grove, California, USA.

Lindberg, A.C., Kelland, A., Nicol, C.J. 1999. Effects of observational learning on acquisition of an operant response in horses. *Applied Animal Behaviour Science*, 61(3), 187–199.

Lindsay, S.R. 2000. Adaptation and learning. In: *Handbook of Applied Dog Behaviour and Training*, Vol. I, pp. 233–288. Blackwell, Iowa, USA.

Linklater, W.L. 2007. Equine learning in a wider context – opportunities for integrative pluralism. *Behavioural Processes*, 76, 53–56.

Linklater, W.L., Cameron, E.Z., Stafford, K.J., Veltman, C.J. 2000. Social and spatial structure and range use by Kaimanawa wild horses (*Equus caballus: Equidae*). *New Zealand Journal of Ecology*, 24(2), 139–152.

Loch, S. 1977. *The Classical Rider: Being at One with Your Horse*. Trafalgar Square, North Pomfret, VT, USA.

Lorenz, K.Z. 1937. The companion in the bird's world. *Auk*, 54, 245–473.

Lovett, T., Hodson-Tole, E., Nankervis, K. 2004. A preliminary investigation of rider position during walk, trot and canter. *Equine and Comparative Exercise Physiology*, 2, 71–76.

Mader, D.R., Price, E.O. 1982. Discrimination learning in horses: effects of breed, age and social dominance. *Journal of Animal Science*, 50, 962–965.

Maier, S.F., Seligman, M.E.P., Solomon, R.L. 1969. Pavlovian fear conditioning and learned helplessness: effects on escape and avoidance behaviour (a) the CS–US contingency and (b) the independence of the US and voluntary responding. In: *Punishment and Aversive Behaviour*. Eds: B. Campbell and R.M. Church. Holt, Rinehart and Winston, New York, pp. 299–343.

Mal, M.E., Friend, T.H., Lay, D.C., Vogelsang, S.G., Jenkins, O.C. 1991. Behavioral responses of mares to short-term confinement and social isolation. *Applied Animal Behaviour Science*, 31, 13–24.

Mal, M.E., McCall, C.A. 1996. The influence of handling during different ages on a halter training test in foals. *Applied Animal Behaviour Science*. 50, 115–120.

Mal, M.E., McCall, C.A., Cummins, K.A., Newland, M.C. 1994. Influence of preweaning handling methods on post-weaning ability and manageability of foals. *Applied Animal Behaviour Science*, 40, 187–195.

Manfredi, J., Clayton, H.M., Derksen, F.J. 2005. Effects of different bits and bridles on frequency of induced swallowing in cantering horses. *Equine and Comparative Exercise Physiology*, 2(4), 241–244.

Manning, A. 1972. *Contemporary Biology*. Edward Arnold, London.

Manteca, X., Deag, J.M. 1993. Use of physiological measures to assess individual differences in reactivity. *Applied Animal Behaviour Science*, 37, 265–270.

Marinier, S., Alexander, A. 1994. The use of a maze in testing learning and memory in horses. *Applied Animal Behaviour Science*, 39, 177–182.

Marks, I. 1977. Phobias and obsessions: clinical phenomena in search of a laboratory model. In: *Psychopathology: Experimental Models*, pp. 174-213. Eds: J.D. Maser and M.E.P. Seligman. W.H. Freeman, San Francisco.

Masserman, J.H. 1950. Experimental neurosis. *Scientific American*, 182, 38–43.

McBane, S. 1987. *How to Cure Problems in Horses*. Wiltshire Book Company, California, USA.

McBride, S.D., Hemmings, A. 2005. Altered mesoaccumbens and nigro-striatal dopamine physiology is associated with stereotypy development in a non-rodent species. *Behavioural Brain Research*, 159, 113–118.

McCall, C.A. 1990. A review of learning behaviour in horses and its application in horse training. *Journal of Animal Science*, 68, 75–81.

McCall, C.A. 2007. Making equine learning research applicable to training procedures. *Behavioural Processes*, 76, 27–28.

McCall, C.A., Burgin, S.E. 2002. Equine utilization of secondary reinforcement during response extinction and acquisition. *Applied Animal Behaviour Science*, 78(2–4), 253–262.

McCall, C.A., Potter, G., Friend, T., Ingram, R. 1981. Learning abilities in yearling horses using the Hebb–Williams closed field maze. *Journal of Animal Science*, 53, 928–933.

McCann, J.S., Heird, J.C., Bell, R.W., Lutherer, L.O. 1988. Normal and more highly reactive horses. I. Heart rate, respiration rate and behavioural observations. *Applied Animal Behaviour Science*, 19, 201–214.

McDonnell, S.M. 2003. *The Equid Ethogram. A Practical Field Guide to Horse Behavior*. The Blood Horse Inc; Lexington, Kentucky.

McDonnell, S.M., Haviland, J.C.S. 1995. Agonistic ethogram of the equid bachelor band. *Applied Animal Behaviour Science*, 43, 147–188.

McDonnell, S.M., Poulin, A. 2001. Equid play ethogram. *Applied Animal Behaviour Science*, 78, 263–295.

McGreevy, P.D. 1996. *Why Does My Horse...?* Souvenir Press, London.

McGreevy, P.D. 2004. *Equine Behaviour: A Guide for Veterinarians and Equine Scientists*. W.B. Saunders, Edinburgh, UK.

McGreevy, P.D. 2007. The advent of equitation science. *The Veterinary Journal*, 174, 492–500.

McGreevy, P.D., Boakes, R.A. 2007. *Carrots and Sticks – Principles of Animal Training*. Cambridge University Press, Cambridge.

McGreevy, P.D., Burton, F.L., McLean, A.N. 2009a. The horse–human dyad: can we align horse training and handling activities with the equid social ethogram? *The Veterinary Journal*, 181(1), 12–18.

McGreevy, P.D., Cripps, P.J., French, N.P., Green, L.E., Nicol, C.J. 1995a. Management factors associated with stereotypic and redirected behaviour in the Thoroughbred horse. *Equine Veterinary Journal*, 27, 86–91.

McGreevy, P.D., French, N.P., Nicol, C.J. 1995b. The prevalence of abnormal behaviours in dressage, eventing and endurance horses in relation to stabling. *Veterinary Record*, 137, 36–37.

McGreevy, P.D., Landrieu, J-P., Malou, P.F.J. 2007. A note on motor laterality in plains zebras (*Equus burchellii*) and impalas (*Aepyceros melampus*). *Laterality*, 12(5), 449–457.

McGreevy, P.D., McLean, A.N. 2005. Behavioural problems with the ridden horse. In: *The Domestic Horse. The Origins, Development, and Management of Its Behaviour*, pp. 196–211. Eds: D.S. Mills and S.M. McDonnell. Cambridge University Press, Cambridge, UK.

McGreevy, P.D., McLean, A.N. 2006. Ethological challenges for the working horse and the limitations of ethological solutions in training. In: Second International Equitation Science Symposium, Milan, Italy. Eds: M. Minero, E. Canali, A. Warren-Smith, A. McLean, D. Goodwin, Mari Zetterqvist and N. Waran, P. McGreevy. Veterinary Faculty of Milano, Italy, p. 11.

McGreevy, P.D., McLean, A.N. 2007. The roles of learning theory and ethology in equitation. *Journal of Veterinary Behavior: Clinical Applications and Research*, 2, 108–118.

McGreevy, P.D., McLean, A.N., Thomson, P.C. 2009b. SMART: Sensitivity Models for Animals in Response to Training. *The Veterinary Journal*, 181(1), 72–73.

McGreevy, P.D., McLean, A.N., Warren-Smith, A.K., Waran, N., Goodwin D. 2005. Defining the terms and processes associated with equitation. In: Proceedings of the 1st International Equitation Science Symposium, Broadford, Victoria. Eds: P. McGreevy,

A. McLean, N. Waran, D. Goodwin and A. Warren-Smith. Post-Graduate Foundation in Veterinary Science, Sydney, pp. 10–43.

McGreevy, P.D., Nicholas, F.W. 1999. Some practical solutions to welfare problems in dog breeding. *Animal Welfare*, 8, 329–341.

McGreevy, P.D., Nicol, C.J. 1998. The effect of short-term prevention on the subsequent rate of crib-biting in horses. *Equine Veterinary Journal Supplement. Clinical Behaviour*, 27, 30–34.

McGreevy, P.D., Rogers, L.J. 2005. Motor and sensory laterality in Thoroughbred horses. *Applied Animal Behaviour Science*, 92(4), 337–352.

McGreevy, P.D., Thomson, P.C. 2006. Differences in motor laterality in breeds of performance horse. *Applied Animal Behaviour Science*, 99(1–2), 183–190.

McLean, A.N. 2001. Cognitive abilities – the result of selective pressures on food acquisition? *Applied Animal Behaviour Science*, 71(3), 241–258.

McLean, A.N. 2003. *The Truth about Horses*, pp. 48–49. Penguin, Melbourne, Australia.

McLean, A.N. 2004. Short-term spatial memory in the domestic horse. *Applied Animal Behaviour Science*, 85, 93–105.

McLean, A.N., 2005a. The positive aspects of correct negative reinforcement. *Anthrozoos: A Multidisciplinary Journal of the Interactions of People & Animals*, 18(3), 245–254.

McLean, A.N. 2005b. The mental processes of the horse and their consequences for training. PhD thesis, University of Melbourne.

McLean, A.N. 2008. Overshadowing: a silver lining to a dark cloud in horse training? *Journal of Applied Animal Welfare Science*, 11, 3, 236–248.

McLean, A.N., McGreevy, P.D. 2004. Training. In: *Equine Behaviour – A Guide for Veterinarians and Equine Scientists*, pp. 291–312. W.B. Saunders, Edinburgh, UK.

McLean, A.N., Mclean, M.M. 2008. *Academic Horse Training: Equitation Science in Practice*. Australian Equine Behaviour Centre, Victoria, Australia.

McMillan, F.D. 2005. *Mental Health and Well-Being in Animals*. Blackwell, Iowa, USA.

Mead, G.H. 1934. *Mind, Self and Society*. University of Chicago Press, Chicago.

Mendl, M., Paul, E.S. 2008. Do animals live in the present? Current evidence and implications for welfare. *Applied Animal Behaviour Science*, 113, 357–382.

Midgley, M. 1983. *Animals and Why They Matter*. University of Georgia Press, Athens, USA.

Midkiff, M.D. 1996. *Fitness, Performance and the Female Equestrian*. Macmillan, New York.

Midkiff, M.D. 2001. *She Flies without Wings: How Horses Touch a Woman's Soul*. Random House, New York.

Miller, R.M. 1991. *Imprint Training of the Newborn Foal*. Western Horseman, Colorado Springs, CO, USA.

Miller, R.M. 1995. Behavior of the horse. 1. The 10 behavioral characteristics unique to the horse. *Journal of Equine Veterinary Science*, 15(1), 13–14.

Miller, R.M. 2001. Fallacious studies of foal imprint training. *Journal of Equine Veterinary Science*, 21(3), 102–103.

Mills, D.S. 1998. Applying learning theory to the management of the horse: the difference between getting it right and getting it wrong. *Equine Veterinary Journal Supplement*, 27, 44–48.

Mills, D.S. 2005a. Repetitive movement problems in the horse. In: *The Domestic Horse. The Origins, Development, and Management of its Behaviour*, pp. 212–227. Eds: D.S. Mills and S.M. McDonnell. Cambridge University Press, Cambridge, UK.

Mills, D.S. 2005b. What's in a word? Recent findings on the attributes of a command on the performance of pet dogs. *Anthrozoös*, 18, 208–221.

Minero, M., Canali, E., Ferrante, V., Verga, M., Ödberg, F.O. 1999. Heart rate and behavioural responses of crib-biting horses to two acute stressors. *The Veterinary Record*, 145(15), 430–433.

Miyashita, Y., Nakajima, S., Imada, H. 2000. Differential outcome effect in the horse. *Journal of Experimental Animal Behaviour*, 74(2), 245–254.

Moberg, G.P., Mench, J.A. 2000. *The Biology of Animal Stress. Basic Principles and Implications for Animal Welfare*. CABI Publishing, Wallingford, UK.

Mohr, E. 1971. *The Asiatic Wild Horse*. Allen, London.

Moore, B.R., Reed, S.M., Biller, D.S., Kohn, C.W., Weisbrode, S.E. 1994. Assessment of vertebral canal diameter and bony malformations of the cervical part of the spine in horses with cervical stenotic myelopathy. *American Journal of Veterinary Research*, 55(1), 5–13.

Morgan, W.G. 1974. The shaping game: a teaching technique. *Behaviour Therapy*, 5, 271–272.

Morris, D. 1988. *Horsewatching*. Jonathan Cape, London.

Murphey, R.M., Moura Duarte, F.A., Torres Penendo, M.C. 1981. Response of cattle to humans in open spaces: breed comparisons and approach–avoidance relationships. *Behaviour Genetics*, 2, 37–47.

Murphy, J. 2007. An innovative approach to equitation foundation training (backing the horse) within an automated horse walker may reduce conflict behavior in the horse. In: Proceedings of the 3rd International Equitation Science Symposium, Michigan. Eds: D. Goodwin, C. Heleski, P. McGreevy, A. McLean, H. Randle, C. Skelly, M. van Dierendonck and N. Waran. MSU, Michigan, p. 13.

Murphy, J., Arkins, S. 2007. Equine learning behaviour. *Behavioural Processes*, 76, 1–13.

Myers, R.D., Mesker, D.C. 1960. Operant responding in a horse under several schedules of reinforcement. *Journal of Experimental Animal Behaviour*, 3, 161–164.

Nadeau, J.A., Andrews, F.M., Mathew, A.G., Argenzio, R.A., Blackford, J.T., Sohtell, M., Saxton, A.M. 2000. Evaluation of diet as a cause of gastric ulcers in horses. *American Journal of Veterinary Research*, 61, 784–790.

Nadel, L., O'Keefe, J., Black, A. 1975. Slam on the brakes: a critique of Altman, Brunner and Bayer's response-inhibition model of hippocampal function. *Behavioral Biology*, 14, 151–162.

Nangalama, A.W., Moberg, G.P. 1991. Interaction between cortisol and arachidonic acid on the secretion of LH from ovine pituitary tissue. *Journal of Endocrinology*, 131, 87–94.

Neveu, P.H., Moya, S. 1997. In the mouse, the corticoid stress response depends on lateralisation. *Brain Research*, 749, 344–346.

Nicol, C.J. 1996. Farm animal cognition. *Journal of Animal Science*, 62, 375–391.

Nicol, C.J. 2002. Equine learning: progress and suggestions for future research. *Applied Animal Behaviour Science*, 78, 193–208.

Nicol, C.J., Badnell-Waters, A.J., Bice, R., Kelland, A., Wilson, A.D., Harris, P.A. 2005. The effects of diet and weaning method on the behaviour of young horses. *Applied Animal Behaviour Science*, 95, 205–221.

O'Brien, J.K., Heffernan, S., Thomson, P.C., McGreevy, P.D. 2008. Effect of positive reinforcement training on physiological and behavioural stress responses in the hamadryas baboon (*Papio hamadryas*). *Animal Welfare*, 17(2), 125–138.

Ödberg, F.O. 1987. Chronic stress in riding horses. *Equine Veterinary Journal*, 18, 268–269.

Ödberg, F.O., Bouissou, M-F. 1999. The development of equestrianism from the Baroque period to the present day and its consequences for the welfare of horses. the role of the horse in Europe. *Equine Veterinary Journal Supplement*, 28, 26–30.

Olsen, S.L. 1996. Horse hunters of the Ice Age. In: *Horses Through Time*, pp. 35–56. Ed: S.L. Olsen. Robert Rinehart Publishers, Boulder, CO, USA.

Parelli, P. 1995. *Natural Horsemanship*. Western Horseman, Colorado Springs, CO, USA.

Parker, M., Redhead, E.S., Goodwin, D., McBride, S.D. 2008. Impaired instrumental choice in crib-biting horses (*Equus caballus*). *Behavioural Brain Research*, 191, 137–140.

Pavlov, I.P. 1927. *Conditioned Reflexes*. Oxford University Press, Oxford, UK.

Pavlov, I.P. 1941. *Lectures on Conditioned Reflexes*. International Publishers, New York.

Peloso, J.G., Mundy, G.D., Cohen, N.D. 1996. Prevalence of, and factors associated with, musculoskeletal racing injuries of Thoroughbreds. *Journal of the American Veterinary Medical Association*, 204(4), 620–626.

Perone, M. 2003. Negative effects of positive reinforcement. *Behaviour Analysis*, 26, 1–14.

Petsche, V.M., Derksen, F.J., Berney, C.E., Robinson, N.E. 1995. Effect of head position on upper airway function in exercising horses. *Equine Veterinary Journal Supplement*, 18, 18–22.

Pfungst, O. 1965. *Clever Hans: (The horse of Mr. von Osten)*. Holt, Rinehard and Winston, Inc., New York.

Pilliner, S., Elmhurst, S., Davies, Z. 2002. *The Horse in Motion*, pp. 65, 150. Blackwell, Oxford, UK.

Pineo, M. 1994. French dressage for the German dressage rider. *Dressage and CT*, June, 25–28.

Pinker, S. 1994. *The Language Instinct*. Norton, New York.

Podhajsky, A. 1966. *The Complete Training of Horse and Rider in the Principles of Classical Horsemanship*. Translated by E. Podhajsky and V.D.S. Williams. Doubleday, Bantam Doubleday Dell, New York.

Pratt, D. 1980. *Alternatives to Pain in Experiments on Animals*. Pratt, Dallas, USA.

Premack, D. 2007. Human and animal cognition: continuity and discontinuity. *Proceedings of the National Academy of Sciences*, 104(35), 13861–13867.

Preuschoft, H., Witte, H., Recknagel, S., Bar, H., Lesch, C., Wuthrich, M. 1999. The effects of various headgears on horses. *Deutsche Tierarztliche Wochenschrift*, 106, 69–175.

Prokasy, W.F., Whaley, F.L. 1963. Inter-trial interval range shift in classical eyelid conditioning. *Psychological Reports*, 12, 55–58.

Proops, L., McComb, K., Reby, D. 2009. Cross-modal individual recognition in domestic horses (*Equus caballus*). *Proceedings of the National Academy of Sciences*, 106, 947–951.

Racklyeft, D.J., Love, D.N. 1990. Influence of head posture on the respiratory tract of healthy horses. *Australian Veterinary Journal*, 67, 402–405.

Ragozzino, M.E. 2007. The contribution of the medial prefrontal cortex, orbitofrontal cortex, and dorsomedial striatum to behavioral flexibility. *Annals of the New York Academy of Science*, 1121, 355–375.

Rees, L. 1977. *The Horse's Mind*. Ebury Press, London.

Regan, T. 1983. *The Case for Animal Rights*. University of California Press, Berkeley, Los Angeles, USA.

Rivera, E., Benjamin, S., Nielsen, B., Shelle, J., Zanella, A.J. 2002. Behavioral and physiological responses of horses to initial training: the comparison between pastured versus stalled horses. *Applied Animal Behaviour Science*, 78(2–4), 235–252.

Rizzolatti, G., Fadiga, L. Gallese, V., Fogassi, L. 1996. Premotor cortex and the recognition of motor actions. *Cognitive Brain Research*, 3, 131–141.

Roberts, J.M., Browning, B.A. 1998. Proximity and threats in highland ponies. *Social Networks*, 20(3), 227–238.

Roberts, M. 1997. *The Man Who Listens to Horses*. Arrow Books, London.

Roberts, M. 2000. *Join-Up – Horse Sense for People*. Harper Collins, London.

Roberts, T. 1992. *Equestrian Technique*. J.A. Allen & Co Ltd, London.

Rollin, B.E. 2000. Equine welfare and emerging social ethics. Animal Welfare Forum: Equine Welfare. *Journal of the American Veterinary Medical Association*, 216(8), 1234–1237.

Rolls, E.T. 2000. Précis of the brain and emotion. *Behavioral and Brain Sciences*, 23, 177–234.

Rose, R.J., Hodgson, D.R. 1993. *Manual of Equine Practice*. W.B. Saunders, Edinburgh, UK.

Sappington, B.K.F., McCall, C.A., Coleman, D.A., Kuhlers, D.L., Lishak, R.S. 1997. A preliminary study of the relationship between discrimination reversal learning and performance tasks in yearling and 2-year-old horses. *Applied Animal Behaviour Science*, 53, 157–166.

Saslow, C.A. 2002. Understanding the perceptual world of horses. *Applied Animal Behaviour Science*, 78, 235–252.

Schilder, M.B.H., van der Borg, J.A.M. 2004. Training dogs with help of the shock collar: short and long term behavioural effects. *Applied Animal Behaviour Science*, 85, 319–334.

Schonholtz, C.M. 2000. Animals in rodeo – a closer look. Animal Welfare Forum: Equine Welfare. *Journal of the American Veterinary Medical Association*, 216(8), 1246–1249.

Schramm, U. 1986. *The Undisciplined Horse – Causes and Corrections*. J.A. Allen, London.

Seligman, M.E.P. 1970. On the generality of the laws of learning. *Psychological Review*, 77, 406–408.

Seligman, M.E.P. 1971. Phobias and preparedness. *Behaviour Therapy*, 2, 307–320.

Seligman, M.E.P. 1975. *Helplessness: On Depression, Development and Death*. W.H. Freeman and Company, San Francisco, USA.

Seligman, M.E.P., Altenor, A., Weinraub, M., Schulman, A. 1980. Coping behavior: learned helplessness, physiological change and learned inactivity. *Behavioural Research and Therapy*, 18, 459–512.

Seligman, M.E.P., Maier, S.F. 1967. Failure to escape traumatic shock. *Journal of Experimental Psychology*, 74, 1–9.

Sewell, A. 1877. *Black Beauty*. Penguin Classics.

Sgoifo, A., de Boer, S.F., Westenbroek, C., Maes, F.W., Beldhuis, H., Suzuki, T., Koolhaas, J.M. 1997. Incidence of arrhythmias and heart rate variability in wild-type rats exposed to social stress. *American Journal of Physiology*, 273(4 Pt 2), 1754–1760.

Shapiro, K.J. 1990. Understanding dogs through kinesthetic empathy, social construction and history. *Anthrozoös*, 3, 184–185.

Shettleworth, S.J. 2001. Animal cognition and animal behaviour. *Animal Behaviour*, 61(2), 277–286.

Sighieri, C., Tedeschi, D., De Andreis, C., Petri, L., Baragli, P. 2003. Behaviour patterns of horses can be used to establish a dominant–subordinate relationship between man and horse. *Animal Welfare*, 12(4), 705–708.

Sigurjonsdottir, H., Gunnarsson, V. 2002. *Controlled study of early handling and training of Icelandic foals*. Eds: S. McDonnell and D. Mills. Dorothy Russell Havemeyer Workshop Horse Behavior and Welfare, Iceland, 13–16 June, pp. 35–39.

Simpson, B. 2002. Neonatal foal handling. *Applied Animal Behaviour Science*, 78, 303–317.

Sivewright, M. 1984. *Thinking Riding, Book 2: In Good Form*. J.A. Allen, London.

Skinner, B.F. 1938. *The Behavior of Organisms*. Appleton-Century-Crofts, New York.

Skinner, B.F. 1953. *Science and Human Behavior*. Macmillan, New York.

Skinner, B.F. 1971. *Beyond Freedom and Dignity*. Hackett publishing, Indianapolis, USA.

Skipper, L. 1999. *Inside Your Horse's Mind: A Study of Equine Intelligence and Human Prejudice*. J.A. Allen, London.

Sloet van Oldruitenborgh-Oosterbaan, M.M., Barneveld, A., Schamhardt, H.C. 1995. Effects of weight and riding on workload and locomotion during treadmill exercise. *Equine Veterinary Journal Supplement*, 18, 413–417.

Solomon, R.L. 1964. Punishment. *American Psychologist*, 19, 239–253.

Søndergaard, E., Halekoh, U. 2003. Young horses' reactions to humans in relation to handling and social environment. *Applied Animal Behaviour Science*, 84, 265–280.

Søndergaard, E., Ladewig, J. 2004. Group housing exerts a positive effect on the behaviour of young horses during training. *Applied Animal Behaviour Science*, 87, 105–118.

Spalding, D. 1873. Instinct: with observations on young animals. *Macmillan's magazine*. 27, 283–293 (Reprinted in the *British Journal of Animal Behaviour*, 2, 1–11.)

Spier, S.J., Pusterla, J.B., Villarroel, A., Pusterla, N. 2004. Outcome of tactile conditioning of neonates, or 'imprint training' on selected handling measures in foals. *Veterinary Journal*, 168, 252–258.

Stoffel-Willame, M., Stoffel-Willame, Y. 1999. Horses of the Namib. *Africa, Environment & Wildlife*, 7(1), 58–67.

Stolba, A., Baker, N., Wood-Gush, D.G.M. 1983. The characterization of stereotyped behaviour in stalled sows by information redundancy. *Behavior*. 87, 157–182.

Stone, S.M. 2001. Specific concept formation in horses: you sure look familiar. PhD thesis, Faculty of the Graduate College of the Oklahoma State University, USA.

Terada, K. 2000. Comparison of head movement and EMG activity of muscles between advanced and novice horseback riders at different gaits. *Journal of Equine Science*, 11, 83–90.

Terada, K., Mullineaux, D.R., Lanovaz, J., Kato, K., Clayton, H.M. 2004. Electromyographic analysis of the rider's muscles at trot. *Equine and Comparative Exercise Physiology*, 1(3), 193–198.

Thomas, R.K. 1986. Vertebrate intelligence: a review of the laboratory research. In: *Animal Intelligence: Insights into the Animal Mind, pp. 37–56*. Eds: R.J. Hoage and L. Goldman. Smithsonian Institution Press, Washington, DC.

Thorndike, E.L. 1911. *Animal Intelligence*. Macmillan, New York.

Thorne, J.B., Goodwin, D., Kennedy, M.J., Davidson, H.P.B., Harris, P. 2005. Foraging enrichment for individually housed horses: practicality and effects on behaviour. *Applied Animal Behaviour Science*, 94, 149–164.

Tobin, T. 1978. A review of the pharmacology of reserpine in the horse. *Journal of Equine Medical Surgery*, 2(10), 433–438.

Tolman, E.C. 1948. Cognitive map in rats and men. *Psychological Review*, 55, 189–209.

Tyler, S.J. 1972. The behaviour and social organization of the New Forest ponies. *Animal Behaviour Monograph*, 5, 85–196.

Ueda, Y., Yoshida, K., Oikawa, M. 1993. Analyses of race accident conditions through use of patrol video. *Journal of Equine Veterinary Science*, 13, 707–710.

USDF, 2002. *Glossary of Dressage Judging Terms*. Compiled by United States Dressage Federation Council of Judges. Lincoln, USA.

Valentine, B.A., Hintz, H.F., Freels, K.M., Reynolds, A.J., Thompson, K.N. 1998. Dietary control of exertional rhabdomyolysis in horses. *Journal of the American Veterinary Association*, 212(10), 1588–1593.

van Breda, E. 2006. A nonnatural head-neck position (Rollkur) during training results in less acute stress in elite, trained, dressage horses. *Journal of Applied Animal Welfare Science*, 9(1), 59–64.

van Dierendonck, M., Goodwin, D. 2005. Social contact in horses: implications for human–horse interactions. In: The human-animal relationship. Eds: F. de Jong, R. van den Bos. *Animals in Philosophy and Science*, 4, 65–81.

van Dierendonck, M.C., Devries, H., Schilder, M.B.H. 1995. An analysis of dominance, its behavioural parameters and possible determinants in a herd of Icelandic horses in captivity. *Netherlands Journal of Zoology*, 45(3–4), 362–385.

van Dierondonck, M. 2006. Assessment of ethological methods as a diagnostic tool to determine early overtraining in horses. In: Proceedings of the 2nd International Equitation Science Symposium, Milan. Eds:

M. Minero, E. Canali, A. Warren-Smith, A. McLean, D. Goodwin, Mari Zetterqvist, N. Waran and P. McGreevy. University of Milan, Milan, p. 13.

van Heel, M.C.V., Kroekenstoel, A.M., Van Dierendonck, M.C., van Weeren, P.R., Back, W. 2006. Uneven feet in a foal may develop as a consequence of lateral grazing behaviour induced by conformational traits. *Equine Veterinary Journal*, 38(7), 646–651.

van Weeren, P.R., Meyer, H., Johnston, C., Roepstorff, L., Weishaupt, M.A. 2006. The effect of different head and neck positions on the thoracolumbar kinematics in the unridden horse. In: Report of the FEI Veterinary and Dressage Committee's Workshop. The use of over-bending ('Rollkur') in FEI Competition, 31 January, during the FEI Veterinary Committee meeting at the Olympic Museum, Lausanne, p. 8.

Visser, E.K. 2002. Horsonality: a study on the personality of the horse. PhD thesis, Wageningen University and Research Center Publications (Netherlands).

Visser, E.K., Ellis, A.D., van Reenen, C.G. 2008. The effect of two different housing conditions on the welfare of young horses stabled for the first time. *Applied Animal Behaviour Science*, 114, 521–533.

Visser, E.K., van Reenen, C.G., Hopster, H., Schilder, M.B.H., Knaap, J.H., Barneveld, A., Blokhuis, H.J. 2001. Quantifying aspects of young horse's temperament: consistency of behavioural variables. *Applied Animal Behaviour Science*, 74(4), 241–258.

Visser, E.K., van Reenen, C.G., Schilder, M.B.H., Barneveld, A., Blokhuis, H.J. 2003. Learning performances in young horses using two different learning tests. *Applied Animal Behaviour Science*, 80, 311–326.

Von Borell, E., Langbein, L., Despres, G., Hansen, S., Leterrier, C., Marchant-Forde, J., Marchant-Forde, R., Minero, M., Mohr, E., Prunier, A., Valance, D., Veissier, I. 2007. Heart rate variability as a measure of autonomic regulation of cardiac activity for assessing stress and welfare in farm animals – a review. *Physiology and Behaviour*, 92, 293–316.

Von Borstel, U.U., Duncan, I.J.H., Shoveller, A.K., Millman, S.T., Keeling, L.J. 2007. Transfer of nervousness from competition rider to the horse. In: Proceedings of the 3rd International Society for Equitation Science, Michigan. Eds: D. Goodwin, C. Heleski, P. McGreevy, A. McLean, H. Randle, C. Skelly, M. van Dierendonck and N. Waran. MSU, Michigan, USA, p. 17.

von Uexküll, J. 1957. A stroll through the worlds of animals and men: a picture book of invisible worlds. In: *Instinctive Behavior: The Develepment of a Modern Concept, pp. 5–80*. Ed. and trans. Claire H. Schiller. International Universities Press, Inc., New York.

Waiblinger, S., Boivin, X., Pedersen, V., Tosi, M.-V., Janczak, A., Visser, K., Jones, R.B. 2006. Assessing the human–animal relationship in farm species: a critical review. *Applied Animal Behaviour Science*, 101, 185–242.

Wallace, J. 1993. *The Less-Than-Perfect Horse*. Methuen, London, UK.

Wanless, M. 2006. *Ride with Your Mind: Essentials*. Kenilworth Press, UK.

Waran, N., McGreevy, P., Casey, R.A. 2002. Training methods and horse welfare. In: *The Welfare of Horses*, pp. 151–180. Ed: N. Waran. Kluwer Academic Publishers, Dordrecht, The Netherlands.

Waring, G.H. 1983. *Horse Behavior: The Behavioral Traits and Adaptations of Domestic and Wild Horses, Including Ponies*. Noyes, Park Ridge, NJ, USA.

Waring, G.H. 2003. *Horse Behavior*. 2nd edn. Noyes/William Andrew, New York, USA.

Warren-Smith, A.K., Curtis, R.A., Greetham, L., McGreevy, P.D. 2007a. Rein contact between horse and handler during specific equitation movements. *Applied Animal Behaviour Science*, 108, 157–169.

Warren-Smith, A.K., Curtis, R.A., McGreevy, P.D. 2005a. A low-cost device for measuring the pressures exerted on domestic horses by riders and handlers. In: Proceedings of the 1st International Equitation Science Symposium, Broadford, Victoria. Eds: P. McGreevy, A. McLean, N. Waran, D. Goodwin and A. Warren-Smith. Post-Graduate Foundation in Veterinary Science, Sydney, pp. 44–55.

Warren-Smith, A.K., Greetham, L., McGreevy, P.D. 2007b. Behavioral and physiological responses of horses (*Equus caballus*) undergoing head lowering. *Journal of Veterinary Behavior: Clinical Applications and Research*, 2–3, 59–67.

Warren-Smith, A.K., McGreevy, P.D. 2005b. The use of head lowering in horses as a method of inducing calmness. In: Proceedings of the 1st International Equitation Science Symposium, Broadford, Victoria. Eds: P. McGreevy, A. McLean, N. Waran, D. Goodwin and A. Warren-Smith. Post-Graduate Foundation in Veterinary Science, Sydney, pp. 75–83.

Warren-Smith, A.K., McGreevy, P.D. 2006. An audit of the application of the principles of equitation science by qualified equestrian instructors in Australia. In: Proceedings of the 2nd International Equitation Science Symposium, Milan. Eds: M. Minero, E. Canali, A. Warren-Smith, A. McLean, D. Goodwin, Mari Zetterqvist, N. Waran and P. McGreevy. University of Milan, Milan, p. 12.

Warren-Smith, A.K., McGreevy, P.D. 2007. The use of blended positive and negative reinforcement in shaping the halt response of horses (*Equus caballus*). *Animal Welfare*, 16, 481–488.

Warren-Smith, A.K., McGreevy, P.D. 2008a. Equestrian coaches' understanding and application of learning theory in horse training. *Anthrozoös*, 21(2), 153–162.

Warren-Smith, A.K., McGreevy, P.D. 2008b. Preliminary investigations into the ethological relevance of round-pen (round-yard) training of horses. *Journal of Applied Animal Welfare Science*, 11(3), 285–298.

Warren-Smith, A.K., McLean, A.N., Nicol, H.I., McGreevy, P.D. 2005b. Variations in the timing of reinforcement as a training technique for foals. *Anthrozoös*, 18(3), 255–272.

Wasilewski, A. 2005. 'Friendship' in ungulates? Sociopositive relationships between non-related herd members of the same species. http://www.staff.uni-marburg.de/~z-phylog/wisstaff/waso-sum.htm. Accessed 16 March 2007.

Waters, A.J., Nicol, C.J., French, N.P. 2002. Factors influencing the development of stereotypic and redirected behaviours in young horses: findings of a four-year prospective epidemiological study. *Equine Veterinary Journal*, 34(6), 572–579.

Watt, L.M., McDonnell, S.M. 2001. Demonstration of concept formation in the horse. Equine Behavior Laboratory, University of Pennsylvania School of Veterinary Medicine, August 2001, Interim Report.

Webster, A.J.F. 1994. *Animal Welfare: A Cool Eye towards Eden*. Blackwell Science, London.

Weeks, J.W., Crowell-Davis, S.L., Caudle, A.B., Heusner, G.L. 2000. Aggression and social spacing in light horse (*Equus caballus*) mares and foals. *Applied Animal Behaviour Science*, 68(4), 319–337.

Weinraub, M., Schulman, A. 1980. Coping behavior: learned helplessness, physiological change and learned inactivity. *Behavioural Research and Therapy*, 18, 459–512.

Weiss, J.M., Glazer, H.I., Pohorecky, L.A., Brick, J., Miller, N.E. 1975. Effects of chronic exposure to stressors on avoidance–escape behavior and on brain norepinephrine. *Psychosomatic Medicine*, 37, 522–534.

Wells, D.L., Hepper, P.G. 1999. Male and female dogs respond differently to men and women. *Applied Animal Behaviour Science*, 61, 341–349.

Wiepkema, P.R. 1987. Behavioural aspects of stress. In: *Biology of Stress in Farm Animals: An Integrative Approach*, pp. 113–133. Eds: P.R. Wiepkema and P.W.M. van Adrichem. Martinus Nijhoff, Leiden, The Netherlands.

Wilewski, K.A., Rubin, L. 1999. Bit seats: a dental procedure for enhancing performance of show horses. *Equine Practise*, 21(4), 16–20.

Williams, D.E., Norris, B.J. 2007. Laterality in stride pattern preferences in racehorses. *Animal Behaviour*, 74, 941–950.

Williams, J.L., Friend, T.H., Collins, M.N., Toscano, M.J., Sisto-Burt, A., Nevill, C.H. 2002. The effects of early training sessions on the reactions of foals at 1, 2 and 3 months of age. *Applied Animal Behaviour Science*, 77, 105–114.

Williams, J.L., Friend, T.H., Collins, M.N., Toscano, M.J., Sisto-Burt, A., Nevill, C.H. 2003. Effects of imprint training procedure at birth on the reactions of foals at age six months. *Equine Veterinary Journal*, 35, 127–132.

Wilson, A. 2004. *Top Horse Training Methods Explored*. David and Charles, Newton Abbot, Devon, UK.

Wittling, W., Roschmann, R. 1993. Emotion-related hemisphere asymmetry: subjective emotional responses to laterally presented films. *Cortex*, 29, 431–448.

Wolff, A., Hausberger, M. 1996. Learning and memorisation of two different tasks in horses: the effects of age, sex and sire. *Applied Animal Behaviour Science*, 46, 137–143.

Wolpe, J. 1958. *Psychotherapy by Reciprocal Inhibition*. Stanford University Press, Palo Alto, CA, USA.

Woodward, A.L. 1999. Infants' ability to distinguish between purposeful and nonpurposeful behav-iors. *Infant Behavior and Development*, 22, 145–160.

Wouters, L., De Moor, A. 1979. Ultrastructure of the pigment epithelium and the photoreceptors in the retina of the horse. *American Journal of Veterinary Research*, 40, 1066–1071.

Wright, M. 1973. *The Jeffery Method of Horse Handling. An Introduction to a New Approach to the Handling of Horses*. R.M. Williams, Prospect, South Australia.

Xenophon. 1962. *The Art of Horsemanship*. Translated by M.H. Morgan. J.A. Allen and Company, London.

Yerkes, R.M., Dodson, J.D. 1908. The relation of strength to stimulus to rapidity of habituation. *Journal of Comparative Neurology and Psychology*, 18, 459–482.

Zeitler-Feicht, M. 2004. *Horse Behaviour Explained. Origins, Treatment and Prevention of Problems*. Manson Publishing, London.

Index

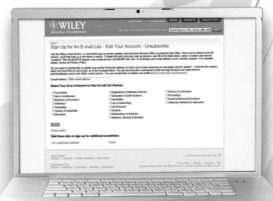
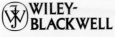